VOLUME ONE HUNDRED AND TWENTY TWO

# INTERNATIONAL REVIEW OF NEUROBIOLOGY

## Omic Studies of Neurodegenerative Disease: Part B

# INTERNATIONAL REVIEW OF NEUROBIOLOGY

VOLUME 122

## SERIES EDITORS


**R. ADRON HARRIS**

*Waggoner Center for Alcohol and Drug Addiction Research*
*The University of Texas at Austin*
*Austin, Texas, USA*

**PETER JENNER**

*Division of Pharmacology and Therapeutics*
*GKT School of Biomedical Sciences*
*King's College, London, UK*

VOLUME ONE HUNDRED AND TWENTY TWO

# INTERNATIONAL REVIEW OF NEUROBIOLOGY

## Omic Studies of Neurodegenerative Disease: Part B

Edited by

**MICHAEL J. HURLEY**
*Imperial College London, London, UK*

ELSEVIER

AMSTERDAM • BOSTON • HEIDELBERG • LONDON
NEW YORK • OXFORD • PARIS • SAN DIEGO
SAN FRANCISCO • SINGAPORE • SYDNEY • TOKYO
Academic Press is an imprint of Elsevier

Academic Press is an imprint of Elsevier
125 London Wall, London, EC2Y 5AS, UK
525 B Street, Suite 1800, San Diego, CA 92101-4495, USA
225 Wyman Street, Waltham, MA 02451, USA
The Boulevard, Langford Lane, Kidlington, Oxford OX5 1GB, UK

First edition 2015



**Notices**

Knowledge and best practice in this field are constantly changing. As new research and experience broaden our understanding, changes in research methods, professional practices, or medical treatment may become necessary.

Practitioners and researchers must always rely on their own experience and knowledge in evaluating and using any information, methods, compounds, or experiments described herein. In using such information or methods they should be mindful of their own safety and the safety of others, including parties for whom they have a professional responsibility.

To the fullest extent of the law, neither the Publisher nor the authors, contributors, or editors, assume any liability for any injury and/or damage to persons or property as a matter of products liability, negligence or otherwise, or from any use or operation of any methods, products, instructions, or ideas contained in the material herein.

ISBN: 978-0-12-804762-0
ISSN: 0074-7742

For information on all Academic Press publications visit our website at http://store.elsevier.com/

# CONTENTS

*Contributors* *vii*
*Preface* *ix*

**1. Utility of Autoantibodies as Biomarkers for Diagnosis and Staging of Neurodegenerative Diseases** **1**

Cassandra DeMarshall, Abhirup Sarkar, Eric P. Nagele, Eric Goldwaser, George Godsey, Nimish K. Acharya, and Robert G. Nagele

1. Introduction: A Brief History of Autoantibodies 3
2. A Causal Role for Autoantibodies Revealed in Well-Known Autoimmune Diseases 4
3. Autoantibodies in Cancer: Byproduct or Biomarker? 8
4. Escalating Involvement of Autoantibodies in Neurological and Neurocognitive Disorders 9
5. Autoantibodies: Abundant, Ubiquitous, and Clinically Useful 19
6. Methods of Autoantibody Detection in Biofluids 24
7. Utility of Autoantibodies as Biomarkers of Disease 29
8. Conclusions and Perspectives 35

Acknowledgments 37
References 37

**2. Metabolomics of Neurodegenerative Diseases** **53**

Alejandro Botas, Hannah Moore Campbell, Xu Han, and Mirjana Maletic-Savatic

1. Metabolomics in Medicine 55
2. Metabolomics Biomarkers of Disease 56
3. Metabolomics Biomarker Discovery in Neurodegenerative Disorders 61
4. Summary 72

Acknowledgments 73
References 73

**3. Parkinson's Disease: *In Vivo* Brain Metabolomics by MRS** **81**

Mario Rango

1. Proton MRS 82
2. 1H MRS: Compounds Detectable *In Vivo* 82
3. Phosphorus MRS 83

4. Mitochondrial Dysfunction 89
5. Other Findings 89
6. High Magnetic Field 90
7. Parkinson's Disease and Solvent Exposure 90
8. Conclusions 91
References 91

**4. Recent Advances and Applications of Metabolomics to Investigate Neurodegenerative Diseases** **95**

Clara Ibáñez, Alejandro Cifuentes, and Carolina Simó

1. Introduction 96
2. Metabolomics and Neurodegenerative Disorders 100
3. Conclusions 123
References 126

**5. Lipidomics of Human Brain Aging and Alzheimer's Disease Pathology** **133**

Alba Naudí, Rosanna Cabré, Mariona Jové, Victoria Ayala, Hugo Gonzalo, Manuel Portero-Otín, Isidre Ferrer, and Reinald Pamplona

1. Introduction 134
2. Lipidomics of Human Brain 136
3. Lipidomics of Human Brain Aging 163
4. Lipidomics of Alzheimer's Disease Pathology 168
5. Summary and Future Prospects 177
Acknowledgments 178
References 178

*Index* *191*
*Contents of Recent Volumes* *195*

# CONTRIBUTORS

**Nimish K. Acharya**
Biomarker Discovery Center, New Jersey Institute for Successful Aging, and Department of Geriatrics and Gerontology, Rowan University School of Osteopathic Medicine, Stratford, New Jersey, USA

**Victoria Ayala**
Department of Experimental Medicine, University of Lleida-Biomedical Research Institute of Lleida, Lleida, Spain

**Alejandro Botas**
BioSciences Department, Rice University, Houston, Texas, USA

**Rosanna Cabré**
Department of Experimental Medicine, University of Lleida-Biomedical Research Institute of Lleida, Lleida, Spain

**Hannah Moore Campbell**
Medical Scientist Training Program, Baylor College of Medicine, Houston, Texas, USA

**Alejandro Cifuentes**
Laboratory of Foodomics, Institute of Food Science Research (CIAL), CSIC, Madrid, Spain

**Cassandra DeMarshall**
Biomarker Discovery Center, New Jersey Institute for Successful Aging; Graduate School of Biomedical Sciences, Rowan University, and Department of Geriatrics and Gerontology, Rowan University School of Osteopathic Medicine, Stratford, New Jersey, USA

**Isidre Ferrer**
Institute of Neuropathology, Bellvitge University Hospital, University of Barcelona, Biomedical Research Institute of Bellvitge, L'Hospitalet de Llobregat, Barcelona, and Center for Biomedical Research on Neurodegenerative Diseases (CIBERNED), ISCIII, Madrid, Spain

**George Godsey**
Graduate School of Biomedical Sciences, Rowan University, and Department of Geriatrics and Gerontology, Rowan University School of Osteopathic Medicine, Stratford, New Jersey, USA

**Eric Goldwaser**
Biomarker Discovery Center, New Jersey Institute for Successful Aging; Graduate School of Biomedical Sciences, Rowan University, and Department of Geriatrics and Gerontology, Rowan University School of Osteopathic Medicine, Stratford, New Jersey, USA

**Hugo Gonzalo**
Department of Experimental Medicine, University of Lleida-Biomedical Research Institute of Lleida, Lleida, Spain

**Xu Han**
Department of Pediatrics, Baylor College of Medicine, and Jan and Dan Duncan Neurological Research Institute at Texas Children's Hospital, Houston, Texas, USA

**Clara Ibáñez**
Laboratory of Foodomics, Institute of Food Science Research (CIAL), CSIC, Madrid, Spain

**Mariona Jové**
Department of Experimental Medicine, University of Lleida-Biomedical Research Institute of Lleida, Lleida, Spain

**Mirjana Maletic-Savatic**
Department of Pediatrics; Jan and Dan Duncan Neurological Research Institute at Texas Children's Hospital; Program in Developmental Biology; Program in Structural and Computational Biology and Molecular Biophysics, and Department of Neuroscience, Baylor College of Medicine, Houston, Texas, USA

**Eric P. Nagele**
Biomarker Discovery Center, New Jersey Institute for Successful Aging, Rowan University School of Osteopathic Medicine, Stratford, and Durin Technologies, Inc., New Brunswick, New Jersey, USA

**Robert G. Nagele**
Biomarker Discovery Center, New Jersey Institute for Successful Aging; Department of Geriatrics and Gerontology, Rowan University School of Osteopathic Medicine, and Durin Technologies, Inc., New Brunswick, New Jersey, USA

**Alba Naudí**
Department of Experimental Medicine, University of Lleida-Biomedical Research Institute of Lleida, Lleida, Spain

**Reinald Pamplona**
Department of Experimental Medicine, University of Lleida-Biomedical Research Institute of Lleida, Lleida, Spain

**Manuel Portero-Otín**
Department of Experimental Medicine, University of Lleida-Biomedical Research Institute of Lleida, Lleida, Spain

**Mario Rango**
Department of Neurological Sciences and Excellence Center for advanced MR studies, IRCCS Ca' Granda-Ospedale Maggiore Policlinico Foundation, University of Milan, Milano, Italy

**Abhirup Sarkar**
Biomarker Discovery Center, New Jersey Institute for Successful Aging; Graduate School of Biomedical Sciences, Rowan University, and Department of Geriatrics and Gerontology, Rowan University School of Osteopathic Medicine, Stratford, New Jersey, USA

**Carolina Simó**
Laboratory of Foodomics, Institute of Food Science Research (CIAL), CSIC, Madrid, Spain

# PREFACE

If you can pass the anathematic word "omic" and choose to read this volume of the *International Review of Neurobiology*, then you will have done yourself a favor. Because nestled within the usual scientific prose is some truly outstanding and innovative work describing state-of-the-art omic investigations into the cause, diagnosis, and treatment of neurodegenerative disorders such as Alzheimer's disease, Parkinson's disease, Huntington's disease, amyotrophic lateral sclerosis, multiple sclerosis, and prion diseases.

The aim of the volume is to bring together diverse work that explores facets of neurodegenerative disease that are often overlooked by traditional hypothesis-driven research and to present such work in a readable format which appeals to researchers and students from a wide range of scientific backgrounds.

The reason for doing so is that neurodegenerative diseases ruin and frequently shorten the life of the patient and place immense strain upon their families and carers of the affected individual. This in turn has a high social and economic cost to society as a whole. Paradoxically, as advances in medicine successfully treat many illnesses and life expectancy increases, the prevalence of neurodegenerative disease is also rising, since the biggest risk factor for the most common neurodegenerative diseases is aging. Consequently, these costs will only get worse as the world population ages and the apparent advantages of a greater life expectancy are less desirable if the reality is that there is a high probability of developing a debilitating disease which renders the individual dependent on constant care. Yet, despite the vast quantities of research that has been conducted over many decades into neurodegenerative diseases, in the majority of cases the cause of neurodegeneration is unknown and treatments, if available, only tackle some symptoms of neurodegeneration and do nothing to slow the progression of the disease.

The chapters in this volume of *International Review of Neurobiology* showcase novel approaches to study the genome, proteome, and metabolome of samples from patients with neurodegenerative disease in the hope of finding clues regarding the causes of neurodegenerative disease, furthering our understanding of mechanisms of neurodegeneration, aiding earlier diagnosis through the detection of biomarkers, and identifying putative therapeutic targets that will allow successful treatment of neurodegenerative diseases or delay their onset.

Finally, I would like to thank the authors of the chapters in this volume for their work and hope that the readers find something within the volume that stimulates them to contribute toward further research into the cause, treatment, and cure of neurodegenerative disease in the future.

Michael J. Hurley
London, April 2015

CHAPTER ONE

# Utility of Autoantibodies as Biomarkers for Diagnosis and Staging of Neurodegenerative Diseases

**Cassandra DeMarshall**[*,†,‡], **Abhirup Sarkar**[*,†,‡], **Eric P. Nagele**[*,§], **Eric Goldwaser**[*,†,‡], **George Godsey**[†,‡], **Nimish K. Acharya**[*,‡], **Robert G. Nagele**[*,‡,§,1]

[*]Biomarker Discovery Center, New Jersey Institute for Successful Aging, Rowan University School of Osteopathic Medicine, Stratford, New Jersey, USA
[†]Graduate School of Biomedical Sciences, Rowan University, Stratford, New Jersey, USA
[‡]Department of Geriatrics and Gerontology, Rowan University School of Osteopathic Medicine, Stratford, New Jersey, USA
[§]Durin Technologies, Inc., New Brunswick, New Jersey, USA
[1]Corresponding author: e-mail address: nagelero@rowan.edu

## Contents

1. Introduction: A Brief History of Autoantibodies 3
2. A Causal Role for Autoantibodies Revealed in Well-Known Autoimmune Diseases 4
   2.1 Role of Autoantibodies and Protein Citrullination in Rheumatoid Arthritis 4
   2.2 SLE, an Autoimmune Disease with Autoantibodies Directed Against Common Nuclear and Cytoplasmic Proteins 5
   2.3 Systemic Sclerosis (Scleroderma) 7
3. Autoantibodies in Cancer: Byproduct or Biomarker? 8
4. Escalating Involvement of Autoantibodies in Neurological and Neurocognitive Disorders 9
   4.1 Introduction 9
   4.2 MG—A Classical Example of Autoantibodies Causing a Neurological Disease 11
   4.3 MS—A Neuroinflammatory Demyelinating Disease Associated with Autoantibodies 13
   4.4 Neuromyelitis Optica—A Neuroinflammatory Demyelinating Disease with a Causative Autoantibody 15
   4.5 Anti-NMDAR Encephalitis—Autoantibodies Targeting Receptors Causing Neuropsychiatric Symptoms 16
   4.6 AD—Evidence that Autoantibodies and Blood–Brain Barrier Breakdown Are Partners in Crime 18

*International Review of Neurobiology*, Volume 122
ISSN 0074-7742
http://dx.doi.org/10.1016/bs.irn.2015.05.005

5. Autoantibodies: Abundant, Ubiquitous, and Clinically Useful 19
5.1 The Rise of Natural Autoantibodies 19
5.2 Prevalence and Stability of Natural Autoantibodies 21
5.3 Isotype and Reactivity of Natural Autoantibodies 21
5.4 Natural Autoantibody Production 22
5.5 Function of Natural Autoantibodies 23
5.6 Implications and Opportunity 24
6. Methods of Autoantibody Detection in Biofluids 24
6.1 Proteomic Approaches for Autoantibody Analysis in Biological Samples 24
6.2 Discovery of Candidate Autoantibody Biomarkers Using the Whole Human Proteome 26
6.3 Autoantibody Discovery by Fluid-Phase Immunoassays 27
6.4 Autoantibody Discovery by Antigen Microarray Technologies 27
6.5 Validation of Biomarker Candidates 29
7. Utility of Autoantibodies as Biomarkers of Disease 29
7.1 Classical Targets Miss the Mark as the Most Useful Diagnostic Biomarkers 30
7.2 Immunoglobulin-Binding Patterns Using Random Peptide Ligands and Mimetics for Biomarker Identification in AD 32
7.3 Disease-Specific Autoantibody Profiles Using Human Protein Microarrays for the Diagnosis and Staging of AD and PD 33
8. Conclusions and Perspectives 35
Acknowledgments 37
References 37

## Abstract

Autoantibodies are self-reactive antibodies that have been widely implicated as causal agents of autoimmune diseases. They are found in the blood of all human sera, regardless of age, gender, or the presence or absence of disease. While the underlying reason for their ubiquity remains unknown, it has been hypothesized that they participate in the clearance of blood-borne cell and tissue debris generated in both healthy and diseased individuals on a daily basis. Although much evidence supports this debris clearance role, recent studies also suggest a causal role for autoantibodies in disease. This chapter first presents well-known examples of autoimmune diseases that emphasize a direct causal role for autoantibodies and then discusses the veritable explosion of evidence now supporting their involvement in a wide variety of other diseases, including cancers and several types of neurological and neurodegenerative diseases. Lastly, translational strategies that take advantage of the "cause and/or effect" role of autoantibodies and recent technological advancements in their detection to exploit autoantibodies as sensitive and specific biomarkers useful for the detection and diagnosis of disease are outlined. Their use in the diagnosis and staging of Alzheimer's and Parkinson's diseases is presented, and future applications in clinical medicine and basic science are highlighted.

## 1. INTRODUCTION: A BRIEF HISTORY OF AUTOANTIBODIES

Autoantibodies, in the most basic conception, are simply antibodies that bind to one's self. The fact that they even exist has been subject to nearly a century of ardent opinion and unanticipated discovery.

Early pioneers of immunology left no room for the existence of autoantibodies. Paul Ehrlich, a father of the modern humoral immune system, was openly antagonistic to the idea. He envisioned that individuals have the capacity to produce antibodies to every possible nonself-antigen upon exposure and that this was a primary mechanism of fighting disease and invasion (Ehrlich, 1899). The lynchpin of this theory, however, was that one could never produce antibodies to one's self—to do this would unleash a cataclysm of immune self-destruction. Organisms therefore must have a tolerance to themselves and an aversion to self-recognition, the *horror autotoxicus*.

Succeeding decades proved more technical in their elaboration of this concept. Sir Frank Macfarlane Burnet provided a tentative mechanism for absolute self-tolerance in his clonal selection theory of acquired immunity (Burnet, 1959). There, he suggested that B lymphocytes with surface receptors responding to foreign antigens would be selectively stimulated to clonally proliferate and thereby increase the capacity for production of a single protective antibody. On the other hand, any B cell that responded to a self-antigen during fetal life would be selectively "deleted," and thus the ability to produce antibodies that recognize and bind to one's self would be eradicated forever.

But the twentieth century was marked by the discovery of dozens of autoimmune diseases clearly mediated by antibodies binding to self. The dogma of strict self-tolerance eventually crumpled under the weight of clinical evidence. Autoantibodies now seemed to be real. Despite this relatively recent admission, it had been known that antibodies react with self-antigens on spermatozoa and erythrocytes for over a century (Avrameas, Ternynck, Tsonis, & Lymberi, 2007). And there had been convincing evidence of autoantibodies and their relationship with disease as early as 1904 (Donath & Landsteiner, 1904). The existence of autoantibodies was finally accepted, but had to be reconciled within the previous framework of immunological thinking. It was postulated that only a condition of gross immune dysregulation would allow for their production, and that is what we now call an autoimmune disease. In this paradigm, the presence of autoantibodies always indicates disease and so they are biomarkers by their very nature.

The past three decades have revealed much about the prevalence of autoantibodies. It is now exceedingly clear that there are natural autoantibodies present outside of the setting of autoimmune disease. In fact, they are ubiquitous in the serum of all individuals, regardless of age, gender, or the presence of disease (Nagele et al., 2013). Self-reactive immunoglobulins have also been shown to be present in all tested mammals and in a variety of biological fluids, including blood, colostrum, saliva, and cerebrospinal fluid (CSF) (Avrameas, 1991; Avrameas & Ternynck, 1995; Bouvet & Dighiero, 1998). Moreover, while the profile of these natural autoantibodies differs from one individual to another, they are remarkably stable over time within a single individual (Lacroix-Desmazes, Mouthon, Kaveri, Kazatchkine, & Weksler, 1999; Mirilas, Fesel, Guilbert, Beratis, & Avrameas, 1999). The truth, it seems, is more strange and wonderful than our immunological forebears could have predicted.

It is now imagined that there are vast networks of self-reactive antibodies (autoantibodies) of multiple isotypes and affinities, working in concert to perform a variety of immunological and homeostatic tasks (Avrameas et al., 2007; Cohen, 2007). It is perhaps in these functions, which we are only now beginning to comprehend, that autoantibodies will have the most potency as biomarkers.

## 2. A CAUSAL ROLE FOR AUTOANTIBODIES REVEALED IN WELL-KNOWN AUTOIMMUNE DISEASES

### 2.1 Role of Autoantibodies and Protein Citrullination in Rheumatoid Arthritis

The relationship between autoantibodies and disease is probably best exemplified by rheumatoid arthritis (RA). RA is a progressive inflammatory disorder and common cause of joint deformity and pain in the aging population (Turk, van Beers-Tas, & van Schaardenburg, 2014). In the last two decades, RA has become widely regarded as an outcome of immune dysfunction in which one's own protein epitopes are targeted by autoantibodies generated by the immune system. Several studies have identified some of the protein targets and causal pathways that lead to the generation of autoantigens. Rheumatoid factor (RF) and anticitrullinated peptide antibodies (ACPAs) are two types of autoantibodies commonly detected in RA patient's sera.

Among these, ACPAs are considered to be more specific to RA as elevated RF levels are also detected in other autoimmune diseases, such as systemic lupus erythematosus (SLE) and Sjögren's syndrome, as well as in several non-autoimmune diseases. ACPAs can also activate complement via both classical and alternative pathways in a dose-dependent manner (Trouw et al., 2009).

Interestingly, it has been discovered that antigens associated with production of ACPAs are generated by protein citrullination, a chemical reaction catalyzed by a group of enzymes known as peptidylarginine deiminases (PADs) in which citrulline is formed from arginine within the protein scaffold. Citrullination of self-proteins appears to render them more antigenic, and proteins such as vimentin, filaggrin, keratin, fibrinogen, and α-enolase are known to undergo this reaction (Sakkas, Bogdanos, Katsiari, & Platsoucas, 2014). Therefore, generation of self-antigenic targets through citrullination results in loss of self-tolerance. Detection of antibodies in patient sera directed against citrullinated versions of the aforementioned proteins has strengthened our knowledge about the role of ACPAs in RA pathogenesis (Fig. 1) (Kinloch et al., 2005; Mathsson et al., 2008; Union et al., 2002). More recently, analysis of sera from RA patients prior to their diagnosis has revealed the presence of autoantibodies against PAD4 during preclinical phases of RA (Kolfenbach et al., 2010). Another study has also suggested that ACPAs may prove useful in diagnosing RA up to 10 years before the emergence of symptoms (Arkema et al., 2013). Additional evidence for the role of protein citrullination in RA comes from a study that demonstrated an increased incidence of the disease in patients with periodontitis (Mercado, Marshall, Klestov, & Bartold, 2001). Patients infected with *Porphyromonas gingivalis*, a common cause of periodontitis display increased levels of PAD expression and protein citrullination (Abdullah, Farmer, Spargo, Logan, & Gully, 2013; Wegner et al., 2010), as well as post-translational citrullination of vimentin and fibrin (Abdullah et al., 2013). In addition to the organ systems involved in RA, increased expression of enzymes catalyzing citrullination, such as PAD2, has also been observed in the bronchial mucosa and alveolar compartment of healthy smokers in comparison to healthy nonsmokers (Makrygiannakis et al., 2008).

## 2.2 SLE, an Autoimmune Disease with Autoantibodies Directed Against Common Nuclear and Cytoplasmic Proteins

SLE is a chronic multisystem inflammatory autoimmune disorder predominantly affecting women. Although the pathogenesis of SLE is not

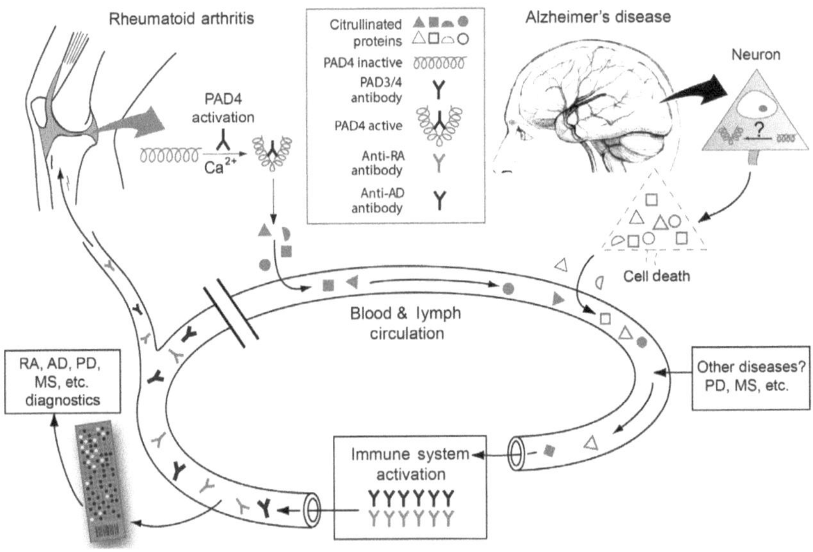


**Figure 1** In chronic diseases, such as rheumatoid arthritis (RA) and Alzheimer's disease (AD), many cells in regions of evolving pathology express PADs. PADs catalyze the post-translational citrullination of proteins, thereby enhancing their antigenicity. Cell death occurring in regions of pathology leads to the release of these proteins and their fragments as disease-associated debris. This debris continually spills into the circulation, and the immune system responds by eliciting the production of cognate autoantibodies. These disease-associated autoantibodies enter the blood, where they can bind to their blood-borne debris targets and where they are useful for detection as diagnostic indicators of disease. Once they enter into the blood, autoantibodies can also gain access to the joints (RA) or brain (AD), where they can react with any directly exposed cell surface-bound or -free antigens. Chronic binding of autoantibodies to their targets in vulnerable organs and tissues like the joints and the brain can exacerbate disease progression and may be a common mediator of a wide variety of diseases.

completely understood, genetic, environmental, and autoimmune factors have been implicated. Both humoral and innate immunity are thought to play a key role in the disease as numerous studies have identified dysfunction of the immune system and loss of tolerance during the pathogenesis of SLE (Ippolito et al., 2011). Several autoantibodies associated with SLE have been identified that target nuclear, cytoplasmic, surface membrane, and extracellular antigens present in various cell types and tissues (Ippolito et al., 2011; Sherer, Gorstein, Fritzler, & Shoenfeld, 2004; Yaniv et al., 2015). One specific type of autoantibody broadly implicated in SLE, antinuclear autoantibody (ANA), is comprised of several subtypes that are primarily directed against nucleic acids and their bound proteins, as well as small nuclear ribonucleoprotein particles (snRNPs), PCNA, and various other nuclear enzymes (Smeenk, 2000). Some ANAs have also been demonstrated to bind cytoplasmic targets, including SSA/Ro (Sjogren's syndrome-related antigen A/Ro) and SSB/La (Sjogren's syndrome type B antigen/lupus La protein) (Smeenk, 2000). Binding of ANAs to these proteins can generate immune complexes capable of triggering complement activation, eventually leading to extensive tissue inflammation.

In addition to ANAs, anti-*N*-methyl-D aspartate receptor (anti-NMDAR) autoantibodies have also been associated with SLE and neuropsychiatric systemic lupus erythematosus (NPSLE) (Hanly et al., 2011; Hirohata, Arinuma, Takayama, & Yoshio, 2007; Yaniv et al., 2015; Yoshio, Hirata, Onda, Nara, & Minota, 2005). A study by DeGiorgio et al. demonstrated cross-reactivity between the NR2A and NR2B subunits of NMDARs and antidouble-stranded (ds)DNA autoantibodies, leading to the loss of neurons both *in vivo* and *in vitro* models (DeGiorgio et al., 2001). Furthermore, studies by Kowal et al. have established the binding of anti-dsDNA autoantibodies directed against NMDAR subunits using a mouse model of NPSLE with a compromised blood–brain barrier (BBB) (Kowal et al., 2006, 2004). These studies demonstrate the role of both anti-NMDAR and anti-dsDNA autoantibodies in triggering neuropsychiatric disorders.

## 2.3 Systemic Sclerosis (Scleroderma)

Systemic sclerosis (SSc) is a chronic disorder characterized by fibrosis of the skin and internal organs. Although the pathogenesis of SSc is not fully understood, several autoantibodies directed against self-antigens have been implicated in the disease. Antitopoisomerase I (anti-topo I) and anticentromere (ACA) autoantibodies are the two most commonly identified ANAs in SSc pathology, with their expression and titer correlating with the course and severity of the disease (Cepeda & Reveille, 2004; Hamaguchi, 2010; Wielosz, Dryglewska, & Majdan, 2014). Furthermore, the presence of ACAs have also been associated with Raynaud's phenomenon; however, it is important to note that they are rarely present in healthy individuals or those with other connective tissue disorders (Kallenberg, Wouda, Hoet, & van Venrooij, 1988; Lee, Tsay, & Tsai, 1993). In addition to the identification of anti-topo I and ACA autoantibodies, anti-RNA polymerase, anti-Th/To, anti-U3RNP, anti-U1RNP, and anti-PM-Sci, as well as six centromeric polypeptides, (CENP-A to -F) were also found to be associated with SSc. Among these, CENP-B was found to be the major autoantigen implicated in the disease (Earnshaw, Machlin, Bordwell, Rothfield, & Cleveland, 1987; Hamaguchi, 2010).

## 3. AUTOANTIBODIES IN CANCER: BYPRODUCT OR BIOMARKER?

Interest surrounding the role of autoantibodies has steadily increased during the past decade, resulting in a more intense focus on their development as early biomarkers of cancer. There have been multiple studies citing increased levels of autoantibodies preceding the development of disease symptoms (Gnjatic et al., 2009; Tan & Zhang, 2008), as well as correlating this with the incidences (Nesterova, Johnson, Cheadle, & Cho-Chung, 2006) for cancers of the lung (Chapman et al., 2011; Diesinger et al., 2002), colon (Scanlan et al., 1998), breast (Disis et al., 1994), prostate (Wang et al., 2005), ovary (Chatterjee et al., 2006), and head and neck (Carey et al., 1983; Smith et al., 2008). Several theories have been offered to explain the mechanisms behind autoantibody production in association with the various types of cancers. Many hypothesize that cancer immunosurveillance, a process by which the body's own immune system recognizes and eliminates foreign pathogens and transformed host cells, initiates the immune response toward tumor-associated antigens during the early stages of tumorigenesis (Anderson & LaBaer, 2005; Caron, Choquet-Kastylevsky, & Joubert-Caron, 2007; Finn, 2005). The immune system may respond to various insults, including mutations, degradation, overexpression/production of proteins, release of protein debris from damaged tissue, or even misfolded proteins (Chen, Gure, & Scanlan, 2005; Jaras & Anderson, 2011; Kazarian & Laird-Offringa, 2011; Scanlan, Simpson, & Old, 2004).

With numerous groups investigating the link between autoantibodies and cancer, there have been many successful studies aimed at developing diagnostic biomarkers. For example, Xie et al. developed a test platform by combining the detection of six autoantibodies directed against prostate cancer with PSA levels, increasing the accuracy of detection from 65% using PSA alone to 81% with both methods (Xie et al., 2011). A similar outcome was achieved in breast cancer diagnosis, where Chapman et al. used a panel of six autoantigens to detect ductal carcinoma *in situ* with a specificity of 85% (Chapman et al., 2007). The heterogeneous nature of lung cancer has long hindered the development of a diagnostic test for early detection. However, with recent advances in autoantibody identification, Chapman et al. were able to test autoantibodies directed against various markers to develop a biomarker panel yielding up to 76% sensitivity and 92% specificity (Chapman et al., 2008). Patel et al. went even further to develop an autoantibody "direct-capture" immunobead assay using selected antigens for successful detection of nonsmall-cell lung carcinoma with a sensitivity and specificity of 94% and 97%, respectively (Patel et al., 2011). Similar advances using panels of autoantibodies have been made for the diagnosis of colon cancer (Belousov et al., 2008; Chen et al., 2007; Cioffi et al., 2004; Yoshizawa et al., 2007), stomach cancer (di Mario & Cavallaro, 2008), and hepatocellular carcinoma (Li, Chen, Yu, Li, & Wang, 2008; Marrero et al., 2003). Studies have demonstrated that the successful development of a single autoantibody biomarker approach for disease diagnostics has so far been hampered by low sensitivity, specificity, and predictive values, as well as poor reproducibility in larger sample cohorts. As a result, investigators are moving toward the use of panels containing multiple autoantibody biomarkers, thus significantly improving overall diagnostic accuracy.

## 4. ESCALATING INVOLVEMENT OF AUTOANTIBODIES IN NEUROLOGICAL AND NEUROCOGNITIVE DISORDERS

### 4.1 Introduction

The immune system consists of a myriad of cells that adapt to an ever-changing environment in order to maintain and optimize homeostasis. The autoimmune spectrum of disease has been attributed to a hyperactive immune system, in which B- and T cells otherwise tasked with surveying and removing foreign matter and cellular debris react to self-antigens or autoantigens. A classic example of this awry system is the "one autoantibody-to-one autoantigen" paradigm. Originally, the presence of an autoantibody was confined solely to the pathoetiology of a particular disease; however, recent evidence has led researchers to question whether or not the presence of an autoantibody faithfully denotes disease. For instance, a vital organ of the endocrine system, the thyroid, is relied on for hormonal effectors of protein, carbohydrate, and lipid metabolic functioning throughout the body, as well as fetal and neonatal brain development. Diseases associated with hyper- or hypofunctioning of this key organ can be caused by certain circulating autoantibody to given thyroid proteins and give rise to Graves' disease or Hashimoto's thyroiditis, respectively (Budenhofer,

Ditsch, Jeschke, Gartner, & Toth, 2013). Detection of the specific autoantibody allows for the existence of claims that describe the pathoetiology, prognostic outcomes, and treatment responsiveness based on autoantibody presence and titers (Chiovato et al., 2003; Dong & Fu, 2014).

The nervous system is no different. Myasthenia gravis (MG), discussed in Section 4.2, is one such disorder that is thought to follow the "one autoantibody-to-one autoantigen" system. Here, specific acetylcholine receptors and other functionally important structural components on and within the postsynaptic membrane are targeted by autoantibodies. This culminates in the pathology and clinical presentation seen in MG patients (Jayam Trouth, Dabi, Solieman, Kurukumbi, & Kalyanam, 2012). Recent findings in immunology research have tremendously altered the direction that the autoimmune field has taken to pathoetiology, prognostic outcomes, and treatment responsiveness. It would appear that the "one autoantibody-to-one autoantigen" hypothesis is an overly simplified model of what is occurring at the level of disease development and progression.

Multiple sclerosis (MS), discussed in detail in Section 4.3, is a central nervous system (CNS) inflammatory demyelinating condition rooted in autoimmune reactivity. This condition falls into this next category where autoantibodies play a largely contentious role in what was once thought to be a clearly defined relationship (Mirshafiey & Kianiaslani, 2013; Terryberry, Thor, & Peter, 1998). Indeed, the immune system effector T cells are integral to the development of this disease, while the presence and detection of autoantibody to various neuronal and myelin proteins have remained scattered from causative, to prognostic, to diagnostic among the medical community (Harris & Sadiq, 2014).

Neuromyelitis optica (NMO) and anti-*N*-methyl-D-aspartate (anti-NMDA) receptor encephalitis, discussed in Sections 4.4 and 4.5, respectively, are examples of another autoantibody model. This model attributes the pathological autoantibody binding to its cognate autoantigen, which in these cases are neuronal surface receptors. These differ largely from MG in that these conditions are housed within the so-called immunoprivileged CNS. Furthermore, these conditions have been found to exist with varying phenomenological descriptions based on autoantibody profiles. In fact, after its discovery, anti-NMDAR encephalitis was named after its reported cause, NMDAR autoantibodies (Kayser & Dalmau, 2014; Needham & Zandi, 2014). Considering that different autoantibodies can be found giving rise to seemingly similar psychiatric conditions, this discovery provides insight into disease prognosis and treatment based on the autoantibody profiles present. Moreover, this allows for a laboratory diagnosis of purely clinical syndromes, and it is now being expanded into other psychiatric conditions like psychosis and schizophrenia (Dahm et al., 2014; Hammer et al., 2014).

Alzheimer's disease (AD), a CNS proteinopathy discussed in Section 4.6, is gaining popularity in the guise of a neuroinflammatory-mediated condition (Needham & Zandi, 2014). Here, the presence of autoantibodies is now given much attention in basic science and translational research attempts for presymptomatic diagnostics and treatment regimens (Terryberry et al., 1998). Recent efforts have implicated autoantibodies in a more causative role. Efforts have been made to demonstrate the relationship between intracellular neuronal Aβ42 deposition, which may coincide with extracellular accumulation and precede amyloid plaque formation, and the binding of autoantibodies to the surfaces of neurons damaged in the wake of these events (D'Andrea & Nagele, 2006; Nagele, D'Andrea, Anderson, & Wang, 2002). Although the cognate receptor to which these candidate autoantibodies bind is not yet known, evidence for such a phenomenon can reshape our current thinking on the pathogenesis of AD. A list of autoantibodies that have the potential for use as blood-based autoantibody biomarkers in various diseases are listed in Table 1.

## 4.2 MG—A Classical Example of Autoantibodies Causing a Neurological Disease

Identified in 1895, "myasthenia gravis pseudoparalytica" is characterized by fluctuating muscle weakness that becomes worse upon exertion (Trouth et al., 2012). Similar symptoms were found between MG patients and those suffering from curare poisoning. Curare, a plant-based chemical native to South American rainforests, competitively inhibits nicotinic acetylcholine receptors (nAChRs) of the neuromuscular junction. Curare poisoning had been effectively treated with the anticholinesterase physostigmine, and this therapy also proved effective for MG patients. Eventually, researchers were able to recapitulate MG in a rabbit model system following injections of acetylcholine receptors. This meant that the disease could successfully be reversed with anticholinesterases, and it defined MG as autoimmune in nature, as autoantibodies directed to nAChR were demonstrated to cause disease pathology (Patrick & Lindstrom, 1973).

Much has been learned about MG since it has been classified as an autoimmune disease. While scientists hoped to develop a laboratory test that could be used for clinical diagnosis, the poor sensitivity of the tests limited the detectable levels of circulating autoantibodies. Also, a group of clinically

**Table 1** Diagnosable Conditions and Their Associated Autoantibodies

| Condition | Associated Autoantibodies | Reference(s) |
|---|---|---|
| Rheumatoid arthritis | Rheumatoid factor<br>Citrullinated peptide antibody | Trouw et al. (2009) |
| Systemic lupus erythematosus | Nuclear antibodies (nucleosomes, snRNP, SSA/Ro, and SSB/La)<br>Smith<br>Phospholipid | Aho, Koskela, Makitalo, Heliovaara, and Palosuo (1992); Smeenk, 2000 |
| | NMDAR | Hanly et al. (2011) |
| | P-ribosomal | Hirohata et al. (2007); Yoshio et al. (2005) |
| | U1RNP | Sato et al. (2010) |
| | dsDNA | Arbuckle et al. (2001); DeGiorgio et al. (2001) |
| Systemic sclerosis (scleroderma) | Topoisomerase I<br>Centromere (CENP) | Earnshaw et al. (1987); Hamaguchi (2010) |
| | RNA polymerase<br>Th/To<br>U3RNP, U1RNP<br>PM-Sci | Hamaguchi (2010) |
| Graves' disease | Thyroid stimulating hormone | Dong and Fu (2014); Sinclair (2008) |
| Hashimoto's thyroiditis | Thyroid peroxidase<br>Thyroglobulin<br>Pendrin | Dong and Fu (2014); Gupta, Sinha, and Dagar (2013) |
| Myasthenia gravis | Nicotinic acetylcholine receptor<br>Muscle-specific tyrosine kinase | Jayam Trouth et al. (2012) |
| Multiple sclerosis | Myelin oligodendrocyte glycoprotein | Fraussen, Claes, de Bock, and Somers (2014); Mirshafiey and Kianiaslani (2013); Weber, Hemmer, and Cepok (2011) |
| | Myelin basic protein | Panitch, Hooper, and Johnson (1980) |

**Table 1** Diagnosable Conditions and Their Associated Autoantibodies—cont'd

| Condition | Associated Autoantibodies | Reference(s) |
|---|---|---|
| | Myelin proteolipid protein Myelin-associated glycoprotein | Johnson et al. (1986) |
| | KIR4.1 | Schirmer, Srivastava, and Hemmer (2014) |
| | GAGA4 | Brettschneider et al. (2009) |
| Neuromyelitis optica | Aquaporin-4 | Lennon, Kryzer, Pittock, Verkman, and Hinson (2005) |
| NMDAR encephalitis | *N*-methyl-D-aspartate receptor | Kayser and Dalmau (2014) |
| Alzheimer's disease | Amyloid-β | Maftei et al. (2013) |
| Parkinson's disease | α-Synuclein | Yanamandra et al. (2011) |
| | Melanin | Double et al. (2009) |

diagnosed MG patients emerged that lacked autoantibodies to nAChR, and this called into question the utility of a laboratory diagnosis that did not support clear clinical diagnoses. Later, other autoantibodies were discovered that had a similar presentation to MG autoantibodies—particularly muscle-specific tyrosine kinase (MuSK) autoantibodies. Studies have revealed that up to 50% of patients with no detectable nAChR autoantibodies (roughly 15% of MG cases) were positive for autoantibodies to MuSK and other postsynaptic neuromuscular junction proteins (Romi, Aarli, & Gilhus, 2005; Trouth et al., 2012). Although the presence and diagnostic implications of these autoantibodies have not yet been defined, it is clear that they possess the capability to incite damage at the postsynaptic neuromuscular junction.

### 4.3 MS—A Neuroinflammatory Demyelinating Disease Associated with Autoantibodies

The identification of MS, today's most common debilitating CNS autoimmune disease, is predated by over 150 years of clinical classification (Harris & Sadiq, 2014). The common early symptoms of extremity muscle weakness and paresthesias, blurred vision, and cognitive decline manifest from CNS neuronal demyelination, which first occurs in the white matter of the brain (including the optic nerve) and spinal cord, but later includes gray matter lesions (Harris & Sadiq, 2014; Jurynczyk, Craner, & Palace, 2015). Lesions are typically found to contain clonal populations of B cells and plasma cells, CD4 + autoreactive T cells, and autoantibodies. Recently, CD8 + cytotoxic T cells have been found in these lesions as well and are implicated in the pathogenesis of characteristic MS lesions. Oligodendrocytic damage defines most of the pathology of MS, as the targets of the reactive immune effectors include antigens on the oligodendrocytes themselves and the myelin sheath (Mirshafiey & Kianiaslani, 2013). The mechanism by which cellular damage is thought to take place includes antibody-dependent cellular cytotoxicity, opsonization, and phagocytosis, complement fixation, activation, and assembly of the membrane attack complex, and even, as most recently reported, antibody-induced cross-linking and demyelination (Marta et al., 2005; Weber et al., 2011). Details of the dynamic interplay of these cells and reactive autoantibodies during disease pathogenesis have yet to be clearly defined.

The autoantibodies linked to MS have been implicated as causative, diagnostic, prognostic, and even treatment-responsiveness forms of blood biomarkers. For example, causative autoantibodies often have been cited as targeting specific myelin surface proteins, namely myelin oligodendrocyte glycoprotein (MOG), myelin basic protein (MBP), myelin proteolipid protein, and myelin-associated glycoprotein (Fraussen et al., 2014; Johnson et al., 1986; Panitch et al., 1980). Autoantibodies of both IgG and IgM types have been detected for these antigens (Fraussen et al., 2014). Berger et al. studied levels of anti-MOG and anti-MBP autoantibodies in patients with clinically isolated syndrome (CIS), often considered by neurologists as preceding overt MS, and found that higher titers of anti-MOG and anti-MBP autoantibodies in CIS patients were predictive of earlier and more frequent relapses of the disease (Berger et al., 2003). Several other studies have supported the use of anti-MOG and anti-MBP antibodies for diagnosis of MS (Greeve et al., 2007; Tomassini et al., 2007), but other reports dispute the utility of anti-MOG and anti-MBP for this purpose (Kuhle et al., 2007; Lim et al., 2005). New research has identified a novel protein target located on astrocytic foot processes and oligodendrocytes—KIR4.1. This potassium channel is seemingly lost on implicated cells in chronic and acute MS lesions and is being thoroughly investigated as to its role in the autoimmune reactivity driving disease pathology. When investigated for its diagnostic utility, it was found that 47% of MS patients had autoantibodies to KIR4.1 protein, which are seldom found in healthy patient samples (Schirmer et al., 2014).

Autoantibodies directed against glycans are also showing promise as diagnostic indicators of MS. Anti-GAGA4 [Glc(α1,4)Glc(α)] antibodies have been used to distinguish patients with the relapsing-remitting form of MS (RRMS) from healthy controls as well as individuals with other neurological diseases (Brettschneider et al., 2009). In addition, anti-GAGA4 antibodies were shown to differentiate patients with RRMS from those with the secondary progressive form of MS (Brettschneider et al., 2009). Similarly, high titers of anti-α-glucose IgM have been reported to be predictive of imminent relapse in first presentation MS patients (Freedman et al., 2009).

The ability for symptoms of MS to remit for periods of time lends very appropriately to an *in vivo* model by which the body is able to regain homeostasis in the face of rampant disease, yet retain the ability to relapse in the future. This feature of MS makes it an ideal situation to gauge for distinguishing biomarkers of remission and relapse, which can be expounded to prognostic outcomes and treatment responsiveness by following such biomarkers over time. Given the CNS compartmentalization of the disease, it makes sense to assay the CSF for markers of ongoing CNS pathology. Present within the CSF in MS patients are abnormally abundant B cells, memory cells, and plasmablasts without plasma cells and increased levels of IgG throughout the course of their disease (Cepok et al., 2005). Additionally, the discovery of electrophoretically isolated oligoclonal species of antibodies in the CSF (accompanying clonotypic B-cell populations in the lesions) has allowed for the advent of a highly sensitive diagnostic test called oligoclonal IgG banding (OCB) (Cole, Beck, Moke, Kaufman, & Tourtellotte, 1998; Link & Huang, 2006), which demonstrates the presence of an ongoing neuroinflammatory B-cell-mediated process (Link & Huang, 2006). Although OCB is found in other conditions associated with neuroinflammation, when compared with the clinical features and autoantibody findings, the specificity of an MS diagnosis becomes highly accurate.

## 4.4 Neuromyelitis Optica—A Neuroinflammatory Demyelinating Disease with a Causative Autoantibody

In 2005, a subset variant of MS known as "optic-spinal" MS was discovered. This group of traditionally "treatment-unresponsive" MS patients was found to possess a unique autoantibody that was largely absent in the "treatment-responsive" population (Lennon et al., 2005, 2004). This autoantibody was found to bind to a specific class of aquaporin channels native to astrocytic foot processes (aqp-4). The advent of highly sensitive assays for the aqp-4 autoantibody in the sera of these patients led to the realization that optic-spinal MS is not a variant of MS; rather, it is a new disease altogether, leading to the discovery of NMO (Lennon et al., 2005).

Although NMO and MS present with very similar symptoms, the presence of aqp-4 autoantibodies in the sera and CSF of NMO patients renders them susceptible to different treatment options and procedures. While some still consider NMO to be under the umbrella of MS, NMO has gained popularity among neurologists as a water-channel targeting, autoantibody-mediated astrocytopathy, giving it a distinct immunopathogenesis, and thus treatment–response profile (Jurynczyk et al., 2015). While NMO can be managed, albeit temporarily, with plasmaphoresis, it seems to contain less of a cellular component and more of a soluble autoantibody factor than MS. Furthermore, NMO patients seropositive for aqp-4 autoantibodies may also possess anti-MOG autoantibody (Kitley et al., 2014). Additionally, aqp-4 seronegative NMO patients may be MOG autoantibody positive, again blurring the lines between the laboratory diagnosis of MS and NMO with the clinical features and presentation. While the autoantibodies of MS remain contentious as to their primary role and purpose, those of NMO are excellent biomarkers of disease progression and response to treatment.

## 4.5 Anti-NMDAR Encephalitis—Autoantibodies Targeting Receptors Causing Neuropsychiatric Symptoms

Anti-NMDAR encephalitis, another type of causative autoantibody-induced neuronal disease, is characterized by autoantibodies directed toward a specific subunit of glutamate receptors found on the neuronal surfaces. What makes this disease unique from many of the other supposedly autoimmune diseases is the specificity by which these autoantibodies can be used as diagnostic and prognostic indicators for disease presence, progression, and treatment responsiveness. Glutamatergic signaling accounts for a large portion of the synaptic transmission in the corticolimbic system of the mammalian brain (Coyle, 2012; Paoletti, Bellone, & Zhou, 2013). While there are several types of ionotropic cation-channel receptors that respond to the neurotransmitter glutamate, the NMDARs are of particularly growing interest in neuropsychiatry. Long predating the discovery of NMDAR autoantibodies, glutamate neurotransmission rose to the forefront of psychotic conditions, including schizophrenia, where it plays a central role in the pathoetiology.

Recently, drug therapies have harnessed the complex networks, by which serotonin mediates its receptor subtypes to act on dopaminergic neurotransmission, and this has replaced the "dopamine hypothesis of schizophrenia." The serotonin circuitry of the limbic system in the midbrain, including the hippocampus, is under glutamatergic and GABAergic regulation (Coyle, 2012; Meltzer, Horiguchi, & Massey, 2011; Paoletti et al., 2013). The aforementioned studies paralleled an ever-growing immunologic theory for psychiatric conditions, which culminated in Dr. Josep Dalmau's landmark 2007 discovery of NMDAR autoantibodies in a patient diagnosed with intractable schizophrenia (Kayser & Dalmau, 2014). In cases of intractable psychosis to conventional therapies, neurological consultation often will involve investigation into organic etiologies, like biomarkers of other pathologies. NMDAR autoantibodies are being considered a highly accurate indicator for this variant of encephalitis-induced psychosis. In many cases, NMDAR autoantibodies are detected and, over 80% of the time, aggressive immunotherapy and steroids will have a positive prognostic outcome (Kayser & Dalmau, 2014). These autoantibodies are detected in much higher titers in the CSF than in the sera, and they can also be followed for treatment responsiveness (Kayser & Dalmau, 2014).

Studies aimed at addressing the cellular and molecular mechanisms of NMDAR encephalitis have shown that, upon autoantibody binding to the cognate receptor, cross-linking of IgG occurs followed by clathrin-mediated endocytosis that leads to subsequent internalization of the autoantibody-bound receptor, and its delivery to the lysosomal compartment (Hammer et al., 2014; Hughes et al., 2010). The decrease in NMDARs on the synaptic terminal reduces synaptic plasticity in the implicated region, most notably the hippocampus where there is a large population of these neurons (Moscato et al., 2014). In essence, autoantibody binding to NMDAR precedes IgG cross-linking and subsequent internalization (Lancaster, Martinez-Hernandez, & Dalmau, 2011; Pollak, Nicholson, Mellers, Vincent, & David, 2014). The ensuing depletion of NMDAR dictates the clinical findings of psychosis that is oftentimes diagnosed as schizophrenia until the blood is assayed for autoantibody presence. Recent efforts have begun assaying large cohorts of schizophrenic patients not otherwise diagnosed as having NMDAR encephalitis, reporting such autoantibodies present in greater than 10% of patients (Hammer et al., 2014). However, these autoantibodies are also found with similar prevalence in controls (Dahm et al., 2014; Hammer et al., 2014). At first glance, this would seem to call into question the utility and exclusivity of NMDAR encephalitis rooted in autoantibody production. However, recent work by Ehrenreich and coworkers has suggested that two factors are required:

the presence of NMDAR autoantibodies and compromise of the BBB, the latter being essential for allowing access of blood-borne autoantibodies to the brain parenchyma to drive the pathology (Dahm et al., 2014; Hammer et al., 2014; Nagele, Clifford, et al., 2011; Nagele, Han, Demarshall, Belinka, & Nagele, 2011).

## 4.6 AD—Evidence that Autoantibodies and Blood–Brain Barrier Breakdown Are Partners in Crime

AD is a progressive and devastating neurodegenerative disorder of the elderly highlighted by dramatic cognitive and memory impairment and linked to a loss of neurons and synapses that causes brain shrinkage and a release of brain debris pertinent to the generation of disease-associated autoantibodies (Fig. 1) (Bertoni-Freddari et al., 2003; D'Andrea, Nagele, Wang, Peterson, & Lee, 2001; Hamos, DeGennaro, & Drachman, 1989; Selkoe, 2002). Well-known pathological features include rampant neuronal loss, deposition of amyloid beta (Aβ) peptides (especially the 42-amino acid peptide (Aβ42)) primarily in pyramidal neurons, amyloid plaques, and in the walls of brain blood vessels as well as the appearance of neurofibrillary tangles, reactive gliosis, and inflammation (Clifford et al., 2008; D'Andrea et al., 2001; Dickson, 1997b; Gouras et al., 2000; Nagele et al., 2002; Schwab & McGeer, 2008). Intraneuronal Aβ deposition occurs early in the disease, preceding the formation of amyloid plaques and tangles, but occurs concurrently with loss of synapses (D'Andrea et al., 2001; Gouras et al., 2000; Nagele, Clifford, et al., 2011; Nagele et al., 2002; Nagele, Han, et al., 2011).

Mechanisms and factors contributing to intraneuronal Aβ deposition and amyloid plaques remain elusive and controversial. However, as shown for many of the diseases described in this review, strong evidence is now emerging that autoantibodies may also play an important role in the initiation and progression of AD (Acharya et al., 2012). For example, it has been previously reported that brain-reactive autoantibodies (IgG) are ubiquitous in human sera (Nagele et al., 2013; Oddo, Caccamo, Kitazawa, Tseng, & LaFerla, 2003). This, along with the consistent presence of IgG-positive neurons in regions of AD pathology, suggests that chronic BBB compromise allows autoantibodies to gain access to their targets on the surfaces of neurons (Levin et al., 2010; Stein, Fedynyshyn, & Kalil, 2002). Soluble Aβ42 is known to preferentially accumulate on the surfaces of certain types of neurons, especially those that abundantly express the α-7 nAChR, for which Aβ42 has strong binding affinity (Nagele et al., 2002; Wang et al., 2000). A study by Nagele et al. used adult mouse hippocampal brain slice cultures as a model system to test the effects of human serum autoantibodies on intraneuronal deposition of soluble Aβ42 peptide (Nagele, Clifford, et al., 2011; Nagele, Han, et al., 2011). Binding of human autoantibodies to pyramidal neurons dramatically increased the rate and extent of Aβ42 internalization and accumulation in these cells, presumably via stimulation of antibody-mediated endocytosis. Importantly, individual sera varied considerably in potency with regard to their capacity to enhance intraneuronal Aβ42 accumulation *in vitro*. This suggests that the presence and titer of specific autoantibodies may be linked to relative risk for AD as well as the expected rate of progression. Although the identities and titers of these putative causal autoantibodies are unknown, work is currently underway to identify them.

It has been proposed that chronic binding of autoantibodies to the surfaces of neurons, made possible by breakdown of BBB integrity, triggers autoantibody-induced endocytosis, and that this drives the observed chronic neuronal internalization and accumulation of cell surface-associated Aβ42 (Acharya, Nagele, Han, & Nagele, 2013; Clifford et al., 2007; Nagele, Clifford, et al., 2011; Nagele, Han, et al., 2011). Under these conditions, intraneuronal Aβ42 accumulations would increase over time by virtue of the fact that Aβ42 is largely nondegradable within the expanding lysosomal compartment (Grbovic et al., 2003). The two-hit mechanism proposed here has chronic breakdown of the BBB as the required trigger and neuron-binding autoantibodies playing the role of key mediators of AD pathology at sites of the BBB breach. This mechanism can account for the clear association of AD with aging, its delayed onset in healthy active individuals (good microvascular health and an intact BBB), and its strong association with vascular trauma such as occurs in stroke, traumatic brain injury, or anesthesia. Given this mechanism, the expected rate of AD progression in patients would be dependent, at least in part, on the identity and titer of certain neuron-binding autoantibodies in their blood, the extent and specific brain location of the BBB breach, and the relative abundance of the target protein on neuronal surfaces in the vicinity of the vascular leak.

## 5. AUTOANTIBODIES: ABUNDANT, UBIQUITOUS, AND CLINICALLY USEFUL

### 5.1 The Rise of Natural Autoantibodies

When the existence of autoantibodies was finally accepted, they were quickly branded as aberrant. It was thought that they could only exist in the setting of a gross immunological dysfunction. They were considered a pathology. And the emerging role of autoantibodies in disease, especially in diseases driven by the direct interaction of single-epitope autoantibodies and their receptor, such as in Graves' disease, MG, and NMO, seemed to bear out this thinking.

Continued investigation demonstrated the diagnostic utility of using autoantibodies as biomarkers to confirm the presence of autoimmune pathology. For example, patients with RA, SLE, and vasculitis are now routinely screened for RF, ANAs, and antineutrophil cytoplasmic antibodies, respectively. But the widespread clinical measurement of these autoantibodies revealed their true prevalence in the population. And it is now clear that traditional autoantibody biomarkers have a specificity problem—that is, a surprising number of people without autoimmune disease appear to have "disease-associated" autoantibodies.

The use of ANAs to screen for lupus encapsulates the dilemma. Despite the high sensitivity of the ANA test to screen for SLE, its specificity is low. These antibodies, which bind to a variety of intracellular nuclear antigens, can also be present in healthy individuals, the elderly, those with thyroid disease, patients with active infections, and others (Kavanaugh, Tomar, Reveille, Solomon, & Homburger, 2000; Marin, Cardiel, Cornejo, & Viveros, 2009; Nilsson et al., 2006). Moreover, ANAs are often present in patients with malignancies, with a prevalence of 5–55%, depending on the particular cancer (Imran, Neelam, & Tariq, 2003; Kavanaugh et al., 2000; Solans-Laque et al., 2004). According to one recent study, even after a 1:80 dilution of serum, the prevalence of ANAs in healthy controls is 8% and more than 12% in those with multiple medical problems (Wichainun et al., 2013). Similar data exist for many of the other autoantibody biomarkers routinely used to screen for and identify rheumatic diseases. These data suggest that autoantibodies exist in far greater swaths of the population than was originally thought.

Given that these results were in direct contradiction of accepted precepts, they were often dismissed as technical errors, background "noise," or due to some inherent "glue-like" property of immunoglobulins (Avrameas et al., 2007). But further investigations proved that the phenomenon was widespread, involving antibodies that react to a multitude of intra- and extracellular autoantigens. These autoantibodies were identified in a variety of biological fluids, including blood, colostrum, saliva, and CSF (Avrameas, 1991; Avrameas & Ternynck, 1995; Bouvet & Dighiero, 1998). And they were identified in all tested mammals, including mice, rats, rabbits, pigs, and cows. They were even found in other nonmammal vertebrates, with sandbar sharks possessing IgM to thyroglobulin and single-stranded DNA (Marchalonis, Hohman, Thomas, & Schluter, 1993). It was becoming evident that the presence of autoantibodies is a normal finding. Therefore, for the first time, researchers began working under the assumption that these autoantibodies were not produced through some dysregulatory pathology, but were perhaps a purposeful product of the immune system. They were termed "natural autoantibodies."

## 5.2 Prevalence and Stability of Natural Autoantibodies

All healthy humans have natural autoantibodies. Early investigations tended to identify these autoantibodies one at a time, usually focused on auto-IgM binding to a particular postapoptotic antigen-like phosphatidyl serine, cardiolipin, or annexin IV (Madi et al., 2009; Mouthon et al., 1995). But, as technology advanced and high-throughput screening methods have become available, the true scale and diversity of serum autoantibodies has come into focus. One recent study, testing the sera of 166 individuals, demonstrated that IgG autoantibodies were present in every subject, and typically numbered in the thousands. Moreover, the number and diversity of autoantigens represented was influenced by age, gender, and the presence of disease (Nagele et al., 2013). Interestingly, the profile of natural autoantibodies, while differing greatly from one individual to the next, appears stable in children and adults over time (Lacroix-Desmazes et al., 1999; Mirilas et al., 1999; Nagele et al., 2013). There is even a forensics company that made clever use of the stability of autoantibody profiles to develop a non-DNA identity test for use at crime scenes (Non-DNA Human Identification Test Announced, 2015). It is now well established that autoantibodies are ubiquitous in human serum, are influenced by age, gender, and disease, and are remarkably stable over time.

## 5.3 Isotype and Reactivity of Natural Autoantibodies

In mammals, natural autoantibodies are of the IgM, IgA, and IgG isotypes (Avrameas et al., 2007). It was once thought that the majority of natural autoantibodies were IgM, but recent studies have highlighted the prominence of auto-IgG as well (Nagele et al., 2013). Part of the difficulty in assessing the relative titer of each isotype is that it seems to depend on the protein environment in which they are being measured. High levels of IgM natural autoantibodies are identified in sera, but not in plasma (Sigounas, Kolaitis, Monell-Torrens, & Notkins, 1994). All isotypes of natural autoantibodies demonstrate a considerable increase in autoreactivity when isolated (Coutinho, Kazatchkine, & Avrameas, 1995; Sigounas et al., 1994). Therefore, it seems that circulating proteins may have some dampening effect on the autoreactivity of natural autoantibodies. And this dampening effect appears to exist in a dynamic equilibrium. For example, normal rats possess various antiglomerular antibodies that do not bind to their epitopes due to nonimmunoglobulin serum proteins. On the other hand, rats with autoimmune glomerulonephritis demonstrate strong autoantibody binding to glomerular antigens that can be inhibited by the addition of serum protein (Druet, Praddaude, Druet, & Dietrich, 1998). Similar natural autoantibodies to glomerular basement membrane type IV collagen were recently found in healthy humans, but their discovery required special unmasking methods from serum protein (Cui, Zhao, Segelmark, & Hellmark, 2010; Jennette & Falk, 2010).

Natural autoantibodies were long thought to be largely weak affinity, polyreactive immunoglobulins. In reality, they are more diverse. Natural autoantibodies can be both mono- and polyreactive, and it has been observed that both can be encoded by nonmutated germline genes (Casali & Schettino, 1996; Notkins, 2004; Ochsenbein & Zinkernagel, 2000). Polyreactive IgM was experimentally found to be more reactive to foreign proteins than autoantigens, and so it may even be likely that the preponderance of natural autoantibodies is skewed toward being monoreactive (Lee et al., 2002). Further research is needed for a more nuanced understanding of natural autoantibody reactivity, but at this point, it is clear that they represent the full spectrum of specificity and affinity.

## 5.4 Natural Autoantibody Production

IgM natural autoantibodies are present in newborn humans as well as in newborn mice reared in germ- and antigen-free conditions. Interestingly, the repertoires of natural autoantibodies produced in both are independent of external antigenic contact (Haury et al., 1997; Hooijkaas, Benner, Pleasants, & Wostmann, 1984; Merbl, Zucker-Toledano, Quintana, & Cohen, 2007). For this reason, it was long postulated that natural autoantibodies were produced by B1 CD5+ lymphocytes residing within the peritoneum, as that particular class of B-cell has a lower threshold for exogenous stimulation to produce immunoglobulins. However, these cells also respond poorly to receptor-mediated activation and have a limited ability to isotype switch (Baumgarth, Tung, & Herzenberg, 2005). Therefore, this class of

B cell alone would be unable to produce the IgG and IgA natural autoantibodies that are also ubiquitous. It has since been demonstrated that numerous subpopulations of B cells contribute to the manufacture of circulating autoantibodies (Zhou & Notkins, 2004). The exact mechanisms by which these B cells produce natural autoantibodies and the intracellular communications required for their regulation remain to be determined.

## 5.5 Function of Natural Autoantibodies

The purview of natural autoantibody function is a matter of active discussion. When viewed in isolation, natural autoantibodies have some surprising effects. Those binding with individual receptors can sometimes mimic the action of its ligand. For example, natural autoantibodies that react with estrogen receptors have some estrogenic activity. Those reacting with opioid receptors have morphine-like properties. And IgG natural autoantibodies directed toward thyrotropin receptors have some thyroid stimulating effect (Latrofa et al., 2004; Mace, Blanpied, Emorine, Druet, & Dietrich, 1999; Tassignon, Haeseleer, & Borkowski, 1997). Other natural autoantibodies recognize intracellular antigens and promote catalytic activities (Paul, 1996; Ruiz-Arguelles, Rivadeneyra-Espinoza, & Alarcon-Segovia, 2003). Still others are known to contribute to host defense against pathogens (Ochsenbein et al., 1999; Ochsenbein & Zinkernagel, 2000).

But given the widespread evolutionary conservation of natural autoantibodies and the vast metabolic expense of maintaining the clonal B-cell populations necessary to support such a stable and complex profile of thousands of autoantibodies, it would appear that the primary role of natural autoantibodies is more fundamental. A clue as to what this function may be comes from IgM. Auto-IgM is known to bind to postapoptotic antigens and markers of cell senescence (Hardy & Hayakawa, 2005; Madi et al., 2009; Mouthon et al., 1995). Moreover, mice experimentally deprived of their auto-IgM develop lupus-like symptoms associated with the build-up of intracellular debris (Boes et al., 2000; Lampropoulou et al., 2010). Thus, it appears that a prominent role of natural autoantibodies is debris-clearance and the maintenance of tissue homeostasis.

The hypothesis that natural autoantibodies have a primary role in the clearance of day-to-day physiologic debris is corroborated by studying the profile of natural autoantibodies in newborns. It has been discovered that newborns share a selected, conserved panel of innate auto-IgM, regardless of the highly variable transplacentally delivered IgG from their mother (Madi,

Bransburg-Zabary, Kenett, Ben-Jacob, & Cohen, 2012; Merbl et al., 2007). It is thought that this panel of IgM natural autoantibodies is "programmed" to represent the most common antigens derived from physiologic debris, such as those indicating apoptosis or cell senescence. But, these innate, class-restricted, low-titer IgMs are suitable only for anticipated debris. The vast amounts of cell and tissue damage resulting from injury or illness would require an adaptable natural autoantibody response. It is this adaptation and specificity to which IgG is best suited.

### 5.6 Implications and Opportunity

It is in their newfound capacity for debris-clearance and the maintenance of homeostasis that autoantibodies may derive their ultimate potency as diagnostic biomarkers. If pathology results in the production of specific cell and tissue damage, it would then also result in the production of specific autoantibodies suited to the clearance of that debris. Thus, the appearance of specific perturbations in one's natural autoantibody profile could be telltale of pathology. It is as if a particular pathology or disease casts a recognizable shadow upon the immune system which is laboring to maintain the interstitial and intracellular *status quo*. If we can learn to recognize particular natural autoantibody profile perturbations and link them to individual pathologies, then autoantibodies may provide very early and specific indicators of disease.

## 6. METHODS OF AUTOANTIBODY DETECTION IN BIOFLUIDS

### 6.1 Proteomic Approaches for Autoantibody Analysis in Biological Samples

Identification of autoantibody biomarkers involves an assortment of technological approaches (Fig. 2). This includes a discovery process, which is unbiased and usually semiquantitative. In this phase, the differential expression of specific proteins or group of proteins is compared between healthy and diseased states. The source of these proteins ranges from human biological materials including blood, to mouse models and cell lines. The number of markers discovered by this approach might range from a few to several hundreds, all requiring further validation.

Among the basic proteomic platforms currently being utilized, mass spectroscopy appears to be a common denominator, with an overview of the general methods for the discovery of autoantibody biomarkers detailed

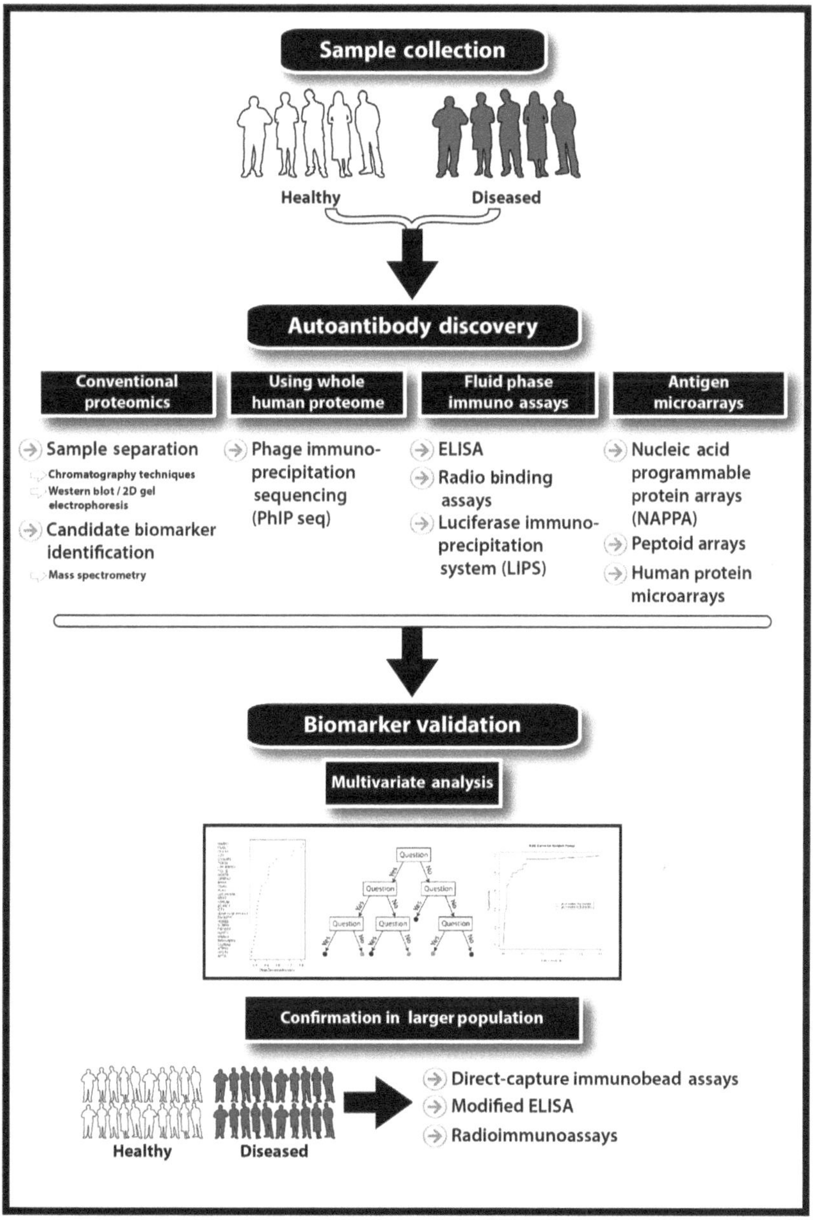


**Figure 2** General schematic displaying various techniques currently employed for discovery of autoantibody-based biomarkers and their further validation.

below. Serum samples are generally collected from two distinct groups: healthy and diseased populations. Commonly employed techniques to identify significant differences in autoantigen expression in the two groups include chromatographic techniques (GC and LC/HPLC) and two-dimensional gel electrophoresis/Western blot analysis. The final output of these steps is a protein map with several proteins segregated into individual spots, visualized using common staining protocols (Candiano et al., 2004; Chevallet et al., 2008) and fluorescent dyes (Berggren et al., 2000). The stained gels are then digitized and analyzed using dedicated software for the estimation of protein amount by comparing the intensities of individually stained spots (Berth, Moser, Kolbe, & Bernhardt, 2007). Proteins of interest are then isolated from the gel using standard enzymatic digestion protocols, giving a mixture of peptides that are ready for mass spectrometry analysis. Commonly employed mass spectrometry techniques include matrix-assisted laser desorption/ionization time of flight analysis (Tambor et al., 2010) and tandem (MS/MS) mass spectrometry (Domon & Aebersold, 2006; Mann, Hendrickson, & Pandey, 2001). The generated mass spectrometry data are then analyzed based on predetermined parameters using bioinformatics tools to compare and identify individual proteins.

## 6.2 Discovery of Candidate Autoantibody Biomarkers Using the Whole Human Proteome

The complete spectrum of autoantibody candidates associated with different pathological states remains unknown. Completion of the human proteome draft has made new strategies possible for the identification of potential autoantibody targets. Phage immunoprecipitation sequencing (PhIP seq) (Larman et al., 2011) employs a T7 bacteriophage system exhibiting greater than 400,000, 36-residue, overlapping peptides derived from the entire human proteome. This method generates a library of phage-expressed human peptides, which is applied to immobilized autoantibodies derived from patient sera. The peptides identified by this method are bound by autoantibodies and subsequently purified by repeated steps of washing and immunoprecipitation. Specific phages encoding the identified antigens are then analyzed directly by high-throughput DNA sequencing. PhIP seq has been previously utilized to identify potentially novel autoantigens in cases of RA (Larman et al., 2013), encephalitis (Larman et al., 2011), and MS (Larman et al., 2013). It has also been used to validate potential antigenic epitopes (Larman et al., 2013) identified in other studies (Srivastava et al., 2012).

## 6.3 Autoantibody Discovery by Fluid-Phase Immunoassays

A significant percentage of human autoantibodies are directed against conformational epitopes rather than their linear counterparts. Conventional immunoassay (solid-phase) methods such as ELISA exhibit low diagnostic efficacy for detecting such epitopes from autoantigens (Liu & Eisenbarth, 2007). Fluid-phase radio binding assays (RBAs) provide a more efficient alternative. In this method, the autoantigens are tested in solution rather than being immobilized on a solid surface. A significant advantage of using RBA as the assay of choice lies in the fact that any protein can be generated in this format, including large and commercially unavailable proteins, since the radiolabeled proteins are synthesized by *in vitro* transcription and translation. This approach has had success with multiple diseases including Type I diabetes, celiac, and thyroid diseases (Liu & Eisenbarth, 2007). Although RBA is a highly sensitive technique, the requirement of radioactivity remains a major drawback for more common use. The Luciferase immunoprecipitation system (LIPS) (Burbelo, Ching, Bren, & Iadarola, 2011) is an alternative fluid-phase immunoassay that bypasses the requirement of radioactivity. This method utilizes light-emitting recombinant antigens in high-throughput immunoprecipitation formats, which generate autoantibody profiles to identify patient subsets. The LIPS technology is able to quantify autoantibody titers over an extensive dynamic range. It has been successfully used to study autoantibody profiles in several disorders including Sjögren's syndrome (Burbelo et al., 2009), SLE (Ching et al., 2012), and idiopathic inflammatory myopathies (Gan et al., 2014).

## 6.4 Autoantibody Discovery by Antigen Microarray Technologies

In most autoimmune disorders and other conditions involving the generation of autoantibodies, patients usually display a more heterogeneous phenotype and divergent autoantibody response. Antigen microarrays present a technique that makes it possible to test for multiple potential autoantigens at the same time, thus increasing the sensitivity of disease detection. Typically, these arrays are comprised of multiple antigens, ranging from 50 to nearly 10,000 in number, spotted onto a membrane or a solid support. They are first incubated with sera, followed by washes to remove unbound antibody and subsequent incubations with secondary anti-IgG antibodies conjugated to reporter molecules, often with a fluorescence-based readout. Thus, antigen microarrays make it possible to simultaneously quantify a much larger number of potential autoantibody candidates on a single platform, generating unique autoantibody profiles for various diseases.

### 6.4.1 Nucleic Acid Programmable Protein Arrays

Nucleic acid programmable protein arrays (NAPPAs) utilize a large number of epitope-tagged recombinant proteins, directly immobilized onto arrays. These proteins are generated using *in vitro* transcription/translation methods. Several reports of utilizing this technology to identify novel autoantibodies for conditions like juvenile arthritis (Gibson et al., 2012), ankylosing spondylitis (Wright et al., 2012), and type 1 diabetes (Miersch et al., 2013) have been published.

### 6.4.2 Peptoid Arrays

Peptoids (*N*-substituted oligoglycines) (Simon et al., 1992) are antigen surrogates that can be used to isolate candidate IgG antibody biomarkers (Reddy et al., 2011). This technology bypasses the requirement to have prior knowledge of native antigens of a diseased state to construct the arrays, and thus provides a more unbiased approach to serum biomarker discovery. Investigators have successfully used this technique to identify antibody–peptoid interactions in a mouse model of MS, as well as in serum samples from patients with AD (Reddy et al., 2011). This platform and strategy will be discussed in greater detail in Section 7.2.

### 6.4.3 Human Protein Microarrays

Human protein microarrays (e.g., ProtoArray®, Life Technologies) make it possible to identify autoantibody biomarker candidates constituting nearly one-third of the human proteome using full-length native human proteins as capture antigens. Similar to other commonly used array protocols, this technology also utilizes patient sera to probe the microarray as the sole source of autoantibodies, as well a secondary antihuman IgG bound to a fluorescent reporter molecule, which is then quantified and analyzed by an array scanner and proprietary software. These arrays have been successfully used to identify biomarkers for multiple diseases, including ovarian (Gunawardana, Memari, & Diamandis, 2009), prostate (Nguyen et al., 2010), bladder (Orenes-Pinero et al., 2010), and lung cancers (Gnjatic et al., 2009) as well as Alzheimer's and Parkinson's diseases (PD) (Han, Nagele, DeMarshall, Acharya, & Nagele, 2012; Nagele, Clifford, et al., 2011; Nagele, Han, et al., 2011).

### 6.5 Validation of Biomarker Candidates

All of the above mentioned technologies have made it possible to efficiently assess and identify panels of potential autoantibody biomarker candidates for a variety of diseases. Once they have been identified in the discovery phase, the next step involves the validation of the practical viability of these biomarkers. This step involves the selection of the least possible number of biomarkers required to maintain the highest diagnostic accuracy for the diagnosis with optimal sensitivity and specificity. The selection process necessitates the use of various multivariate statistical methods like *Random Forest*. Typically, the validation process involves the use of the identified biomarkers to classify a much larger, blinded cohort of samples into disease and nondisease groups, using a practical platform that can be further developed into a clinical assay. Several platforms including, but not limited to, direct-capture immunobead assays, modified ELISAs, and radioimmunoassays have been developed for this purpose.

## 7. UTILITY OF AUTOANTIBODIES AS BIOMARKERS OF DISEASE

The utility of self-reactive autoantibodies for the diagnosis of diseases has previously been limited to traditional autoimmune diseases, such as RA, SLE, and insulin-dependent (type 1) diabetes, among others. Individuals with traditional autoimmune diseases possess either a single autoantibody or a combination of several autoantibodies that serve as diagnostic and/or prognostic biomarkers. In some cases, the characterization of autoantibody biomarkers helps to shed light on previously unknown pathogenic mechanisms and pathways in certain diseases.

The identification of autoantibodies present in diseases not previously classified as autoimmune in nature remains a controversial field of study. Recently, the focus has shifted mainly from a proteomic standpoint to include a relatively new field of study, termed "antibody-omics," suggesting that perturbations in circulating antibody titers, in this case self-reactive autoantibody titers, can be indicative of specific disease states. Current research by several groups has not only established the presence of autoantibodies in several neurodegenerative diseases but also that they have the potential to be used as biomarkers capable of diagnosis and staging various degrees of pathology. These studies demonstrate the ubiquity of autoantibodies across a broad spectrum of neurodegenerative diseases, possibly underlying a common pathogenic mechanism among many of these diseases.

Heralded as the "gold standard" in disease detection and diagnosis, the identification of blood-borne biomarkers for neurodegenerative diseases has reached a fever pitch in the scientific and medical communities. A routine medical procedure, blood collection, is a relatively simple, inexpensive, and minimally invasive method that bears little overall risk to the patient when compared to other biofluid collection procedures, such as a lumbar puncture. For these reasons, the pursuit of candidate blood-borne autoantibody biomarkers for neurodegenerative diseases is of the utmost priority. Researchers around the world have identified numerous serum autoantibody targets in a number of diseases, including AD, PD, MS, and autism spectrum disorder, among others. The following sections highlight some of the more prominent autoantibody biomarker discoveries in the aforementioned diseases, illustrating the broad scope of these molecules in this new diagnostic approach.

## 7.1 Classical Targets Miss the Mark as the Most Useful Diagnostic Biomarkers

### *7.1.1 Alzheimer's Disease*

Biomarker discovery efforts for progressive neurodegenerative brain disorders such as AD have become increasingly important as projections for the elderly population most susceptible to this disease are expected to exceed 20% of the total population of United States by 2050 (Wiener & Tilly, 2002). Diagnosis of AD remains exceptionally difficult, and preclinical pathology is estimated to begin nearly a decade before afflicted individuals experience the telltale symptoms of the disease (Gandy & DeKosky, 2013). Pathological hallmarks of AD include amyloid plaques, cerebral amyloid angiopathy, tau hyperphosphorylation, and neurofibrillary tangles, ultimately resulting in the death of neurons and loss of synaptic connections (Dickson, 1997a; Serrano-Pozo, Frosch, Masliah, & Hyman, 2011). In several studies, increased serum autoantibody titers to amyloid-β peptide have been demonstrated in AD patients relative to controls, although there is much disagreement regarding whether the autoantibody is better detected disassociated or bound to the antigen in a complex (Gustaw-Rothenberg et al., 2010; Maftei et al., 2013; Nath et al., 2003). To confound this data, conflicting studies have also been published citing lower serum amyloid-β autoantibody levels in patients with AD compared to their healthy control counterparts (Qu et al., 2014; Weksler et al., 2002). Increased levels of amyloid-β autoantibodies in CSF of AD patients have also been reported (Boncoraglio et al., 2014; Maftei et al., 2013). On a more positive note, much effort is now being expended on the standardization of AD sample collection and handling procedures (O'Bryant et al., 2014; Snyder et al., 2014). For example, the Alzheimer's Disease Neuroimaging Initiative has focused on building large repositories of high-quality samples, defined by extensive clinical documentation supporting each sample diagnosis (Carrillo, Bain, Frisoni, & Weiner, 2012).

### 7.1.2 Parkinson's Disease

PD is the second most common neurodegenerative disease worldwide, affecting roughly 1%of people aged 60 years and older, demonstrating an increase in disease prevalence with each passing decade (de Lau & Breteler, 2006). PD results from the death of dopaminergic neurons in the substantia nigra pars compacta (Thomas & Beal, 2007). One extensively characterized pathological hallmark of PD is the abnormal aggregation of α-synuclein protein into structures known as Lewy bodies, presumably causing widespread disruption of neuronal homeostasis and synaptic dysfunction (Antony, Diederich, Kruger, & Balling, 2013). Similar to biomarker discovery efforts in AD, autoantibodies to established biomarkers of PD have also been reported with inconsistent results. Some studies claim an increase in α-synuclein autoantibodies in PD patients relative to controls, while others find decreased levels, or simply no differential expression between the two groups (Besong-Agbo et al., 2013; Papachroni et al., 2007; Smith, Schiess, Coffey, Klaver, & Loeffler, 2012; Yanamandra et al., 2011). Another study by Double et al. (2009) found significantly higher titers of autoantibodies directed against melanin in the sera of PD patients in earlier stages of disease; however, no additional data validating this observation have been reported by this group or others since its publication (Double et al., 2009).

### 7.1.3 Multiple Sclerosis

As described above, MS is an inflammatory disorder characterized by progressive demyelination and subsequent scarring of axon tracks, ultimately resulting in the inability of affected neurons to properly conduct electrical signals (Compston & Coles, 2008). Traditionally classified as an autoimmune disease, autoantibodies directed against myelin constituents, such as MBP and MOG have been identified in MS patients as potential biomarkers (Egg, Reindl, Deisenhammer, Linington, & Berger, 2001). Researchers have attempted to evaluate the efficacy of using autoantibodies against

MBP and MOG to predict the progression to MS of patients experiencing a primary demyelinating event. Studies by Tomassini et al. and Berger et al. found that patients seropositive for either one or both autoantibodies had an increased risk for relapse and experienced shorter intervals between subsequent relapses than seronegative patients (Berger et al., 2003; Tomassini et al., 2007). Conflicting studies found no association between the presence of MBP and MOG autoantibodies and progression to MS (Kuhle et al., 2007; Pelayo et al., 2007). Additional studies have sought to identify nonmyelin autoantibodies in both serum and CSF as useful diagnostic biomarkers (Levin et al., 2013; Mirshafiey & Kianiaslani, 2013; Querol et al., 2013). Thus far, the inability to identify one or more autoantibody biomarkers for MS that show high sensitivity and specificity using more conventional methods has been disappointing. Perhaps new approaches such as those described below will achieve more favorable results.

## 7.2 Immunoglobulin-Binding Patterns Using Random Peptide Ligands and Mimetics for Biomarker Identification in AD

For many diseases, identification of potentially diagnostic autoantibody biomarkers has been problematic, largely due to the fact that their target antigen(s) remain unknown. To circumvent this apparent limitation, a study by Reddy et al. employed combinatorial library screening using a microarray comprised of thousands of unnatural synthetic molecules to bind antibodies present in higher concentrations in individuals with AD compared to healthy controls (Reddy et al., 2011). These unnatural synthetic molecules, termed "peptoids" are *N*-substituted oligoglycines that serve to mimic native autoantigens, thus forming a complex with antibodies believed to be the causal agents or otherwise involved in the disease.

In this study, three candidate peptoids were chosen as top differentiators that displayed a minimum threefold difference in bound IgG from six AD subjects compared to the same number of age-matched nondemented control subjects. These peptoids were then verified in a larger blinded cohort of samples, differentiating AD subjects from controls with an overall accuracy ranging from 93% to 96%, a sensitivity of 93.7%, and a specificity of 93.7–100%. While the use of these candidate peptoids shows great diagnostic promise, validation studies in a much larger group of subjects with longitudinal samples are needed, and such studies are currently underway. Additionally, identification of the native autoantigen mimicked by the bound peptoids could provide valuable insight into pathogenic disease mechanisms as well as identify new targets for therapeutic intervention.

In a later study by some members of the same group, Quan et al. used peptoid microarrays to diagnose SLE subjects from healthy controls with 70.0% sensitivity and 97.5% specificity, thus demonstrating the diagnostic efficacy of this platform for multiple diseases (Quan et al., 2014).

Similar to the previous work by Reddy et al., Restrepo et al. have also created an array-based platform consisting of mimetic molecules for the purpose of binding AD-specific autoantibodies (Restrepo, Stafford, Magee, & Johnston, 2011). Instead of synthetic peptoids, these arrays consist of 10,000 random-sequence peptides, each composed of 17 residues with a carboxyl glycine–serine–cysteine linker for spacing purposes. Using these custom arrays, the authors were able to detect a single common IgG binding pattern in plasma samples from eight subjects with AD that were distinct from two patterns present in nine age-matched control subjects without dementia, eight cognitively normal, and one subject with progressive supranuclear palsy (PSP). Interestingly, it was noted that the binding pattern of the PSP subject was different from both the AD subjects as well as the nondemented controls, but upon analysis, cosegregated with one of the control patterns. Although the authors have not speculated on the possible reasons for this difference, it suggests that distinct disease-specific autoantibody binding profiles exist for both AD and PSP, and potentially for other diseases as well. Using the aforementioned antibody-binding patterns established for the AD subjects and controls, the authors tested the predictive capacity of each pattern in a blinded cohort, correctly identifying six out of eight total samples, validating the specificity of the patterns for their respective diagnoses.

## 7.3 Disease-Specific Autoantibody Profiles Using Human Protein Microarrays for the Diagnosis and Staging of AD and PD

Little is known regarding the purpose and dynamics of an individual's autoantibody profile. Previous work by Nagele et al. has demonstrated the ubiquitous presence of autoantibodies in all mammals and has shown that their titer is influenced by a variety of variables, including age, gender, and disease state (Nagele et al., 2013). While the exact function of these autoantibodies remains unknown, we have hypothesized that they function as a debris-clearing mechanism, acting to clear the daily debris generated by the body from the blood. If true, we would further predict that the presence of disease in a particular organ would lead to a dramatic and selective increase in the subset of autoantibodies charged with removal of this disease-specific debris (Fig. 1). Based on this supposition, we believe that it is possible to detect and quantify this selective increase in disease-specific autoantibody titers, thus creating a veritable diagnostic "blueprint" for each individual disease. Since the vast majority of known diseases exhibit at least some cell and tissue destruction, identification and detection of the resulting debris-clearing autoantibodies associated with each of these diseases suggest the potential for a multidisease diagnostic strategy.

Recently, the advancement of a number of high-throughput and multiplexed assays has made possible mass-scale screening for the unbiased identification of autoantibodies and their target antigens. For example, using Invitrogen's human protein microarray, a platform containing 9486 full-length native human proteins, equating to an estimated one-third of the total human proteome, an additional study identified a panel of 10 autoantibody biomarkers for the accurate detection and diagnosis of mild–moderate stage AD (Nagele, Clifford, et al., 2011; Nagele, Han, et al., 2011). Unlike the previously mentioned studies by Reddy et al. and Restrepo et al., the identity of both the autoantigen and autoantibody are determined using this approach. In this study, 50 AD samples and 40 nondemented control samples were randomly split into equal Training and Testing Sets, each containing 25 AD samples and 20 control samples. M-statistical analysis was performed on the Training Set using the program *Prospector* to determine the top 10 most differentially expressed autoantibody biomarkers demonstrating the greatest prevalence difference in the AD sample group compared to the controls. These 10 chosen markers were then reverified as significant in the Training Set samples using the *Random Forest* package in the R statistical software platform as well as *Predictive Analysis for Microarrays*.

Using the logic created by *Random Forest* from the Training Set samples, the Testing Set samples, which played no role in the biomarker selection process, were classified with an accuracy of 93.3%. Combining both the Training and Testing Set samples, AD subjects were classified with an overall accuracy of 94.4%, a sensitivity of 96.0%, and a specificity of 92.5%. To rule out the possibility of diagnostic bias toward disease, the 50 AD samples were compared to 30 breast cancer serum samples, differentiating them with an accuracy of 92.5% using the chosen panel of 10 biomarkers. To further demonstrate the ability of this diagnostic strategy to differentiate between closely related neurodegenerative diseases, 29 PD subjects were distinguished from the original 50 AD subjects with over 86% accuracy, using an independent panel of just five autoantibody biomarkers. These results indicate no diagnostic bias toward disease, neurodegenerative, or otherwise.

In addition to mild–moderate stage AD, we have also demonstrated that the same diagnostic strategy can be used to successfully differentiate mild–moderate stage PD from nondemented control subjects with comparable results (Han et al., 2012). Twenty-nine PD samples and 40 nondemented control samples were again randomly divided into a Training and Testing Set, and the top 10 most differentially expressed autoantibodies in the PD Training Set sample group were chosen as the final biomarker panel. Testing Set samples were classified with an accuracy of 97.1%, and the combined Training and Testing Set achieved an overall accuracy of 97.0%, a sensitivity of 93.1%, and a specificity of 100.0%. Using the panel of 10 biomarkers, PD was further differentiated from 10 MS samples with 100.0% accuracy and from 30 breast cancer samples with 96.6% accuracy. PD was also successfully differentiated from AD using a smaller set of biomarkers, as mentioned above (Nagele, Clifford, et al., 2011; Nagele, Han, et al., 2011). Recently, we have also demonstrated the efficacy of this diagnostic strategy for use in early detection by successfully distinguishing early-stage PD from both age- and sex-matched nondemented controls, as well from later stages of the disease (*manuscript submitted for publication*). Using a panel of 50 autoantibody biomarkers, a Testing Set of 51 early-stage PD samples were differentiated from 55 control samples with a sensitivity and specificity of 94.1% and 85.5%, respectively. Furthermore, the same panel of 50 biomarkers was capable of differentiating 51 early-stage PD samples from 29 mild–moderate stage PD samples with an overall accuracy of 97.5%. To our knowledge, this is the first blood-borne biomarker panel capable of effectively discriminating between different stages of the same neurodegenerative disease.

The results described above establish the efficacy of serum autoantibody biomarker panels for the accurate diagnosis of AD and PD and demonstrate that this strategy can be applied to a broad spectrum of neurodegenerative diseases. Additionally, a study published by May et al. (2014), using the same microarray platform as well as a similar biomarker discovery strategy identified 20 differentially expressed autoantibodies with the potential to distinguish amyotrophic lateral sclerosis (ALS) samples from healthy controls. Twenty ALS serum samples were differentiated from 20 control samples with a sensitivity of 99.9%, and a specificity of 100.0%, thus validating the use of Invitrogen's human protein microarray as a biomarker discovery platform as well as confirming the utility of *Random Forest* in biomarker verification (May et al., 2014).

## 8. CONCLUSIONS AND PERSPECTIVES

A preponderance of evidence now supports the abundance and ubiquity of autoantibodies in the blood of humans, and their "cause and effect" role in many different types of disease. A number of studies have now demonstrated specific and consistent perturbations in circulating autoantibody titers in individuals afflicted with a wide variety of diseases, opening the door to making use of such disease-related alterations for early detection. Although it has not yet been proved experimentally, there is considerable indirect evidence that disease-related changes in autoantibody profiles are linked to the ongoing and specific pathology and thus result from the immune system's response to the generation of debris from the organ(s) or tissues affected by the disease.

Undoubtedly, the most exciting beneficial use of this new tool comes from the potential for early disease detection and diagnosis in clinical situations that would otherwise rely on conclusions derived from subjective assessments which are dependent on the presentation of characteristic symptoms. The latter are often apparent only after the disease is well underway. A diagnosis based on the immune system's response to early pathology means that it may be possible to arrive at a conclusive diagnosis long before symptoms emerge. Early detection and diagnosis raises the possibility of earlier treatments, thus greatly increasing the chances for a favorable outcome if treatment is administered before the disease has progressed past the point of therapeutic efficacy. In diseases with exceptionally long prodromal periods preceding overt clinical symptoms, as in AD, early diagnosis would allow patients to avail themselves of treatments much sooner than was previously possible, potentially altering the traditional course of the disease in their favor. Our hope is that early detection of Alzheimer's pathology at some point during the long prodromal phase of this disease via blood-based autoantibody biomarkers will make it possible to enroll patients into clinical trials and treat them at a much earlier point in their disease. In addition, the ability to develop specific biomarker panels for different stages of disease should enable monitoring of disease progression in patients under treatment by their physicians or participating as subjects in clinical trials.

On the research front, identification of useful disease-specific autoantibody biomarkers and their targets may shed light on new disease-relevant molecular pathways that could lead to identification of novel, previously unrecognized therapeutic targets. In addition, the demonstration of the ubiquitous presence of numerous autoantibodies in the blood should spark new research investigating their normal functional role in the body as well as their possible participation in the initiation and/or progression of other diseases. Lastly, it would also suggest that concepts of central tolerance in the field of immunology may need to be revisited and possibly revised. The outcome of these revisions may lead to the recognition of a new function for the immune system (i.e., clearance of cell/tissue debris) in both healthy individuals and those afflicted with disease, potentially opening the door to new therapeutic strategies and targets.

On the practical side, the use of serum autoantibody biomarkers is a simple, minimally invasive, and relatively low cost alternative to other diagnostic methods that require expensive equipment and specialized personnel that may not be widely available. Future directions utilizing disease-specific autoantibody biomarkers could potentially involve the development of a multidisease diagnostic platform, perhaps capable of screening for the presence of any number of assorted maladies utilizing only a single drop of blood. Thus, the continued discovery of blood-based autoantibody biomarkers for diseases amenable to this approach and development of highly accurate blood-based assays for their detection and quantification could have a profound impact on the future of clinical medicine and effect a major change in the approach to disease diagnostics.

Overall, the autoantibody-disease field has grown from its inception to become a very complicated meshwork of laboratory data and clinical observations. By glancing at several of the diseases that are pivotal to autoantibodies, we are able to better see the future directions that research may take. Much is left to discover as new doors open up for all facets of disease that were not long ago considered far removed from the genre of autoimmunity in the classical sense of the word. As this field progresses, a redefinition of autoimmunity may be warranted, and it is necessary to keep this in mind as new explorations embark into the role that autoantibodies play in disease discovery and stratification.

## ACKNOWLEDGMENTS

The authors would like to thank Bob McBride for his help with Fig. 1 and the Michael J. Fox Foundation and Osteopathic Heritage Foundation for supporting our studies on Parkinson's and Alzheimer's diseases.

## REFERENCES

Abdullah, S. N., Farmer, E. A., Spargo, L., Logan, R., & Gully, N. (2013). Porphyromonas gingivalis peptidylarginine deiminase substrate specificity. *Anaerobe*, *23*, 102–108. http://dx.doi.org/10.1016/j.anaerobe.2013.07.001.

Acharya, N. K., Nagele, E. P., Han, M., Coretti, N. J., DeMarshall, C., Kosciuk, M. C., et al. (2012). Neuronal PAD4 expression and protein citrullination: Possible role in production of autoantibodies associated with neurodegenerative disease. *Journal of Autoimmunity*, *38*(4), 369–380. http://dx.doi.org/10.1016/j.jaut.2012.03.004.

Acharya, N. K., Nagele, E. P., Han, M., & Nagele, R. G. (2013). Autoantibodies: Double agents in human disease. *Science Translational Medicine*, *5*(186), 22–24. http://dx.doi.org/10.1126/scitranslmed.3006288, 186fs119.

Aho, K., Koskela, P., Makitalo, R., Heliovaara, M., & Palosuo, T. (1992). Antinuclear antibodies heralding the onset of systemic lupus erythematosus. *The Journal of Rheumatology*, *19*(9), 1377–1379.

Anderson, K. S., & LaBaer, J. (2005). The sentinel within: Exploiting the immune system for cancer biomarkers. *Journal of Proteome Research*, *4*(4), 1123–1133. http://dx.doi.org/10.1021/pr0500814.

Antony, P. M., Diederich, N. J., Kruger, R., & Balling, R. (2013). The hallmarks of Parkinson's disease. *FEBS Journal*, *280*(23), 5981–5993. http://dx.doi.org/10.1111/febs.12335.

Arbuckle, M. R., James, J. A., Kohlhase, K. F., Rubertone, M. V., Dennis, G. J., & Harley, J. B. (2001). Development of anti-dsDNA autoantibodies prior to clinical diagnosis of systemic lupus erythematosus. *Scandinavian Journal of Immunology*, *54*(1–2), 211–219.

Arkema, E. V., Goldstein, B. L., Robinson, W., Sokolove, J., Wagner, C. A., Malspeis, S., et al. (2013). Anti-citrullinated peptide autoantibodies, human leukocyte antigen shared epitope and risk of future rheumatoid arthritis: A nested case–control study. *Arthritis Research and Therapy*, *15*(5), R159. http://dx.doi.org/10.1186/ar4342.

Avrameas, S. (1991). Natural autoantibodies: From 'horror autotoxicus' to 'gnothi seauton'. *Immunology Today*, *12*(5), 154–159. http://dx.doi.org/10.1016/S0167-5699(05)80045-3.

Avrameas, S., & Ternynck, T. (1995). Natural autoantibodies: The other side of the immune system. *Research in Immunology*, *146*(4–5), 235–248.

Avrameas, S., Ternynck, T., Tsonis, I. A., & Lymberi, P. (2007). Naturally occurring B-cell autoreactivity: A critical overview. *Journal of Autoimmunity*, *29*(4), 213–218. http://dx.doi.org/10.1016/j.jaut.2007.07.010.

Baumgarth, N., Tung, J. W., & Herzenberg, L. A. (2005). Inherent specificities in natural antibodies: A key to immune defense against pathogen invasion. *Springer Seminars in Immunopathology*, *26*(4), 347–362. http://dx.doi.org/10.1007/s00281-004-0182-2.

Belousov, P. V., Kuprash, D. V., Sazykin, A. Y., Khlgatian, S. V., Penkov, D. N., Shebzukhov, Y. V., et al. (2008). Cancer-associated antigens and antigen arrays in serological diagnostics of malignant tumors. *Biochemistry (Mosc)*, *73*(5), 562–572.

Berger, T., Rubner, P., Schautzer, F., Egg, R., Ulmer, H., Mayringer, I., et al. (2003). Antimyelin antibodies as a predictor of clinically definite multiple sclerosis after a first demyelinating event. *New England Journal of Medicine*, *349*(2), 139–145. http://dx.doi.org/10.1056/NEJMoa022328.

Berggren, K., Chernokalskaya, E., Steinberg, T. H., Kemper, C., Lopez, M. F., Diwu, Z., et al. (2000). Background-free, high sensitivity staining of proteins in one- and two-dimensional sodium dodecyl sulfate-polyacrylamide gels using a luminescent ruthenium complex. *Electrophoresis*, *21*(12), 2509–2521. http://dx.doi.org/10.1002/1522-2683(20000701)21:12<2509::AID-ELPS2509>3.0.CO;2-9.

Berth, M., Moser, F. M., Kolbe, M., & Bernhardt, J. (2007). The state of the art in the analysis of two-dimensional gel electrophoresis images. *Applied Microbiology and Biotechnology*, *76*(6), 1223–1243. http://dx.doi.org/10.1007/s00253-007-1128-0.

Bertoni-Freddari, C., Fattoretti, P., Solazzi, M., Giorgetti, B., Di Stefano, G., Casoli, T., et al. (2003). Neuronal death versus synaptic pathology in Alzheimer's disease. *The Annals of the New York Academy of Sciences*, *1010*, 635–638.

Besong-Agbo, D., Wolf, E., Jessen, F., Oechsner, M., Hametner, E., Poewe, W., et al. (2013). Naturally occurring alpha-synuclein autoantibody levels are lower in patients with Parkinson disease. *Neurology*, *80*(2), 169–175. http://dx.doi.org/10.1212/WNL.0b013e31827b90d1.

Boes, M., Schmidt, T., Linkemann, K., Beaudette, B. C., Marshak-Rothstein, A., & Chen, J. (2000). Accelerated development of IgG autoantibodies and autoimmune disease in the absence of secreted IgM. *Proceedings of the National Academy of Sciences of the United States of America*, *97*(3), 1184–1189.

Boncoraglio, G. B., Piazza, F., Savoiardo, M., Farina, L., DiFrancesco, J. C., Prioni, S., et al. (2014). Prodromal Alzheimer's disease presenting as cerebral amyloid angiopathy-related inflammation with spontaneous amyloid-related imaging abnormalities and high cerebrospinal fluid anti-abeta autoantibodies. *Journal of Alzheimer's Disease*, *45*, 363–367. http://dx.doi.org/10.3233/JAD-142376.

Bouvet, J. P., & Dighiero, G. (1998). From natural polyreactive autoantibodies to a la carte monoreactive antibodies to infectious agents: Is it a small world after all? *Infection and Immunity*, *66*(1), 1–4.

Brettschneider, J., Jaskowski, T. D., Tumani, H., Abdul, S., Husebye, D., Seraj, H., et al. (2009). Serum anti-GAGA4 IgM antibodies differentiate relapsing remitting and secondary progressive multiple sclerosis from primary progressive multiple sclerosis and other neurological diseases. *Journal of Neuroimmunology*, *217*(1–2), 95–101. http://dx.doi.org/10.1016/j.jneuroim.2009.07.017.

Budenhofer, B. K., Ditsch, N., Jeschke, U., Gartner, R., & Toth, B. (2013). Thyroid (dys-) function in normal and disturbed pregnancy. *Archives of Gynecology and Obstetrics*, *287*(1), 1–7. http://dx.doi.org/10.1007/s00404-012-2592-z.

Burbelo, P. D., Ching, K. H., Bren, K. E., & Iadarola, M. J. (2011). Searching for biomarkers: Humoral response profiling with luciferase immunoprecipitation systems. *Expert Review of Proteomics*, *8*(3), 309–316. http://dx.doi.org/10.1586/epr.11.23.

Burbelo, P. D., Leahy, H. P., Issa, A. T., Groot, S., Baraniuk, J. N., Nikolov, N. P., et al. (2009). Sensitive and robust luminescent profiling of anti-La and other autoantibodies in Sjogren's syndrome. *Autoimmunity*, *42*(6), 515–524. http://dx.doi.org/10.1080/08916930902911738.

Burnet, S. F. M. (1959). *The clonal selection theory of acquired immunity*. Cambridge, UK: University Press Cambridge.

Candiano, G., Bruschi, M., Musante, L., Santucci, L., Ghiggeri, G. M., Carnemolla, B., et al. (2004). Blue silver: A very sensitive colloidal Coomassie G-250 staining for proteome analysis. *Electrophoresis*, *25*(9), 1327–1333. http://dx.doi.org/10.1002/elps.200305844.

Carey, T. E., Kimmel, K. A., Schwartz, D. R., Richter, D. E., Baker, S. R., & Krause, C. J. (1983). Antibodies to human squamous cell carcinoma. *Otolaryngology and Head and Neck Surgery*, *91*(5), 482–491.

Caron, M., Choquet-Kastylevsky, G., & Joubert-Caron, R. (2007). Cancer immunomics using autoantibody signatures for biomarker discovery. *Molecular and Cellular Proteomics*, *6*(7), 1115–1122. http://dx.doi.org/10.1074/mcp.R600016-MCP200.

Carrillo, M. C., Bain, L. J., Frisoni, G. B., & Weiner, M. W. (2012). Worldwide Alzheimer's disease neuroimaging initiative. *Alzheimers Dement*, *8*(4), 337–342. http://dx.doi.org/10.1016/j.jalz.2012.04.007.

Casali, P., & Schettino, E. W. (1996). Structure and function of natural antibodies. *Current Topics in Microbiology and Immunology*, *210*, 167–179.

Cepeda, E. J., & Reveille, J. D. (2004). Autoantibodies in systemic sclerosis and fibrosing syndromes: Clinical indications and relevance. *Current Opinion in Rheumatology*, *16*(6), 723–732.

Cepok, S., Rosche, B., Grummel, V., Vogel, F., Zhou, D., Sayn, J., et al. (2005). Short-lived plasma blasts are the main B cell effector subset during the course of multiple sclerosis. *Brain*, *128*(Pt. 7), 1667–1676. http://dx.doi.org/10.1093/brain/awh486.

Chapman, C., Murray, A., Chakrabarti, J., Thorpe, A., Woolston, C., Sahin, U., et al. (2007). Autoantibodies in breast cancer: Their use as an aid to early diagnosis. *Annals of Oncology*, *18*(5), 868–873. http://dx.doi.org/10.1093/annonc/mdm007.

Chapman, C. J., Murray, A., McElveen, J. E., Sahin, U., Luxemburger, U., Tureci, O., et al. (2008). Autoantibodies in lung cancer: Possibilities for early detection and subsequent cure. *Thorax*, *63*(3), 228–233. http://dx.doi.org/10.1136/thx.2007.083592.

Chapman, C. J., Thorpe, A. J., Murray, A., Parsy-Kowalska, C. B., Allen, J., Stafford, K. M., et al. (2011). Immunobiomarkers in small cell lung cancer: Potential early cancer signals. *Clinical Cancer Research*, *17*(6), 1474–1480. http://dx.doi.org/10.1158/1078-0432.CCR-10-1363.

Chatterjee, M., Mohapatra, S., Ionan, A., Bawa, G., Ali-Fehmi, R., Wang, X., et al. (2006). Diagnostic markers of ovarian cancer by high-throughput antigen cloning and detection on arrays. *Cancer Research*, *66*(2), 1181–1190. http://dx.doi.org/10.1158/0008-5472.CAN-04-2962.

Chen, Y. T., Gure, A. O., & Scanlan, M. J. (2005). Serological analysis of expression cDNA libraries (SEREX): An immunoscreening technique for identifying immunogenic tumor antigens. *Methods in Molecular Medicine*, *103*, 207–216.

Chen, Y., Lin, P., Qiu, S., Peng, X. X., Looi, K., Farquhar, M. G., et al. (2007). Autoantibodies to Ca2+ binding protein Calnuc is a potential marker in colon cancer detection. *International Journal of Oncology*, *30*(5), 1137–1144.

Chevallet, M., Luche, S., Diemer, H., Strub, J. M., Van Dorsselaer, A., & Rabilloud, T. (2008). Sweet silver: A formaldehyde-free silver staining using aldoses as developing agents, with enhanced compatibility with mass spectrometry. *Proteomics*, *8*(23–24), 4853–4861. http://dx.doi.org/10.1002/pmic.200800321.

Ching, K. H., Burbelo, P. D., Tipton, C., Wei, C., Petri, M., Sanz, I., et al. (2012). Two major autoantibody clusters in systemic lupus erythematosus. *PLoS One*, 7(2), e32001. http://dx.doi.org/10.1371/journal.pone.0032001.

Chiovato, L., Latrofa, F., Braverman, L. E., Pacini, F., Capezzone, M., Masserini, L., et al. (2003). Disappearance of humoral thyroid autoimmunity after complete removal of thyroid antigens. *Annals of Internal Medicine*, *139*(5 Pt 1), 346–351.

Cioffi, M., Riegler, G., Vietri, M. T., Pilla, P., Caserta, L., Carratu, R., et al. (2004). Serum p53 antibodies in patients affected with ulcerative colitis. *Inflammatory Bowel Diseases*, *10*(5), 606–611.

Clifford, P. M., Siu, G., Kosciuk, M., Levin, E. C., Venkataraman, V., D'Andrea, M. R., et al. (2008). Alpha7 nicotinic acetylcholine receptor expression by vascular smooth muscle cells facilitates the deposition of Abeta peptides and promotes cerebrovascular amyloid angiopathy. *Brain Research*, *1234*, 158–171. http://dx.doi.org/10.1016/j.brainres.2008.07.092.

Clifford, P. M., Zarrabi, S., Siu, G., Kinsler, K. J., Kosciuk, M. C., Venkataraman, V., et al. (2007). Abeta peptides can enter the brain through a defective blood–brain barrier and bind selectively to neurons. *Brain Research*, *1142*, 223–236. http://dx.doi.org/10.1016/j.brainres.2007.01.070.

Cohen, I. R. (2007). Biomarkers, self-antigens and the immunological homunculus. *Journal of Autoimmunity*, *29*(4), 246–249. http://dx.doi.org/10.1016/j.jaut.2007.07.016.

Cole, S. R., Beck, R. W., Moke, P. S., Kaufman, D. I., & Tourtellotte, W. W. (1998). The predictive value of CSF oligoclonal banding for MS 5 years after optic neuritis. Optic Neuritis Study Group. *Neurology*, *51*(3), 885–887.

Compston, A., & Coles, A. (2008). Multiple sclerosis. *Lancet*, *372*(9648), 1502–1517. http://dx.doi.org/10.1016/S0140-6736(08)61620-7.

Coutinho, A., Kazatchkine, M. D., & Avrameas, S. (1995). Natural autoantibodies. *Current Opinion in Immunology*, 7(6), 812–818.

Coyle, J. T. (2012). NMDA receptor and schizophrenia: A brief history. *Schizophrenia Bulletin*, *38*(5), 920–926. http://dx.doi.org/10.1093/schbul/sbs076.

Cui, Z., Zhao, M. H., Segelmark, M., & Hellmark, T. (2010). Natural autoantibodies to myeloperoxidase, proteinase 3, and the glomerular basement membrane are present in normal individuals. *Kidney International*, *78*(6), 590–597. http://dx.doi.org/10.1038/ki.2010.198.

Dahm, L., Ott, C., Steiner, J., Stepniak, B., Teegen, B., Saschenbrecker, S., et al. (2014). Seroprevalence of autoantibodies against brain antigens in health and disease. *Annals of Neurology*, *76*(1), 82–94. http://dx.doi.org/10.1002/ana.24189.

D'Andrea, M. R., & Nagele, R. G. (2006). Targeting the alpha 7 nicotinic acetylcholine receptor to reduce amyloid accumulation in Alzheimer's disease pyramidal neurons. *Current Pharmaceutical Design*, *12*(6), 677–684.

D'Andrea, M. R., Nagele, R. G., Wang, H. Y., Peterson, P. A., & Lee, D. H. (2001). Evidence that neurones accumulating amyloid can undergo lysis to form amyloid plaques in Alzheimer's disease. *Histopathology*, *38*(2), 120–134.

de Lau, L. M., & Breteler, M. M. (2006). Epidemiology of Parkinson's disease. *Lancet Neurology*, *5*(6), 525–535. http://dx.doi.org/10.1016/S1474-4422(06)70471-9.

DeGiorgio, L. A., Konstantinov, K. N., Lee, S. C., Hardin, J. A., Volpe, B. T., & Diamond, B. (2001). A subset of lupus anti-DNA antibodies cross-reacts with the NR2 glutamate receptor in systemic lupus erythematosus. *Nature Medicine*, *7*(11), 1189–1193. http://dx.doi.org/10.1038/nm1101-1189.

di Mario, F., & Cavallaro, L. G. (2008). Non-invasive tests in gastric diseases. *Digestive and Liver Disease*, *40*(7), 523–530. http://dx.doi.org/10.1016/j.dld.2008.02.028.

Dickson, D. W. (1997a). Neuropathological diagnosis of Alzheimer's disease: A perspective from longitudinal clinicopathological studies. *Neurobiology of Aging*, *18*(4 Suppl.), S21–S26.

Dickson, D. W. (1997b). The pathogenesis of senile plaques. *Journal of Neuropathology and Experimental Neurology*, *56*(4), 321–339.

Diesinger, I., Bauer, C., Brass, N., Schaefers, H. J., Comtesse, N., Sybrecht, G., et al. (2002). Toward a more complete recognition of immunoreactive antigens in squamous cell lung carcinoma. *International Journal of Cancer*, *102*(4), 372–378. http://dx.doi.org/10.1002/ijc.10714.

Disis, M. L., Calenoff, E., McLaughlin, G., Murphy, A. E., Chen, W., Groner, B., et al. (1994). Existent T-cell and antibody immunity to HER-2/neu protein in patients with breast cancer. *Cancer Research*, *54*(1), 16–20.

Domon, B., & Aebersold, R. (2006). Mass spectrometry and protein analysis. *Science*, *312*(5771), 212–217. http://dx.doi.org/10.1126/science.1124619.

Donath, J., & Landsteiner, K. (1904). Uber paroxysmale haemoglobinurie. *Münchener Medizinische Wochenschrift (1950)*, *51*, 1590–1593.

Dong, Y. H., & Fu, D. G. (2014). Autoimmune thyroid disease: Mechanism, genetics and current knowledge. *European Review for Medical and Pharmacological Sciences*, *18*(23), 3611–3618.

Double, K. L., Rowe, D. B., Carew-Jones, F. M., Hayes, M., Chan, D. K., Blackie, J., et al. (2009). Anti-melanin antibodies are increased in sera in Parkinson's disease. *Experimental Neurology*, *217*(2), 297–301. http://dx.doi.org/10.1016/j.expneurol.2009.03.002.

Druet, E., Praddaude, F., Druet, P., & Dietrich, G. (1998). Non-immunoglobulin serum proteins prevent the binding of IgG from normal rats and from rats with Th2-mediated autoimmune glomerulonephritis to various autoantigens including glomerular antigens. *European Journal of Immunology*, *28*(1), 183–192. http://dx.doi.org/10.1002/(SICI)1521-4141(199801)28:01<183::AID-IMMU183>3.0.CO;2-O.

Earnshaw, W. C., Machlin, P. S., Bordwell, B. J., Rothfield, N. F., & Cleveland, D. W. (1987). Analysis of anticentromere autoantibodies using cloned autoantigen CENP-B. *Proceedings of the National Academy of Sciences of the United States of America*, *84*(14), 4979–4983.

Egg, R., Reindl, M., Deisenhammer, F., Linington, C., & Berger, T. (2001). Anti-MOG and anti-MBP antibody subclasses in multiple sclerosis. *Multiple Sclerosis*, *7*(5), 285–289.

Ehrlich, P. (1899). Croonian lecture: On immunity with special reference to cell life. *Proceedings of the Royal Society of London*, *66*(424–433), 424–448.

Finn, O. J. (2005). Immune response as a biomarker for cancer detection and a lot more. *New England Journal of Medicine*, *353*(12), 1288–1290. http://dx.doi.org/10.1056/NEJMe058157.

Fraussen, J., Claes, N., de Bock, L., & Somers, V. (2014). Targets of the humoral autoimmune response in multiple sclerosis. *Autoimmunity Reviews*, *13*(11), 1126–1137. http://dx.doi.org/10.1016/j.autrev.2014.07.002.

Freedman, M. S., Laks, J., Dotan, N., Altstock, R. T., Dukler, A., & Sindic, C. J. (2009). Anti-alpha-glucose-based glycan IgM antibodies predict relapse activity in multiple sclerosis after the first neurological event. *Multiple Sclerosis*, *15*(4), 422–430. http://dx.doi.org/10.1177/1352458508101944.

Gan, L., O'Hanlon, T. P., Gordon, A. S., Rider, L. G., Miller, F. W., & Burbelo, P. D. (2014). Twins discordant for myositis and systemic lupus erythematosus show markedly enriched autoantibodies in the affected twin supporting environmental influences in pathogenesis. *BMC Musculoskeletal Disorders*, *15*, 67. http://dx.doi.org/10.1186/1471-2474-15-67.

Gandy, S., & DeKosky, S. T. (2013). Toward the treatment and prevention of Alzheimer's disease: Rational strategies and recent progress. *Annual Review of Medicine*, *64*, 367–383. http://dx.doi.org/10.1146/annurev-med-092611-084441.

Gibson, D. S., Qiu, J., Mendoza, E. A., Barker, K., Rooney, M. E., & LaBaer, J. (2012). Circulating and synovial antibody profiling of juvenile arthritis patients by nucleic acid programmable protein arrays. *Arthritis Research and Therapy*, *14*(2), R77. http://dx.doi.org/10.1186/ar3800.

Gnjatic, S., Wheeler, C., Ebner, M., Ritter, E., Murray, A., Altorki, N. K., et al. (2009). Seromic analysis of antibody responses in non-small cell lung cancer patients and healthy donors using conformational protein arrays. *Journal of Immunological Methods*, *341*(1–2), 50–58. http://dx.doi.org/10.1016/j.jim.2008.10.016.

Gouras, G. K., Tsai, J., Naslund, J., Vincent, B., Edgar, M., Checler, F., et al. (2000). Intraneuronal Abeta42 accumulation in human brain. *American Journal of Pathology*, *156*(1), 15–20.

Grbovic, O. M., Mathews, P. M., Jiang, Y., Schmidt, S. D., Dinakar, R., Summers-Terio, N. B., et al. (2003). Rab5-stimulated up-regulation of the endocytic pathway increases intracellular beta-cleaved amyloid precursor protein carboxyl-terminal fragment levels and Abeta production. *Journal of Biological Chemistry*, *278*(33), 31261–31268. http://dx.doi.org/10.1074/jbc.M304122200.

Greeve, I., Sellner, J., Lauterburg, T., Walker, U., Rosler, K. M., Mattle, H. P., et al. (2007). Anti-myelin antibodies in clinically isolated syndrome indicate the risk of multiple sclerosis in a Swiss cohort. *Acta Neurologica Scandinavica*, *116*(4), 207–210. http://dx.doi.org/10.1111/j.1600-0404.2007.00872.x.

Gunawardana, C. G., Memari, N., & Diamandis, E. P. (2009). Identifying novel autoantibody signatures in ovarian cancer using high-density protein microarrays. *Clinical Biochemistry*, *42*(4–5), 426–429. http://dx.doi.org/10.1016/j.clinbiochem.2008.11.008.

Gupta, S. C., Sinha, S. K., & Dagar, A. B. (2013). Evaluation of the effectiveness of diagnostic & management decision by teleophthalmology using indigenous equipment in comparison with in-clinic assessment of patients. *The Indian Journal of Medical Research*, *138*(4), 531–535.

Gustaw-Rothenberg, K. A., Siedlak, S. L., Bonda, D. J., Lerner, A., Tabaton, M., Perry, G., et al. (2010). Dissociated amyloid-beta antibody levels as a serum biomarker for the progression of Alzheimer's disease: A population-based study. *Experimental Gerontology*, *45*(1), 47–52. http://dx.doi.org/10.1016/j.exger.2009.10.003.

Hamaguchi, Y. (2010). Autoantibody profiles in systemic sclerosis: Predictive value for clinical evaluation and prognosis. *Journal of Dermatology*, *37*(1), 42–53. http://dx.doi.org/10.1111/j.1346-8138.2009.00762.x.

Hammer, C., Stepniak, B., Schneider, A., Papiol, S., Tantra, M., Begemann, M., et al. (2014). Neuropsychiatric disease relevance of circulating anti-NMDA receptor autoantibodies depends on blood–brain barrier integrity. *Molecular Psychiatry*, *19*(10), 1143–1149. http://dx.doi.org/10.1038/mp.2013.110.

Hamos, J. E., DeGennaro, L. J., & Drachman, D. A. (1989). Synaptic loss in Alzheimer's disease and other dementias. *Neurology*, *39*(3), 355–361.

Han, M., Nagele, E., DeMarshall, C., Acharya, N., & Nagele, R. (2012). Diagnosis of Parkinson's disease based on disease-specific autoantibody profiles in human sera. *PLoS One*, 7(2), e32383. http://dx.doi.org/10.1371/journal.pone.0032383.

Hanly, J. G., Urowitz, M. B., Su, L., Bae, S. C., Gordon, C., Clarke, A., et al. (2011). Autoantibodies as biomarkers for the prediction of neuropsychiatric events in systemic lupus erythematosus. *Annals of the Rheumatic Diseases*, *70*(10), 1726–1732. http://dx.doi.org/10.1136/ard.2010.148502.

Hardy, R. R., & Hayakawa, K. (2005). Development of B cells producing natural autoantibodies to thymocytes and senescent erythrocytes. *Springer Seminars in Immunopathology*, *26*(4), 363–375. http://dx.doi.org/10.1007/s00281-004-0183-1.

Harris, V. K., & Sadiq, S. A. (2014). Biomarkers of therapeutic response in multiple sclerosis: Current status. *Molecular Diagnosis & Therapy*, *18*(6), 605–617. http://dx.doi.org/10.1007/s40291-014-0117-0.

Haury, M., Sundblad, A., Grandien, A., Barreau, C., Coutinho, A., & Nobrega, A. (1997). The repertoire of serum IgM in normal mice is largely independent of external antigenic contact. *European Journal of Immunology*, *27*(6), 1557–1563. http://dx.doi.org/10.1002/eji.1830270635.

Hirohata, S., Arinuma, Y., Takayama, M., & Yoshio, T. (2007). Association of cerebrospinal fluid anti-ribosomal p protein antibodies with diffuse psychiatric/neuropsychological syndromes in systemic lupus erythematosus. *Arthritis Research and Therapy*, *9*(3), R44. http://dx.doi.org/10.1186/ar2184.

Hooijkaas, H., Benner, R., Pleasants, J. R., & Wostmann, B. S. (1984). Isotypes and specificities of immunoglobulins produced by germ-free mice fed chemically defined ultrafiltered "antigen-free" diet. *European Journal of Immunology*, *14*(12), 1127–1130. http://dx.doi.org/10.1002/eji.1830141212.

Hughes, E. G., Peng, X., Gleichman, A. J., Lai, M., Zhou, L., Tsou, R., et al. (2010). Cellular and synaptic mechanisms of anti-NMDA receptor encephalitis. *Journal of Neuroscience*, *30*(17), 5866–5875. http://dx.doi.org/10.1523/JNEUROSCI.0167-10.2010.

Imran, A., Neelam, F., & Tariq, M. (2003). Incidence of circulating antinuclear antibodies in cancer patients. *Indian Journal of Medical Sciences*, *57*(3), 113–116.

Ippolito, A., Wallace, D. J., Gladman, D., Fortin, P. R., Urowitz, M., Werth, V., et al. (2011). Autoantibodies in systemic lupus erythematosus: Comparison of historical and current assessment of seropositivity. *Lupus*, *20*(3), 250–255. http://dx.doi.org/10.1177/0961203310385738.

Jaras, K., & Anderson, K. (2011). Autoantibodies in cancer: Prognostic biomarkers and immune activation. *Expert Review of Proteomics*, *8*(5), 577–589. http://dx.doi.org/10.1586/epr.11.48.

Jayam Trouth, A., Dabi, A., Solieman, N., Kurukumbi, M., & Kalyanam, J. (2012). Myasthenia gravis: A review. *Autoimmune Diseases*, *2012*, 874680. http://dx.doi.org/10.1155/2012/874680.

Jennette, J. C., & Falk, R. J. (2010). The rise and fall of horror autotoxicus and forbidden clones. *Kidney International*, *78*(6), 533–535. http://dx.doi.org/10.1038/ki.2010.237.

Johnson, D., Hafler, D. A., Fallis, R. J., Lees, M. B., Brady, R. O., Quarles, R. H., et al. (1986). Cell-mediated immunity to myelin-associated glycoprotein, proteolipid protein, and myelin basic protein in multiple sclerosis. *Journal of Neuroimmunology*, *13*(1), 99–108.

Jurynczyk, M., Craner, M., & Palace, J. (2015). Overlapping CNS inflammatory diseases: Differentiating features of NMO and MS. *Journal of Neurology, Neurosurgery, and Psychiatry, 86*(1), 20–25. http://dx.doi.org/10.1136/jnnp-2014-308984.
Kallenberg, C. G., Wouda, A. A., Hoet, M. H., & van Venrooij, W. J. (1988). Development of connective tissue disease in patients presenting with Raynaud's phenomenon: A six year follow up with emphasis on the predictive value of antinuclear antibodies as detected by immunoblotting. *Annals of the Rheumatic Diseases, 47*(8), 634–641.
Kavanaugh, A., Tomar, R., Reveille, J., Solomon, D. H., & Homburger, H. A. (2000). Guidelines for clinical use of the antinuclear antibody test and tests for specific autoantibodies to nuclear antigens. American College of Pathologists. *Archives of Pathology & Laboratory Medicine, 124*(1), 71–81. http://dx.doi.org/10.1043/0003-9985(2000)124<0071:GFCUOT>2.0.CO;2.
Kayser, M. S., & Dalmau, J. (2014). Anti-NMDA receptor encephalitis, autoimmunity, and psychosis. *Schizophrenia Research.* http://dx.doi.org/10.1016/j.schres.2014.10.007.
Kazarian, M., & Laird-Offringa, I. A. (2011). Small-cell lung cancer-associated autoantibodies: Potential applications to cancer diagnosis, early detection, and therapy. *Molecular Cancer, 10*, 33. http://dx.doi.org/10.1186/1476-4598-10-33.
Kinloch, A., Tatzer, V., Wait, R., Peston, D., Lundberg, K., Donatien, P., et al. (2005). Identification of citrullinated alpha-enolase as a candidate autoantigen in rheumatoid arthritis. *Arthritis Research and Therapy*, 7(6), R1421–R1429. http://dx.doi.org/10.1186/ar1845.
Kitley, J., Waters, P., Woodhall, M., Leite, M. I., Murchison, A., George, J., et al. (2014). Neuromyelitis optica spectrum disorders with aquaporin-4 and myelin-oligodendrocyte glycoprotein antibodies: A comparative study. *JAMA Neurology, 71*(3), 276–283. http://dx.doi.org/10.1001/jamaneurol.2013.5857.
Kolfenbach, J. R., Deane, K. D., Derber, L. A., O'Donnell, C. I., Gilliland, W. R., Edison, J. D., et al. (2010). Autoimmunity to peptidyl arginine deiminase type 4 precedes clinical onset of rheumatoid arthritis. *Arthritis and Rheumatism, 62*(9), 2633–2639. http://dx.doi.org/10.1002/art.27570.
Kowal, C., Degiorgio, L. A., Lee, J. Y., Edgar, M. A., Huerta, P. T., Volpe, B. T., et al. (2006). Human lupus autoantibodies against NMDA receptors mediate cognitive impairment. *Proceedings of the National Academy of Sciences of the United States of America, 103*(52), 19854–19859. http://dx.doi.org/10.1073/pnas.0608397104.
Kowal, C., DeGiorgio, L. A., Nakaoka, T., Hetherington, H., Huerta, P. T., Diamond, B., et al. (2004). Cognition and immunity; antibody impairs memory. *Immunity, 21*(2), 179–188. http://dx.doi.org/10.1016/j.immuni.2004.07.011.
Kuhle, J., Pohl, C., Mehling, M., Edan, G., Freedman, M. S., Hartung, H. P., et al. (2007). Lack of association between antimyelin antibodies and progression to multiple sclerosis. *New England Journal of Medicine, 356*(4), 371–378. http://dx.doi.org/10.1056/NEJMoa063602.
Lacroix-Desmazes, S., Mouthon, L., Kaveri, S. V., Kazatchkine, M. D., & Weksler, M. E. (1999). Stability of natural self-reactive antibody repertoires during aging. *Journal of Clinical Immunology, 19*(1), 26–34.
Lampropoulou, V., Calderon-Gomez, E., Roch, T., Neves, P., Shen, P., Stervbo, U., et al. (2010). Suppressive functions of activated B cells in autoimmune diseases reveal the dual roles of Toll-like receptors in immunity. *Immunological Reviews, 233*(1), 146–161. http://dx.doi.org/10.1111/j.0105-2896.2009.00855.x.
Lancaster, E., Martinez-Hernandez, E., & Dalmau, J. (2011). Encephalitis and antibodies to synaptic and neuronal cell surface proteins. *Neurology*, 77(2), 179–189. http://dx.doi.org/10.1212/WNL.0b013e318224afde.
Larman, H. B., Laserson, U., Querol, L., Verhaeghen, K., Solimini, N. L., Xu, G. J., et al. (2013). PhIP-Seq characterization of autoantibodies from patients with multiple

sclerosis, type 1 diabetes and rheumatoid arthritis. *Journal of Autoimmunity, 43*, 1–9. http://dx.doi.org/10.1016/j.jaut.2013.01.013.

Larman, H. B., Zhao, Z., Laserson, U., Li, M. Z., Ciccia, A., Gakidis, M. A., et al. (2011). Autoantigen discovery with a synthetic human peptidome. *Nature Biotechnology, 29*(6), 535–541. http://dx.doi.org/10.1038/nbt.1856.

Latrofa, F., Chazenbalk, G. D., Pichurin, P., Chen, C. R., McLachlan, S. M., & Rapoport, B. (2004). Affinity-enrichment of thyrotropin receptor autoantibodies from Graves' patients and normal individuals provides insight into their properties and possible origin from natural antibodies. *Journal of Clinical Endocrinology and Metabolism, 89*(9), 4734–4745. http://dx.doi.org/10.1210/jc.2003-032068.

Lee, W., Gaca, J. G., Edwards, L. A., Braedehoeft, S. J., Parker, W., & Davis, R. D. (2002). Binding of polyreactive antibodies to self versus foreign antigens. *Immunobiology, 205*(1), 95–107. http://dx.doi.org/10.1078/0171-2985-00113.

Lee, S. L., Tsay, G. J., & Tsai, R. T. (1993). Anticentromere antibodies in subjects with no apparent connective tissue disease. *Annals of the Rheumatic Diseases, 52*(8), 586–589.

Lennon, V. A., Kryzer, T. J., Pittock, S. J., Verkman, A. S., & Hinson, S. R. (2005). IgG marker of optic-spinal multiple sclerosis binds to the aquaporin-4 water channel. *Journal of Experimental Medicine, 202*(4), 473–477. http://dx.doi.org/10.1084/jem.20050304.

Lennon, V. A., Wingerchuk, D. M., Kryzer, T. J., Pittock, S. J., Lucchinetti, C. F., Fujihara, K., et al. (2004). A serum autoantibody marker of neuromyelitis optica: Distinction from multiple sclerosis. *Lancet, 364*(9451), 2106–2112. http://dx.doi.org/10.1016/S0140-6736(04)17551-X.

Levin, E. C., Acharya, N. K., Han, M., Zavareh, S. B., Sedeyn, J. C., Venkataraman, V., et al. (2010). Brain-reactive autoantibodies are nearly ubiquitous in human sera and may be linked to pathology in the context of blood–brain barrier breakdown. *Brain Research, 1345*, 221–232. http://dx.doi.org/10.1016/j.brainres.2010.05.038.

Levin, M. C., Lee, S., Gardner, L. A., Shin, Y., Douglas, J. N., & Cooper, C. (2013). Autoantibodies to non-myelin antigens as contributors to the pathogenesis of multiple sclerosis. *Journal of Clinical and Cellular Immunology, 4*. http://dx.doi.org/10.4172/2155-9899.1000148.

Li, L., Chen, S. H., Yu, C. H., Li, Y. M., & Wang, S. Q. (2008). Identification of hepatocellular-carcinoma-associated antigens and autoantibodies by serological proteome analysis combined with protein microarray. *Journal of Proteome Research, 7*(2), 611–620. http://dx.doi.org/10.1021/pr070525r.

Lim, E. T., Berger, T., Reindl, M., Dalton, C. M., Fernando, K., Keir, G., et al. (2005). Anti-myelin antibodies do not allow earlier diagnosis of multiple sclerosis. *Multiple Sclerosis, 11*(4), 492–494.

Link, H., & Huang, Y. M. (2006). Oligoclonal bands in multiple sclerosis cerebrospinal fluid: An update on methodology and clinical usefulness. *Journal of Neuroimmunology, 180*(1–2), 17–28. http://dx.doi.org/10.1016/j.jneuroim.2006.07.006.

Liu, E., & Eisenbarth, G. S. (2007). Accepting clocks that tell time poorly: Fluid-phase versus standard ELISA autoantibody assays. *Clinical Immunology, 125*(2), 120–126. http://dx.doi.org/10.1016/j.clim.2007.08.005.

Mace, G., Blanpied, C., Emorine, L. J., Druet, P., & Dietrich, G. (1999). Isolation and characterization of natural human IgG with a morphine-like activity. *European Journal of Immunology, 29*(3), 997–1003. http://dx.doi.org/10.1002/(SICI)1521-4141(199903)29:03<997::AID-IMMU997>3.0.CO;2-1.

Madi, A., Bransburg-Zabary, S., Kenett, D. Y., Ben-Jacob, E., & Cohen, I. R. (2012). The natural autoantibody repertoire in newborns and adults: A current overview. *Advances in Experimental Medicine & Biology, 750*, 198–212. http://dx.doi.org/10.1007/978-1-4614-3461-0_15.

Madi, A., Hecht, I., Bransburg-Zabary, S., Merbl, Y., Pick, A., Zucker-Toledano, M., et al. (2009). Organization of the autoantibody repertoire in healthy newborns and adults revealed by system level informatics of antigen microarray data. *Proceedings of the National Academy of Sciences of the United States of America, 106*(34), 14484–14489. http://dx.doi.org/10.1073/pnas.0901528106.

Maftei, M., Thurm, F., Schnack, C., Tumani, H., Otto, M., Elbert, T., et al. (2013). Increased levels of antigen-bound beta-amyloid autoantibodies in serum and cerebrospinal fluid of Alzheimer's disease patients. *PLoS One, 8*(7), e68996. http://dx.doi.org/10.1371/journal.pone.0068996.

Makrygiannakis, D., Hermansson, M., Ulfgren, A. K., Nicholas, A. P., Zendman, A. J., Eklund, A., et al. (2008). Smoking increases peptidylarginine deiminase 2 enzyme expression in human lungs and increases citrullination in BAL cells. *Annals of the Rheumatic Diseases, 67*(10), 1488–1492. http://dx.doi.org/10.1136/ard.2007.075192.

Mann, M., Hendrickson, R. C., & Pandey, A. (2001). Analysis of proteins and proteomes by mass spectrometry. *Annual Review of Biochemistry, 70*, 437–473. http://dx.doi.org/10.1146/annurev.biochem.70.1.437.

Marchalonis, J. J., Hohman, V. S., Thomas, C., & Schluter, S. F. (1993). Antibody production in sharks and humans: A role for natural antibodies. *Developmental and Comparative Immunology, 17*(1), 41–53.

Marin, G. G., Cardiel, M. H., Cornejo, H., & Viveros, M. E. (2009). Prevalence of antinuclear antibodies in 3 groups of healthy individuals: Blood donors, hospital personnel, and relatives of patients with autoimmune diseases. *Journal of Clinical Rheumatology, 15*(7), 325–329. http://dx.doi.org/10.1097/RHU.0b013e3181bb971b.

Marrero, J. A., Su, G. L., Wei, W., Emick, D., Conjeevaram, H. S., Fontana, R. J., et al. (2003). Des-gamma carboxyprothrombin can differentiate hepatocellular carcinoma from nonmalignant chronic liver disease in american patients. *Hepatology, 37*(5), 1114–1121. http://dx.doi.org/10.1053/jhep.2003.50195.

Marta, C. B., Montano, M. B., Taylor, C. M., Taylor, A. L., Bansal, R., & Pfeiffer, S. E. (2005). Signaling cascades activated upon antibody cross-linking of myelin oligodendrocyte glycoprotein: Potential implications for multiple sclerosis. *Journal of Biological Chemistry, 280*(10), 8985–8993. http://dx.doi.org/10.1074/jbc.M413174200.

Mathsson, L., Mullazehi, M., Wick, M. C., Sjoberg, O., van Vollenhoven, R., Klareskog, L., et al. (2008). Antibodies against citrullinated vimentin in rheumatoid arthritis: Higher sensitivity and extended prognostic value concerning future radiographic progression as compared with antibodies against cyclic citrullinated peptides. *Arthritis and Rheumatism, 58*(1), 36–45. http://dx.doi.org/10.1002/art.23188.

May, C., Nordhoff, E., Casjens, S., Turewicz, M., Eisenacher, M., Gold, R., et al. (2014). Highly immunoreactive IgG antibodies directed against a set of twenty human proteins in the sera of patients with amyotrophic lateral sclerosis identified by protein array. *PLoS One, 9*(2), e89596. http://dx.doi.org/10.1371/journal.pone.0089596.

Meltzer, H. Y., Horiguchi, M., & Massey, B. W. (2011). The role of serotonin in the NMDA receptor antagonist models of psychosis and cognitive impairment. *Psychopharmacology, 213*(2–3), 289–305. http://dx.doi.org/10.1007/s00213-010-2137-8.

Merbl, Y., Zucker-Toledano, M., Quintana, F. J., & Cohen, I. R. (2007). Newborn humans manifest autoantibodies to defined self molecules detected by antigen microarray informatics. *Journal of Clinical Investigation, 117*(3), 712–718. http://dx.doi.org/10.1172/JCI29943.

Mercado, F. B., Marshall, R. I., Klestov, A. C., & Bartold, P. M. (2001). Relationship between rheumatoid arthritis and periodontitis. *Journal of Periodontology, 72*(6), 779–787. http://dx.doi.org/10.1902/jop.2001.72.6.779.

Miersch, S., Bian, X., Wallstrom, G., Sibani, S., Logvinenko, T., Wasserfall, C. H., et al. (2013). Serological autoantibody profiling of type 1 diabetes by protein arrays. *Journal of Proteomics, 94*, 486–496. http://dx.doi.org/10.1016/j.jprot.2013.10.018.

Mirilas, P., Fesel, C., Guilbert, B., Beratis, N. G., & Avrameas, S. (1999). Natural antibodies in childhood: Development, individual stability, and injury effect indicate a contribution to immune memory. *Journal of Clinical Immunology, 19*(2), 109–115.

Mirshafiey, A., & Kianiaslani, M. (2013). Autoantigens and autoantibodies in multiple sclerosis. *Iranian Journal of Allergy, Asthma, and Immunology, 12*(4), 292–303.

Moscato, E. H., Peng, X., Jain, A., Parsons, T. D., Dalmau, J., & Balice-Gordon, R. J. (2014). Acute mechanisms underlying antibody effects in anti-N-methyl-D-aspartate receptor encephalitis. *Annals of Neurology, 76*(1), 108–119. http://dx.doi.org/10.1002/ana.24195.

Mouthon, L., Nobrega, A., Nicolas, N., Kaveri, S. V., Barreau, C., Coutinho, A., et al. (1995). Invariance and restriction toward a limited set of self-antigens characterize neonatal IgM antibody repertoires and prevail in autoreactive repertoires of healthy adults. *Proceedings of the National Academy of Sciences of the United States of America, 92*(9), 3839–3843.

Nagele, R. G., Clifford, P. M., Siu, G., Levin, E. C., Acharya, N. K., Han, M., et al. (2011). Brain-reactive autoantibodies prevalent in human sera increase intraneuronal amyloid-beta(1–42) deposition. *Journal of Alzheimer's Disease, 25*(4), 605–622. http://dx.doi.org/10.3233/JAD-2011-110098.

Nagele, R. G., D'Andrea, M. R., Anderson, W. J., & Wang, H. Y. (2002). Intracellular accumulation of beta-amyloid(1–42) in neurons is facilitated by the alpha 7 nicotinic acetylcholine receptor in Alzheimer's disease. *Neuroscience, 110*(2), 199–211.

Nagele, E. P., Han, M., Acharya, N. K., DeMarshall, C., Kosciuk, M. C., & Nagele, R. G. (2013). Natural IgG autoantibodies are abundant and ubiquitous in human sera, and their number is influenced by age, gender, and disease. *PLoS One, 8*(4), e60726. http://dx.doi.org/10.1371/journal.pone.0060726.

Nagele, E., Han, M., Demarshall, C., Belinka, B., & Nagele, R. (2011). Diagnosis of Alzheimer's disease based on disease-specific autoantibody profiles in human sera. *PLoS One, 6*(8), e23112. http://dx.doi.org/10.1371/journal.pone.0023112.

Nath, A., Hall, E., Tuzova, M., Dobbs, M., Jons, M., Anderson, C., et al. (2003). Autoantibodies to amyloid beta-peptide (Abeta) are increased in Alzheimer's disease patients and Abeta antibodies can enhance Abeta neurotoxicity: Implications for disease pathogenesis and vaccine development. *Neuromolecular Medicine, 3*(1), 29–39.

Needham, E., & Zandi, M. S. (2014). Recent advances in the neuroimmunology of cell-surface CNS autoantibody syndromes, Alzheimer's disease, traumatic brain injury and schizophrenia. *Journal of Neurology, 261*(10), 2037–2042. http://dx.doi.org/10.1007/s00415-014-7473-x.

Nesterova, M., Johnson, N., Cheadle, C., & Cho-Chung, Y. S. (2006). Autoantibody biomarker opens a new gateway for cancer diagnosis. *Biochimica et Biophysica Acta, 1762*(4), 398–403. http://dx.doi.org/10.1016/j.bbadis.2005.12.010.

Nguyen, M. C., Tu, G. H., Koprivnikar, K. E., Gonzalez-Edick, M., Jooss, K. U., & Harding, T. C. (2010). Antibody responses to galectin-8, TARP and TRAP1 in prostate cancer patients treated with a GM-CSF-secreting cellular immunotherapy. *Cancer Immunology, Immunotherapy, 59*(9), 1313–1323. http://dx.doi.org/10.1007/s00262-010-0858-5.

Nilsson, B. O., Skogh, T., Ernerudh, J., Johansson, B., Lofgren, S., Wikby, A., et al. (2006). Antinuclear antibodies in the oldest-old women and men. *Journal of Autoimmunity, 27*(4), 281–288. http://dx.doi.org/10.1016/j.jaut.2006.10.002.

Non-DNA Human Identification Test Announced. (2015).

Notkins, A. L. (2004). Polyreactivity of antibody molecules. *Trends in Immunology, 25*(4), 174–179. http://dx.doi.org/10.1016/j.it.2004.02.004.

O'Bryant, S. E., Gupta, V., Henriksen, K., Edwards, M., Jeromin, A., & Lista, S. (2014). Guidelines for the standardization of preanalytic variables for blood-based biomarker studies in Alzheimer's disease research. *Alzheimers Dement, 11*, 549–560. http://dx.doi.org/10.1016/j.jalz.2014.08.099.

Ochsenbein, A. F., Fehr, T., Lutz, C., Suter, M., Brombacher, F., Hengartner, H., et al. (1999). Control of early viral and bacterial distribution and disease by natural antibodies. *Science*, *286*(5447), 2156–2159.

Ochsenbein, A. F., & Zinkernagel, R. M. (2000). Natural antibodies and complement link innate and acquired immunity. *Immunology Today*, *21*(12), 624–630.

Oddo, S., Caccamo, A., Kitazawa, M., Tseng, B. P., & LaFerla, F. M. (2003). Amyloid deposition precedes tangle formation in a triple transgenic model of Alzheimer's disease. *Neurobiology of Aging*, *24*(8), 1063–1070.

Orenes-Pinero, E., Barderas, R., Rico, D., Casal, J. I., Gonzalez-Pisano, D., Navajo, J., et al. (2010). Serum and tissue profiling in bladder cancer combining protein and tissue arrays. *Journal of Proteome Research*, *9*(1), 164–173. http://dx.doi.org/10.1021/pr900273u.

Panitch, H. S., Hooper, C. J., & Johnson, K. P. (1980). CSF antibody to myelin basic protein. Measurement in patients with multiple sclerosis and subacute sclerosing panencephalitis. *Archives of Neurology*, *37*(4), 206–209.

Paoletti, P., Bellone, C., & Zhou, Q. (2013). NMDA receptor subunit diversity: Impact on receptor properties, synaptic plasticity and disease. *Nature Reviews. Neuroscience*, *14*(6), 383–400. http://dx.doi.org/10.1038/nrn3504.

Papachroni, K. K., Ninkina, N., Papapanagiotou, A., Hadjigeorgiou, G. M., Xiromerisiou, G., Papadimitriou, A., et al. (2007). Autoantibodies to alpha-synuclein in inherited Parkinson's disease. *Journal of Neurochemistry*, *101*(3), 749–756. http://dx.doi.org/10.1111/j.1471-4159.2006.04365.x.

Patel, K., Farlow, E. C., Kim, A. W., Lee, B. S., Basu, S., Coon, J. S., et al. (2011). Enhancement of a multianalyte serum biomarker panel to identify lymph node metastases in non-small cell lung cancer with circulating autoantibody biomarkers. *International Journal of Cancer*, *129*(1), 133–142. http://dx.doi.org/10.1002/ijc.25644.

Patrick, J., & Lindstrom, J. (1973). Autoimmune response to acetylcholine receptor. *Science*, *180*(4088), 871–872.

Paul, S. (1996). Natural catalytic antibodies. *Molecular Biotechnology*, *5*(3), 197–207.

Pelayo, R., Tintore, M., Montalban, X., Rovira, A., Espejo, C., Reindl, M., et al. (2007). Antimyelin antibodies with no progression to multiple sclerosis. *New England Journal of Medicine*, *356*(4), 426–428. http://dx.doi.org/10.1056/NEJMc062467.

Pollak, T. A., Nicholson, T. R., Mellers, J. D., Vincent, A., & David, A. S. (2014). Epilepsy-related psychosis: A role for autoimmunity? *Epilepsy and Behavior*, *36*, 33–38. http://dx.doi.org/10.1016/j.yebeh.2014.04.022.

Qu, B. X., Gong, Y., Moore, C., Fu, M., German, D. C., Chang, L. Y., et al. (2014). Beta-amyloid auto-antibodies are reduced in Alzheimer's disease. *Journal of Neuroimmunology*, *274*(1–2), 168–173. http://dx.doi.org/10.1016/j.jneuroim.2014.06.017.

Quan, J., Lakhanpal, A., Reddy, M. M., Zaman, S., Li, Q. Z., German, D. C., et al. (2014). Discovery of biomarkers for systemic lupus erythematosus using a library of synthetic autoantigen surrogates. *Journal of Immunological Methods*, *402*(1–2), 23–34. http://dx.doi.org/10.1016/j.jim.2013.11.004.

Querol, L., Clark, P. L., Bailey, M. A., Cotsapas, C., Cross, A. H., Hafler, D. A., et al. (2013). Protein array-based profiling of CSF identifies RBPJ as an autoantigen in multiple sclerosis. *Neurology*, *81*(11), 956–963. http://dx.doi.org/10.1212/WNL.0b013e3182a43b48.

Reddy, M. M., Wilson, R., Wilson, J., Connell, S., Gocke, A., Hynan, L., et al. (2011). Identification of candidate IgG biomarkers for Alzheimer's disease via combinatorial library screening. *Cell*, *144*(1), 132–142. http://dx.doi.org/10.1016/j.cell.2010.11.054.

Restrepo, L., Stafford, P., Magee, D. M., & Johnston, S. A. (2011). Application of immunosignatures to the assessment of Alzheimer's disease. *Annals of Neurology*, *70*(2), 286–295. http://dx.doi.org/10.1002/ana.22405.

Romi, F., Aarli, J. A., & Gilhus, N. E. (2005). Seronegative myasthenia gravis: Disease severity and prognosis. *European Journal of Neurology, 12*(6), 413–418. http://dx.doi.org/10.1111/j.1468-1331.2005.01137.x.

Ruiz-Arguelles, A., Rivadeneyra-Espinoza, L., & Alarcon-Segovia, D. (2003). Antibody penetration into living cells: Pathogenic, preventive and immuno-therapeutic implications. *Current Pharmaceutical Design, 9*(23), 1881–1887.

Sakkas, L. I., Bogdanos, D. P., Katsiari, C., & Platsoucas, C. D. (2014). Anti-citrullinated peptides as autoantigens in rheumatoid arthritis-relevance to treatment. *Autoimmunity Reviews, 13*(11), 1114–1120. http://dx.doi.org/10.1016/j.autrev.2014.08.012.

Sato, T., Fujii, T., Yokoyama, T., Fujita, Y., Imura, Y., Yukawa, N., et al. (2010). Anti-U1 RNP antibodies in cerebrospinal fluid are associated with central neuropsychiatric manifestations in systemic lupus erythematosus and mixed connective tissue disease. *Arthritis and Rheumatism, 62*(12), 3730–3740. http://dx.doi.org/10.1002/art.27700.

Scanlan, M. J., Chen, Y. T., Williamson, B., Gure, A. O., Stockert, E., Gordan, J. D., et al. (1998). Characterization of human colon cancer antigens recognized by autologous antibodies. *International Journal of Cancer, 76*(5), 652–658.

Scanlan, M. J., Simpson, A. J., & Old, L. J. (2004). The cancer/testis genes: Review, standardization, and commentary. *Cancer Immunity, 4*, 1.

Schirmer, L., Srivastava, R., & Hemmer, B. (2014). To look for a needle in a haystack: The search for autoantibodies in multiple sclerosis. *Multiple Sclerosis, 20*(3), 271–279. http://dx.doi.org/10.1177/1352458514522104.

Schwab, C., & McGeer, P. L. (2008). Inflammatory aspects of Alzheimer disease and other neurodegenerative disorders. *Journal of Alzheimer's Disease, 13*(4), 359–369.

Selkoe, D. J. (2002). Alzheimer's disease is a synaptic failure. *Science, 298*(5594), 789–791. http://dx.doi.org/10.1126/science.1074069.

Serrano-Pozo, A., Frosch, M. P., Masliah, E., & Hyman, B. T. (2011). Neuropathological alterations in Alzheimer disease. *Cold Spring Harbor Perspectives in Medicine, 1*(1), a006189. http://dx.doi.org/10.1101/cshperspect.a006189.

Sherer, Y., Gorstein, A., Fritzler, M. J., & Shoenfeld, Y. (2004). Autoantibody explosion in systemic lupus erythematosus: More than 100 different antibodies found in SLE patients. *Seminars in Arthritis and Rheumatism, 34*(2), 501–537.

Sigounas, G., Kolaitis, N., Monell-Torrens, E., & Notkins, A. L. (1994). Polyreactive IgM antibodies in the circulation are masked by antigen binding. *Journal of Clinical Immunology, 14*(6), 375–381.

Simon, R. J., Kania, R. S., Zuckermann, R. N., Huebner, V. D., Jewell, D. A., Banville, S., et al. (1992). Peptoids: A modular approach to drug discovery. *Proceedings of the National Academy of Sciences of the United States of America, 89*(20), 9367–9371.

Sinclair, D. (2008). Analytical aspects of thyroid antibodies estimation. *Autoimmunity, 41*(1), 46–54. http://dx.doi.org/10.1080/08916930701619466.

Smeenk, R. J. (2000). Antinuclear antibodies: Cause of disease or caused by disease? *Rheumatology (Oxford), 39*(6), 581–584.

Smith, E. M., Rubenstein, L. M., Ritchie, J. M., Lee, J. H., Haugen, T. H., Hamsikova, E., et al. (2008). Does pretreatment seropositivity to human papillomavirus have prognostic significance for head and neck cancers? *Cancer Epidemiology, Biomarkers and Prevention, 17*(8), 2087–2096. http://dx.doi.org/10.1158/1055-9965.EPI-08-0054.

Smith, L. M., Schiess, M. C., Coffey, M. P., Klaver, A. C., & Loeffler, D. A. (2012). alpha-Synuclein and anti-alpha-synuclein antibodies in Parkinson's disease, atypical Parkinson syndromes, REM sleep behavior disorder, and healthy controls. *PLoS One*, 7(12), e52285. http://dx.doi.org/10.1371/journal.pone.0052285.

Snyder, H. M., Carrillo, M. C., Grodstein, F., Henriksen, K., Jeromin, A., Lovestone, S., et al. (2014). Developing novel blood-based biomarkers for Alzheimer's disease. *Alzheimers Dement, 10*(1), 109–114. http://dx.doi.org/10.1016/j.jalz.2013.10.007.

Solans-Laque, R., Perez-Bocanegra, C., Salud-Salvia, A., Fonollosa-Pla, V., Rodrigo, M. J., Armadans, L., et al. (2004). Clinical significance of antinuclear antibodies in malignant diseases: Association with rheumatic and connective tissue paraneoplastic syndromes. *Lupus*, *13*(3), 159–164.

Srivastava, R., Aslam, M., Kalluri, S. R., Schirmer, L., Buck, D., Tackenberg, B., et al. (2012). Potassium channel KIR4.1 as an immune target in multiple sclerosis. *New England Journal of Medicine*, *367*(2), 115–123. http://dx.doi.org/10.1056/NEJMoa1110740.

Stein, T. D., Fedynyshyn, J. P., & Kalil, R. E. (2002). Circulating autoantibodies recognize and bind dying neurons following injury to the brain. *Journal of Neuropathology and Experimental Neurology*, *61*(12), 1100–1108.

Tambor, V., Fucikova, A., Lenco, J., Kacerovsky, M., Rehacek, V., Stulik, J., et al. (2010). Application of proteomics in biomarker discovery: A primer for the clinician. *Physiological Research*, *59*(4), 471–497.

Tan, E. M., & Zhang, J. (2008). Autoantibodies to tumor-associated antigens: Reporters from the immune system. *Immunological Reviews*, *222*, 328–340. http://dx.doi.org/10.1111/j.1600-065X.2008.00611.x.

Tassignon, J., Haeseleer, F., & Borkowski, A. (1997). Natural antiestrogen receptor autoantibodies in man with estrogenic activity in mammary carcinoma cell culture: Study of their mechanism of action; evidence for involvement of estrogen-like epitopes. *Journal of Clinical Endocrinology and Metabolism*, *82*(10), 3464–3470. http://dx.doi.org/10.1210/jcem.82.10.4313.

Terryberry, J. W., Thor, G., & Peter, J. B. (1998). Autoantibodies in neurodegenerative diseases: Antigen-specific frequencies and intrathecal analysis. *Neurobiology of Aging*, *19*(3), 205–216.

Thomas, B., & Beal, M. F. (2007). Parkinson's disease. *Human Molecular Genetics*, *16*(Spec No. 2), R183–R194. http://dx.doi.org/10.1093/hmg/ddm159.

Tomassini, V., De Giglio, L., Reindl, M., Russo, P., Pestalozza, I., Pantano, P., et al. (2007). Anti-myelin antibodies predict the clinical outcome after a first episode suggestive of MS. *Multiple Sclerosis*, *13*(9), 1086–1094. http://dx.doi.org/10.1177/1352458507077622.

Trouw, L. A., Haisma, E. M., Levarht, E. W., van der Woude, D., Ioan-Facsinay, A., Daha, M. R., et al. (2009). Anti-cyclic citrullinated peptide antibodies from rheumatoid arthritis patients activate complement via both the classical and alternative pathways. *Arthritis and Rheumatism*, *60*(7), 1923–1931. http://dx.doi.org/10.1002/art.24622.

Turk, S. A., van Beers-Tas, M. H., & van Schaardenburg, D. (2014). Prediction of future rheumatoid arthritis. *Rheumatic Diseases Clinics of North America*, *40*(4), 753–770. http://dx.doi.org/10.1016/j.rdc.2014.07.007.

Union, A., Meheus, L., Humbel, R. L., Conrad, K., Steiner, G., Moereels, H., et al. (2002). Identification of citrullinated rheumatoid arthritis-specific epitopes in natural filaggrin relevant for antifilaggrin autoantibody detection by line immunoassay. *Arthritis and Rheumatism*, *46*(5), 1185–1195. http://dx.doi.org/10.1002/art.10229.

Wang, H. Y., Lee, D. H., D'Andrea, M. R., Peterson, P. A., Shank, R. P., & Reitz, A. B. (2000). beta-Amyloid(1–42) binds to alpha7 nicotinic acetylcholine receptor with high affinity. Implications for Alzheimer's disease pathology. *Journal of Biological Chemistry*, *275*(8), 5626–5632.

Wang, X., Yu, J., Sreekumar, A., Varambally, S., Shen, R., Giacherio, D., et al. (2005). Autoantibody signatures in prostate cancer. *New England Journal of Medicine*, *353*(12), 1224–1235. http://dx.doi.org/10.1056/NEJMoa051931.

Weber, M. S., Hemmer, B., & Cepok, S. (2011). The role of antibodies in multiple sclerosis. *Biochimica et Biophysica Acta*, *1812*(2), 239–245. http://dx.doi.org/10.1016/j.bbadis.2010.06.009.

Wegner, N., Wait, R., Sroka, A., Eick, S., Nguyen, K. A., Lundberg, K., et al. (2010). Peptidylarginine deiminase from Porphyromonas gingivalis citrullinates human fibrinogen and alpha-enolase: Implications for autoimmunity in rheumatoid arthritis. *Arthritis and Rheumatism*, *62*(9), 2662–2672. http://dx.doi.org/10.1002/art.27552.

Weksler, M. E., Relkin, N., Turkenich, R., LaRusse, S., Zhou, L., & Szabo, P. (2002). Patients with Alzheimer disease have lower levels of serum anti-amyloid peptide antibodies than healthy elderly individuals. *Experimental Gerontology*, *37*(7), 943–948.

Wichainun, R., Kasitanon, N., Wangkaew, S., Hongsongkiat, S., Sukitawut, W., & Louthrenoo, W. (2013). Sensitivity and specificity of ANA and anti-dsDNA in the diagnosis of systemic lupus erythematosus: A comparison using control sera obtained from healthy individuals and patients with multiple medical problems. *Asian Pacific Journal of Allergy and Immunology*, *31*(4), 292–298. http://dx.doi.org/10.12932/AP0272.31.4.2013.

Wielosz, E., Dryglewska, M., & Majdan, M. (2014). Serological profile of patients with systemic sclerosis. *Postępy Higieny i Medycyny Doświadczalnej (Online)*, *68*, 987–991. http://dx.doi.org/10.5604/17322693.1117543.

Wiener, J. M., & Tilly, J. (2002). Population ageing in the United States of America: Implications for public programmes. *International Journal of Epidemiology*, *31*(4), 776–781.

Wright, C., Sibani, S., Trudgian, D., Fischer, R., Kessler, B., LaBaer, J., et al. (2012). Detection of multiple autoantibodies in patients with ankylosing spondylitis using nucleic acid programmable protein arrays. *Molecular and Cellular Proteomics*, *11*(2). http://dx.doi.org/10.1074/mcp.M9.00384, M9 00384.

Xie, C., Kim, H. J., Haw, J. G., Kalbasi, A., Gardner, B. K., Li, G., et al. (2011). A novel multiplex assay combining autoantibodies plus PSA has potential implications for classification of prostate cancer from non-malignant cases. *Journal of Translational Medicine*, *9*, 43. http://dx.doi.org/10.1186/1479-5876-9-43.

Yanamandra, K., Gruden, M. A., Casaite, V., Meskys, R., Forsgren, L., & Morozova-Roche, L. A. (2011). alpha-synuclein reactive antibodies as diagnostic biomarkers in blood sera of Parkinson's disease patients. *PLoS One*, *6*(4), e18513. http://dx.doi.org/10.1371/journal.pone.0018513.

Yaniv, G., Twig, G., Shor, D. B., Furer, A., Sherer, Y., Mozes, O., et al. (2015). A volcanic explosion of autoantibodies in systemic lupus erythematosus: A diversity of 180 different antibodies found in SLE patients. *Autoimmunity Reviews*, *14*(1), 75–79. http://dx.doi.org/10.1016/j.autrev.2014.10.003.

Yoshio, T., Hirata, D., Onda, K., Nara, H., & Minota, S. (2005). Antiribosomal P protein antibodies in cerebrospinal fluid are associated with neuropsychiatric systemic lupus erythematosus. *Journal of Rheumatology*, *32*(1), 34–39.

Yoshizawa, S., Matsuoka, K., Inoue, N., Takaishi, H., Ogata, H., Iwao, Y., et al. (2007). Clinical significance of serum p53 antibodies in patients with ulcerative colitis and its carcinogenesis. *Inflammatory Bowel Diseases*, *13*(7), 865–873. http://dx.doi.org/10.1002/ibd.20112.

Zhou, Z. H., & Notkins, A. L. (2004). Polyreactive antigen-binding B (PAB-) cells are widely distributed and the PAB population consists of both B-1 + and B-1- phenotypes. *Clinical and Experimental Immunology*, *137*(1), 88–100. http://dx.doi.org/10.1111/j.1365-2249.2004.02511.x.

CHAPTER TWO

# Metabolomics of Neurodegenerative Diseases

**Alejandro Botas*,[1], Hannah Moore Campbell†,[1], Xu Han‡,§, Mirjana Maletic-Savatic‡,§,¶,||,#,[2]**

*BioSciences Department, Rice University, Houston, Texas, USA
†Medical Scientist Training Program, Baylor College of Medicine, Houston, Texas, USA
‡Department of Pediatrics, Baylor College of Medicine, Houston, Texas, USA
§Jan and Dan Duncan Neurological Research Institute at Texas Children's Hospital, Houston, Texas, USA
¶Program in Developmental Biology, Baylor College of Medicine, Houston, Texas, USA
||Program in Structural and Computational Biology and Molecular Biophysics, Baylor College of Medicine, Houston, Texas, USA
#Department of Neuroscience, Baylor College of Medicine, Houston, Texas, USA
[1]Equal contribution.
[2]Corresponding author: e-mail address: maletics@bcm.edu

## Contents

1. Metabolomics in Medicine 55
2. Metabolomics Biomarkers of Disease 56
   2.1 Metabolomics Platforms for Biomarker Discovery 58
3. Metabolomics Biomarker Discovery in Neurodegenerative Disorders 61
   3.1 Alzheimer's Disease 61
   3.2 Parkinson's Disease 65
   3.3 Huntington's Disease 66
   3.4 Multiple Sclerosis 68
   3.5 Amyotrophic Lateral Sclerosis 71
4. Summary 72
Acknowledgments 73
References 73

## Abstract

Neurodegenerative diseases are progressive, devastating, and terminal, carrying both personal and societal burden. Currently, their diagnosis depends on their clinical presentation. No quantitative biomarkers exist to enable early verdict and commencement of therapy. The lack of diagnostic biomarkers stems from the unavailability of brain tissue, the complexity and heterogeneity of the brain and neurodegenerative pathology, and the fact that peripheral tissues such as blood, urine, and even cerebrospinal fluid might not reflect early stages of brain pathology. Moreover, accumulated evidence indicates the majority of these diseases are not genetically inherited; rather, the genes bring about the risk to develop them, but the trigger is not known. As metabolites are at the intersection between the genetic background of a cell or a tissue and the

*International Review of Neurobiology*, Volume 122
ISSN 0074-7742
http://dx.doi.org/10.1016/bs.irn.2015.05.006

environmental effects on the same, metabolomics has emerged as a field with great promise to deliver new, biologically, and clinically relevant biomarkers for neurodegenerative disorders. Here, we review the basic principles of metabolomics and focus on studies performed in most common neurodegenerative diseases, such as Alzheimer's, Parkinson's, and Huntington's diseases, Multiple sclerosis, and Amyotrophic lateral sclerosis.

The notion that changes in biological fluids can be "read" to reveal an organism's state of health or disease has been with us since ancient Greek physicians observed that ants were attracted to the sweet urine of diabetics. More recent, non-formican technologies such as nuclear magnetic resonance (NMR) spectroscopy and mass spectrometry have furthered our ability to identify specific metabolites and quantify the products of cellular metabolism (de Graaf, 2007). The large-scale study of the small-molecule compounds (<2 kDa) or metabolites in a particular biological sample is termed metabolomics (Dunn, Bailey, & Johnson, 2005; Hollywood, Brison, & Goodacre, 2006; Metz, 2011). The sum of all metabolites in the sample composes the metabolome, and the human metabolome is thought to contain about 42,000 metabolites (Wishart, 2007). These consist of both endogenous (products of the enzymatic reactions within the cell) and exogenous (ingested xenobiotic chemicals) small molecules that human body generates or comes in contact with. The level of each metabolite within the metabolome depends on the specific physiological, developmental, and pathological state of a cell or tissue (Weckwerth & Morgenthal, 2005). Therefore, the metabolome reflects the phenotype of a cell or tissue, which resulted in direct response to different genetic or environmental influences (Fiehn, 2002).

As a field, metabolomics is a systems biology science similar to genomics, transcriptomics, proteomics, and other 'omics sciences, focusing on the metabolome as a whole (Fig. 1). Metabolomics has a few advantages compared to other 'omics studies. First, humans have far fewer metabolites than genes, RNA transcripts, or proteins. With fewer variables, it is easier to identify biologically meaningful patterns. Second, metabolites tend to be more conserved across species, from bacteria to mammals, and thus insights gained from metabolomic studies in model organisms can be more readily translated to human data. Further, metabolomics builds on more than 100 years of knowledge in biochemistry (German, Hammock, & Watkins, 2005), and thus, pathway mapping faces less difficulty compared to other 'omics fields. Additionally, since metabolism is the product not just of an organism's

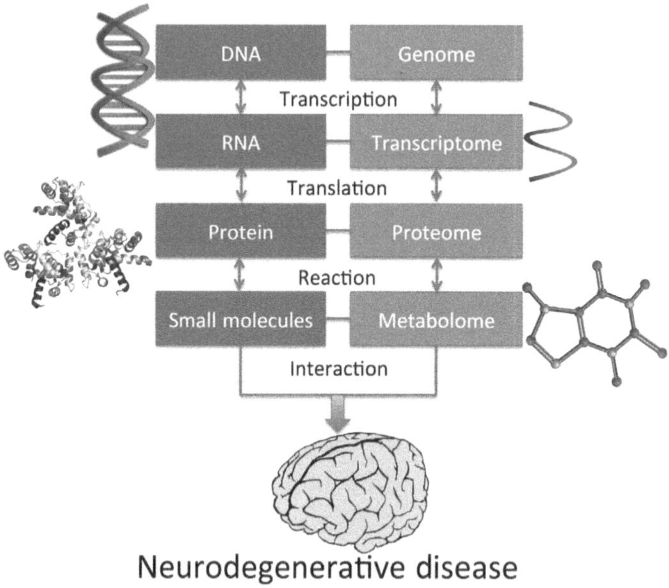


**Figure 1** Metabolomics is an integral part of several 'omics systems biology approaches for studies of cellular function.

native processes, but also of its interactions with the environment, we may glean information from metabolomics that cannot be found using other modes of study. Finally, metabolites are easily accessible *in vivo*, allowing the assessment of organismal health in real time, indispensable for medical diagnostics.

## 1. METABOLOMICS IN MEDICINE

In the field of medicine, metabolomics has two prime objectives: (1) identification of aberrant metabolites and metabolic pathways to generate hypotheses about the *etiology* of a given disease (Jove, Portero-Otin, Naudi, Ferrer, & Pamplona, 2014) and (2) identification of aberrant metabolites for discovery of reliable and reproducible biomarkers for *early diagnosis* of disease or for *therapeutic monitoring*. The logic and practicality behind the first goal is relatively straightforward—metabolomics is a new field and rapidly progressing technologies and data analysis tools are increasingly allowing a new dimension for studies of disease pathology. Importantly, metabolomics also provides the unique opportunity for discovery of new biomarkers. Identification of clinically relevant biomarkers of neurological diseases, including neurodegenerative diseases, has been notoriously challenging due to the unavailability of the human brain tissue for investigations, the complexity and heterogeneity of the brain, and the deficiency of models for functional validation of candidate biomarkers. A recent review of metabolomics and human brain aging (Jove et al., 2014), pointed to a study revealing that of 900 patients in the United States with Alzheimer's disease (AD), the most prevalent of neurodegenerative diseases, clinical diagnosis was inconsistent with autopsy diagnosis 17–30% of the time (Beach, Monsell, Phillips, & Kukull, 2012). In addition, diagnosis often comes too late because in most cases it relies on clinical and/or radiological presentation. However, the underlying pathology of many neurodegenerative diseases precedes the appearance of symptoms, sometimes by years or even decades (Trushina & Mielke, 2014). As metabolome is a dynamic and sensitive biological system, reflective of both innate processes and environmental influences, it encodes to a great extent an organism's health and homeostasis. Thus, early or even presymptomatic diagnosis could be possible by metabolomics biomarkers of disease, as some studies have demonstrated. However, research in this field faces several challenges, both technological and biological.

## 2. METABOLOMICS BIOMARKERS OF DISEASE

A *biomarker* is "a measurable substance in an organism whose presence is indicative of some phenomenon such as disease, infection, or environmental exposure." In the field of metabolomics, however, a biomarker may frequently be a composite of several molecules as metabolites are in constant flux. In addition, as the human metabolome comprises both endogenous and exogenous compounds whose concentrations heavily depend on the tissue being analyzed, it is very important to link the metabolomics biomarker not only to a given disease but also to the tissue where it is found. As illustrated in Fig. 2, the search for metabolomics biomarkers of disease starts from the sample that is analyzed by a chosen platform, followed by complex analytical approaches that can be divided into two main types: chemometric analysis and targeted metabolic profiling (Richards et al., 2010; Wishart, 2007). The aim of chemometric analysis is to discern the spectral profiles of biofluids and tissues in normal and disease states, not to identify metabolites *per se* (Wishart, 2007). In contrast, the aim of targeted metabolic profiling is to identify and quantify metabolites in a sample by comparison with a

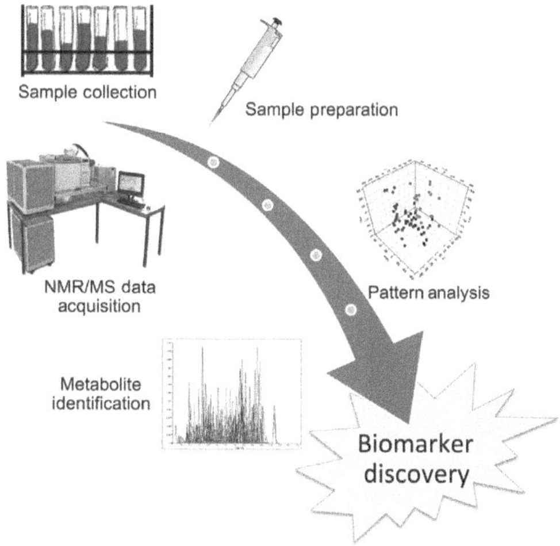


**Figure 2** Schematic representation of metabolomics flow, from samples to biomarker discovery.

reference library of experimentally acquired pure compound spectra (Weljie, Newton, Mercier, Carlson, & Slupsky, 2006). Eventually, both pattern analysis and identification of a specific metabolite may lead to biomarker discovery (Maletic-Savatic et al., 2008).

The choice of tissue sample for metabolomics biomarker discovery in neurodegenerative diseases is critical. The biggest challenge is that neurodegeneration starts locally and is confined to a small region of the brain until pathology expands and causes neuroinflammation, leakage of blood brain barrier, and spillover of the molecules into the cerebrospinal fluid (CSF) and blood. Access to brain tissue *in vivo* is exceptionally limited and thus, for biomarker discovery we rely on peripheral sources such as CSF, blood, urine, and saliva, or postmortem tissue. Both sources have pitfalls—metabolic abnormalities observed in the brain are more likely to be reflective of disease etiology than abnormalities found in peripheral biofluids. CSF is the most commonly analyzed biofluid as it is in close proximity to the pathological tissue, but it is difficult to obtain from healthy subjects and many studies that use it as a sample source suffer from their lack of a healthy control group. On the other hand, rapid degradation of small-molecules postmortem produces a substantial roadblock for data interpretation, as molecules identified may not reflect the pathology *in vivo*. Magnetic resonance spectroscopy (MRS), a noninvasive platform for metabolite identification and quantification, allows noninvasive metabolomics studies of the human brain *in vivo* (Ma, Li, Djurić, & Maletić-Savatić, 2011; Maletic-Savatic et al., 2008; Vingara et al., 2013); however, MRS is sufficiently sensitive to study only a handful of the most concentrated metabolites. Further, clinical data can be greatly affected based on collection procedures. Contamination as well as degradation of the metabolites in a sample can impact results of metabolomics studies. For this reason, the establishment of standard operating procedures to ensure sample quality is critical (Yin & Xu, 2014). When investigating the metabolome in neurodegeneration, one needs to be aware of these roadblocks.

## 2.1 Metabolomics Platforms for Biomarker Discovery

Once the biological sample is obtained, two primary platforms are typically used for metabolic profiling: mass spectrometry (Han, Datla, Chan, & Borchers, 2009) and NMR spectroscopy (Ebbels & Cavill, 2009). *Mass spectrometry* is an analytical chemistry technique that can be used to identify small molecules based on mass to charge ($m/z$) ratio. A mass spectrum of a sample can be obtained by direct injection or in tandem with separation techniques, such as liquid or gas chromatography. In metabolomics, mass spectrometry coupled to liquid chromatography (LC-MS) or gas chromatography (GC-MS) is more commonly utilized as chromographic separation reduces matrix effects and the complexity of the sample (Gika, Theodoridis, Plumb, & Wilson, 2014). A variety of methodologies, instruments, and separation columns are available. Although LC-MS is emerging as the more predominant platform in metabolomics, no individual method is capable of detecting all metabolites, making a variety of instrumentation necessary to more fully characterize the metabolome (Yin & Xu, 2014). Mass spectrometry is most commonly used for targeted metabolomics, as many challenges exist that are necessary to overcome in order to optimize the nontargeted metabolomics approach. Additionally, sample preparation procedures, which can be time consuming and the most error prone aspect of mass spectrometry-based metabolomics, also need to be optimized to allow for greater metabolome coverage as well as reduced sample preparation time and sample loss (Ramos, 2012). Effective sample preparation with minimal sample loss is particularly important in the study of the metabolomics of neurodegenerative disease where CSF samples may be limited to only a few milliliters. To address these challenges, methods such as solid-phase microextraction have been developed (Cudjoe, Bojko, de Lannoy, Saldivia, & Pawliszyn, 2013) as well as ion mobility spectrometry (Castro-Perez et al., 2011; Sowell Koeniger, Valentine, Moon, & Clemmer, et al., 2004; Zinnel, Pai, & Russell, 2012) and capillary electrophoresis-mass spectrometry (Nevedomskaya et al., 2010; Takeuchi et al., 2013).

Additionally, unlike targeted metabolomics where a single internal standard can be utilized for analysis validation, a simple approach is not possible with untargeted metabolomics where data must be extracted from a large array of metabolites of various concentrations. To enable untargeted mass spectrometry-based metabolomics, the strategies include use of multiple internal standards simultaneously as well as the use of quality control samples, which are typically composed of aliquots from the test samples (Gika et al., 2014). Currently, identification of unknown metabolites is greatly limited, making it difficult to effectively identify important biomarkers. Nevertheless, Web-based spectral databases for LC-MS continue to develop (Yin & Xu, 2014), which is expected to accelerate the scope of targeted analysis. It is clear that some obstacles must still be overcome in mass spectrometry-based metabolomics.

NMR is another platform frequently used for metabolite identification and quantification. NMR is a physical phenomenon whereby nuclei in a magnetic field absorb and re-emit electromagnetic energy at a specific resonance frequency depending on the strength of the magnetic field and the magnetic properties of the atoms (de Graaf, 2007). It provides highly reproducible and resolved spectra in a short period of time, which makes it very suitable for clinical diagnostics. In addition, compared to mass spectrometry, the NMR data are quantitative and untargeted. However, the analysis of NMR data is cumbersome, operator biased, and time consuming. This stems from the complex nature of the data and numerous factors that influence the signals, such as those inherent to the molecules, the environment, and the magnetic field used to obtain the spectra. In addition, the spectra contain thousands of resonances that may belong to hundreds of metabolites. To break this complex signal high-dimensional dataset down into its proper components, metabolites, the data must be subjected to mathematical analysis and meaningful dimensions that represent chemical, structural, or metabolic pathway information (Allen & Maletic-Savatic, 2011; Allen, Peterson, Vannucci, & Maletić-Savatić, 2013; Coen, Holmes, Lindon, & Nicholson, 2008; Dunn et al., 2005; Goodacre, Vaidyanathan, Dunn, Harrigan, & Kell, 2004; Weckwerth & Morgenthal, 2005).

Metabolites in the NMR data can be identified by query of metabolomic databases, such as the human metabolome database (Ulrich et al., 2008; Wishart et al., 2007), or by using commercial software, such as *Chenomx* (Weljie et al., 2006), which includes a library of spectral signatures of pure compounds and computer-assisted procedures that require several inputs from the user, including manual adjustment of the peaks' shapes. Metabolite quantification relies on peak integrals being proportional to the concentration of the corresponding metabolites in the sample. The accuracy of the quantification can be affected by variations in the chemical shift of the NMR signals, mainly because of small differences in solution chemistry between samples (Cloarec et al., 2005). Finally, identified metabolites can be explored in the context of metabolic networks, through existing databases such as KEGG.

In summary, the advances in high-throughput technologies have enabled biomedical scientists to interrogate the entire transcriptome, as well as significant portions of the proteome and metabolome, to obtain insights into biological mechanisms associated with cellular function. Until recently, the analysis focused on identifying a list of differentially expressed molecules that may play a significant role in a biological process or determine phenotype. However, most often such a list fails to provide mechanistic insights into the underlying biology of the condition under study. Hence, over the years attention has shifted from lists of molecules to sets of functionally related coordinated alterations, that constitute pathways or bioprocesses, that in concert orchestrate the underlying biology at cellular or organismal level. In other words, this so-called pathway-centric approach results in reduction of data dimensionality while preserving the interaction between the components within an experiment (Glazko & Emmert-Streib, 2009; Peterson et al., 2013). There are different approaches to define pathways using metabolomics data, some of which involve mapping metabolites to existing pathway maps and rely on enrichment methods, while others are much more sophisticated in that they explore enrichments across a larger compendia of molecular processes assembled within databases without the prerequisite for predefined pathway maps. Overall, the analytical path from data acquisition to network discovery in metabolomics involves numerous steps, computational and statistical analysis, as well as bioinformatics approaches necessary to produce accurate and biologically meaningful data. Such complex high-dimensional analysis is now paving the way toward discovery of biologically and clinically important biomarkers in a wide variety of medical pathology, such as in neurodegenerative disorders.

## 3. METABOLOMICS BIOMARKER DISCOVERY IN NEURODEGENERATIVE DISORDERS

### 3.1 Alzheimer's Disease

AD is a neurodegenerative disorder causing progressive and irreversible memory loss and cognitive impairment in the elderly, eventually resulting in death. It is characterized by accumulation of plaques of β-amyloid protein as well as neurofibrillary tangles containing hyperphosphorylated tau protein. These aggregates are found throughout the cortex and the hippocampus, in centers for learning and memory, resulting in progressive dementia (Di Carlo, Giacomazza, & San Biagio, 2012).

It has been more than 100 years since AD was described by German psychiatrist and neuropathologist Alois Alzheimer in 1906 (Zilka & Novak, 2006). While substantial progress has been made toward the understanding of etiology, pathology, and pathophysiology of AD, much work still remains to be done. Currently, it is estimated that more than 35.6 million patients exist worldwide, and further predicted that 115.4 million people will be affected by AD by 2050 (Alzheimer's Disease International, 2010). There are no effective treatments for AD and only very recently have biomarkers begun to show promise in predicting AD before symptoms appear (Andreasson, Vanmechelen, Shaw, Zetterberg, Vanderstichel, 2012; Mishur & Rea, 2012). Such predictive biomarkers are desperately needed as current clinical diagnosis of AD is not always accurate and is only possible well after the pathological process has begun (Graham et al., 2013; Greenberg, Grassano, Thambisetty, Lovestone, & Legido-Quigley, 2009; Hampel, Lista, & Khachaturian, 2012; Li et al., 2010). Further, genetic, epigenetic, and environmental roles in development of AD must all be considered toward a comprehensive, clinically valuable biomarker (Elias-Sonnenschein, Bertram, & Visser, 2012).

Accumulated data points to metabolism, particularly lipid and sugar metabolism, as a main component of AD (see Table 1 for summary; Kaddurah-Daouk et al., 2011; Grimm et al., 2011). It is well established that the presence of the *ApoE 4* allele is associated with an increased risk of cerebral AD pathology and age-related cognitive decline during normal aging (Alonso Vilatela, López-López, & Yescas-Gómez, 2012; Kline, 2012; Liu, Kanekiyo, Xu, & Bu, 2013). ApoE is a major cholesterol carrier that supports

**Table 1** A Summary of Metabolomics Studies in Alzheimer's Disease

| Organism | Sample Tissue/Fluid | Platform | Findings | References |
|---|---|---|---|---|
| Human | Plasma | Mass spec. | Identified a set of 10 phospholipids that predict with 90% accuracy phenoconversion of older adults to AD or amnestic MCI within 2–3 years | Mapstone et al. (2014) |
| Human | CSF | Capillary electrophoresis-mass spec. | Identified a set of metabolites (choline, dimethylarginine, arginine, valine, proline, serine, histidine, creatine, carnitine, and four unidentified), which are able to classify patients and controls into diagnostic groups with 97–100% accuracy. A small follow-up double-blind study had 83% accuracy | Ibanez et al. (2012) |
| Human | CSF | Mass spec. | Female AD patients show greater metabolic deviances from controls than male AD patients. Increased cortisol and cysteine levels in AD | Czech et al. (2012) |
| Human | Plasma | LC-mass spec. | Decreased desmosterol and desmosterol/cholesterol ratio in AD. Correlation between desmosterol and cognitive performance. Metabolite differences in female AD patients show greater significance compared to those of male AD patients | Sato et al. (2012) |
| Human | CSF | LC-ECA | Increased methionine (homocysteine precursor), 5-hydroxyindoleacetic acid, vanillylmandelic acid, and xanthosine in AD. Alterations in one-carbon metabolism, tyrosine, tryptophan, and purine pathways were identified in AD and MCI patients | Kaddurah-Daouk et al. (2013) |

| | | | | |
|---|---|---|---|---|
| Human | Plasma | Mass spec. | Decreased levels of sphingomyelin lipids with long aliphatic chains. Increased levels of ceramide species N16:0 and N21:0. Levels of many sphingomyelin and ceramide species were correlated with AD severity | Han et al. (2011) |
| Human | Plasma, CSF | LC-mass spec. | Cholesterol and sphingolipid transport were altered in both CSF and plasma. Lysine altered in plasma. Krebs cycle metabolites altered in CSF | Trushina, Dutta, Persson, Mielke, and Petersen (2013) |
| Human | Serum | LC-mass spec. | AD patients had diminished ether phospholipids, phosphatidylcholines, sphingomyelins, and sterols. 2,4-dihydroxybutanoic acid is predictive of progression from MCI to AD. Metabolic findings indicative of hypoxia, oxidative stress, as well as membrane lipid remodeling during progression to AD | Oresic et al. (2011) |
| Human | Postmortem CSF | LC-targeted electrochemistry | AD patients had alterations in tyrosine, tryptophan, purine, and tocopherol pathways. Reduced norepinephrine | Kaddurah-Daouk et al. (2011) |
| CRND8 mouse | Hippocampus, cortex, midbrain and cerebellum tissues | NMR | AD patients had decreased NAA, glutamate, glutamine, taurine (except in hippocampus), gamma-amino butyric acid, choline and phosphocholine, creatine, phosphocreatine and succinate, and increased lactate, aspartate, glycine (except in midbrain), and other amino acids including alanine in hippocampus, cortex, frontal cortex (exception frontal cortex), leucine, iso-leucine, valine, and water-soluble free fatty acids | Salek et al. (2010) |

*Continued*

**Table 1** A Summary of Metabolomics Studies in Alzheimer's Disease—cont'd

| Organism | Sample Tissue/Fluid | Platform | Findings | References |
|---|---|---|---|---|
| APP-PS1 mouse | Cortex, hippocampus | MRS | Reduced NAA and glutamate relative to creatine as age increased. Increased myo-inositol as age increased in APP-PS1 mice | Marjanska et al. (2005) |
| FAD mouse | Hippocampal tissue | GC-Mass spec. | Perturbations in nucleotide, Krebs cycle, energy transfer, carbohydrate neurotransmitter, and amino acid metabolic pathways, indicative of mitochondrial stress | Trushina et al. (2012) |

AD, Alzheimer's disease; MCI, mild cognitive impairment; CSF, cerebral spinal fluid; LC, liquid chromatography; GC, gas chromatography; ECA, electrochemical array; NMR, nuclear magnetic resonance; MRS, magnetic resonance spectroscopy; APP-PS1, amyloid precursor protein-presenilin-1; FAD, familial Alzheimer's disease; NAA, *N*-acetyl aspartate.

lipid transport and injury repair in the brain. Graham et al. (2013) investigated the human brain metabolome in an effort to identify potential low-molecular-weight molecules in the brains of AD patients (Graham et al., 2013). Unfortunately, they did not succeed, pointing to the complexity of brain tissue which differs based on the region, pathological examination, and genetics (Graham et al., 2013). A more targeted lipidomics study showed that stearoyl-CoA desaturase and sphingolipids were elevated in the AD brain (Astarita et al., 2011; Hejazi et al., 2011; Oresic et al., 2011; Trushina et al., 2013) as well as plasma (Han et al., 2011), suggesting that fundamental aberrations in lipid metabolism may contribute to AD pathogenesis (Chan et al., 2012). In a most recent study, Mapstone et al. (2014) demonstrated that changes in lipids and specifically phospholipids in plasma can identify antecedent memory loss with 90% accuracy. This report generated great interest because plasma is easy to obtain, and thus identified phospholipids may be routinely tested in the clinical evaluation of elderly at risk.

The impairment in cerebral glucose metabolism is also a consistent pathophysiological feature in AD. Several studies of glucose metabolism aberrations indicated that these may precede cognitive dysfunction, leading to a comparison of AD with diabetes (Cunnane et al., 2011; Jack et al., 2010; Small et al., 1995). The wealth of new research demonstrating the importance of aerobic glycolysis in the brain holds promise that activation of this form of metabolism may offer a new therapeutic strategy for the treatment of AD and other neurodegenerative diseases.

Finally, several attempts have been made to investigate metabolic biomarkers in AD using CSF analysis (Fagan & Perrin, 2012; Myint, Aoshima, Tanaka, Nakamura, & Oda, 2009). Ibanez et al. (2012) were able to classify patients into subgroups (MCI, AD, control) with high accuracy. However, variability of all the metabolomics data is high. This may depend on gender—women show higher metabolomic differences from controls in AD (Czech et al., 2012; Sato et al., 2012). In summary, while progress has been made and numerous potential biomarkers of AD have been identified through metabolomics, further studies and independent validation of these putative biomarkers are needed.

## 3.2 Parkinson's Disease

Parkinson's disease (PD) is a neurodegenerative disorder characterized by the gradual development of bradykinesia, a resting tremor, rigidity, and postural instability (Jankovic, 2003). Although the exact mechanism is not known, dopamine depletion in the basal ganglia secondary to degeneration of the substantia nigra is the cause of disease progression. Disease progression is variable and diagnosis is based on clinical symptomatology, established when neurodegeneration in the substantia nigra reaches a critical point and more than 50% of dopaminergic neurons are lost (Jankovic, 2003). Today, it is estimated that between 7 and 10 million people live with PD worldwide and prevalence increases with age (Pringsheim, Jette, Frolkis, & Steeves, 2014). To better understand the genetic, biochemical, and other factors contributing to the pathophysiology of this disease, much work is being done, including investigations in the field of metabolomics.

In PD, metabolic abnormalities may be underlined by variations in several genes (Funayama et al., 2007; Hauser et al., 2003; Paisán-Ruíz et al., 2004; Scherzer et al., 2007). Indeed, differences in amino acid levels in both plasma and CSF have been reported decades ago—both decreases and increases in glutamate; decreases in iso-leucine, alanine, lysine, arginine, and methionine (Iwasaki, Ikeda, Shiojima, & Kinoshita, 1992; Mally, Szalai, & Stone, 1997); and increases in glycine, aspartate, and valine (Jimenez-Jimenez et al., 1996; Mally et al., 1997). Several reports also indicate that there is a reduction of complex 1 activity in the electron transport chain of PD, suggesting that mitochondrial function is impaired (Haas et al., 1995; Penn et al., 1995). Most recent studies, however, point to homovanillic acid/xanthine ratio as a promising potential biomarker of PD (LeWitt, 2012; LeWitt, Schultz, Auinger, Lu, & Parkinson Study Group, 2011). While metabolomics has started to make some strides in the field of PD (Table 2), much more needs to be done to make an impact relevant for disease diagnosis and/or management.

## 3.3 Huntington's Disease

Huntington disease (HD) is a lethal neurodegenerative disorder characterized by progressive dementia, psychiatric problems, and involuntary movements or chorea (Walker, 2007). The disease is inherited in an autosomal dominant fashion and is caused by a trinucleotide (CAG) repeat expansion of the gene encoding the huntingtin protein. The resultant mutant protein is believed to be neurotoxic although the exact pathophysiology of this disease has yet to be understood. With current treatments being solely symptomatic, better understanding of the disease mechanism and the subsequent development of novel therapies is desperately needed (Mason & Barker, 2015). As reviewed in Table 3, very few metabolomics studies have been done in HD

**Table 2** A Summary of Metabolomics Studies in Parkinson's Disease

| Organism | Sample Tissue/Fluid | Platform | Findings | References |
|---|---|---|---|---|
| Human | Postmortem lateral ventricular CSF | LC and GC-mass spec. | Reduced oxidized glutathione | Amara and Standaert (2013) |
| Human | Serum | Mass spec. | *N*8-acetyl spermidine increased in individuals with rapidly progressing PD compared to individuals with slow progressing PD. Altered polyamine metabolism in PD | Roede et al. (2013) |
| Human | Plasma | LC-ECA | 8-Hydroxy-2-deoxyguanosine levels and glutathione significantly increased in PD patients. Uric acid was significantly reduced | Bogdanov et al. (2008) |
| Human | Postmortem CSF | LC and GC-mass spec. | Increased 3-hydroxykynurenine (33%) and decreased glutathione (40%) concentration in PD | Lewitt et al. (2013) |
| Human | CSF, serum | LC electrochemical detection | Higher concentration of urate in CSF and serum correlated with slower PD progression | Ascherio et al. (2009) |

PD, Parkinson's disease; CSF, cerebral spinal fluid; LC, liquid chromatography; GC, gas chromatography; ECA, electrochemical array; NAA, *N*-acetyl aspartate.

**Table 3** A Summary of Metabolomics Studies in Huntington's Disease

| Organism | Sample Tissue/ Fluid | Platform | Findings | References |
|---|---|---|---|---|
| Presymptomatic HD transgenic rat | Serum and CSF | NMR | Decreased NAA. Increased glutamine, succinic acid, glucose, and lactate in serum. Increased lactate and glucose in CSF | Verwaest et al. (2011) |
| Human and mouse (HD-N171-N82Q) | Serum | GC-mass spec. | Increased malonate in humans and mice. Suggests change to procatabolic phenotype in presymptomatic HD | Underwood et al. (2006) |
| HD mouse (R6/2) | Striatum | NMR | Decreased NAA, γ-aminobutyric acid, aspartate, alanine, acetate, choline, and phosphocholine in R6/2 mice. Increased glycerophosphocholine, scyllo-inositol, glutamine, taurine, myo-inositol, lactate, and creatine | Tsang et al. (2006) |

HD, Huntington's disease; CSF, cerebral spinal fluid; LC, liquid chromatography; GC, gas chromatography; NMR, nuclear magnetic resonance.

and most were in animal models of the disease (Tsang et al., 2006; Underwood et al., 2006; Verwaest et al., 2011). The most recent study (Kumar et al., 2015) indicates the role of manganese in pathophysiology of HD and supports the observation that there is an impairment of energy metabolism in HD that ultimately affects the function of neurons. Metabolomics studies in HD thus are driven more toward hypothesis generation for disease pathology and potential treatment rather than toward finding diagnostic biomarkers.

### 3.4 Multiple Sclerosis

Multiple sclerosis (MS) is an autoimmune-mediated disease affecting the central nervous system. The disease mechanism involves inflammatory damage of the myelin sheaths in the brain as well as spinal cord by a T-cell-mediated attack of either oligodendrocytes or the myelin protein itself (Compston & Coles, 2008). The disease is usually relapsing and remitting in character, with many symptoms resolving between attacks although permanent neurological damage eventually ensues (Manganas & Maletic-Savatic, 2005). Metabolomic research in MS is complicated by this clinical course, because patients have different phenotypes at different times, and their metabolic profiles most likely differ before and after an attack. Nevertheless, metabolomics studies in MS are quite abundant (Table 4) as scientists attempt to discern each step of the disease (Lutz et al., 2007). Most studies are

**Table 4** A Summary of Metabolomics Studies in Multiple Sclerosis

| Organism | Sample Tissue/ Fluid | Platform | Findings | References |
|---|---|---|---|---|
| Human | CSF | NMR | Increased choline, myo-inositol, threonate, and decreased 3-hydroxybutyrate, citrate, phenylalanine, 2-hydroxyisovalerate, and mannose | Reinke et al. (2014) |
| Mouse (relapsing remitting-experimental autoimmune encephalomyelitis) | Plasma | LC and GC–mass spec. | Increased free fatty acid levels. Impacted metabolic pathways included: bile acid biosynthesis, taurine metabolism, tryptophan and histidine metabolism, linoleic acid, and D-arginine metabolism pathways | Mangalam et al. (2013) |
| Human | CSF | NMR | Elevated acetate levels in MS patients; reduced formate levels | Lynch, Peeling, Auty, & Sutherland (1993) |
| Human | CSF | NMR | Increased lactate and fructose concentrations, decreased creatinine and phenylalanine concentrations | Nicoli et al. (1996) |
| Human | CSF | MRS | Increased lactate levels | Simone et al. (1996) |

*Continued*

**Table 4** A Summary of Metabolomics Studies in Multiple Sclerosis—cont'd

| Organism | Sample Tissue/ Fluid | Platform | Findings | References |
|---|---|---|---|---|
| Human | CSF | NMR | Reduced lactate and glutamine | Aasly et al. (1997) |
| Human | CSF | MRS | CSF analysis performed only in untreated MS patients at the time of the first attack. Correlation between CSF lactate concentration and the number of inflammatory MS brain plaques. Increased fructose in MS patients with and without inflammatory plaques | Lutz et al. (2007) |
| Human | CSF | NMR | CSF metabolite profile identified and used to predict MS with 80% accuracy | Sinclair et al. (2010) |
| Human | CSF | GC-mass spec. | Increased sorbitol, fructose, and lactate in MS, particularly secondary progressive MS. Sorbitol and fructose concentrations correlated positively and significantly with neurological disability | Regenold, Phatak, Makley, Stone, and Kling (2008) |
| Rat experimental autoimmune encephalomyelitis | CSF | LC and GC-mass spec. | Decreases in arginine, alanine, and branched amino acid levels at onset of disease. At peak of disease, increases in glutamine, *O*-phosphoethanolamine, branched-chain amino acids, and putrescine | Noga et al. (2012) |

MS, multiple sclerosis; CSF, cerebral spinal fluid; LC, liquid chromatography; GC, gas chromatography; NMR, nuclear magnetic resonance; MRS, magnetic resonance spectroscopy.

done in CSF, which in MS is more easily obtained as patients undergo spinal taps more routinely than in other neurodegenerative diseases. The heterogeneity of patients' clinical status with different lesion burden as well as temporal progression of the disease is reflected in published reports, as some data are contradictory (Aasly et al., 1997; Nicoli et al., 1996; Regenold et al., 2008; Simone et al., 1996). A recent study has indicated changes in phospholipids in CSF of patients with MS (Pieragostino et al., 2015), while other studies also point to lipid and sugar metabolism (Lutz et al., 2007; Mangalam et al., 2013; Regenold et al., 2008). These findings are not surprising, as the accumulation of certain fatty acids in the CSF may reflect degradation of myelin and the neuronal membrane, particularly if found soon after an attack. Overall, the metabolomics studies in MS are promising despite challenges that come mostly from its clinical presentation.

## 3.5 Amyotrophic Lateral Sclerosis

Amyotrophic lateral sclerosis (ALS), also known as Lou Gehrig's disease, is a progressive and fatal disease characterized by degeneration of both upper and lower motor neurons (Kiernan et al., 2011). Symptoms include progressive weakness leading to paralysis and death, most often from respiratory failure. 90% of cases have no known cause, while about 10% are associated with a genetic mutation, most often in superoxide dismutase 1 (*SOD1*) gene. Disease progression is believed to be associated with excitotoxicity. As current diagnosis is solely clinical, much research is being done to discover biomarkers that may lead to earlier diagnosis within a therapeutic window as well as better understanding of the clinical heterogeneity and possible therapeutic targets.

Given the long-standing observation that there is an impairment in reactive oxygen species handling by the diseased neurons as well as an increase in the release of glutamate that eventually leads to excitotoxic cell death, there have been increasing attempts to delineate the metabolic signature of ALS. Several studies have been done, both by mass spectrometry and NMR analysis of CSF, and the results are sometimes contradictory (Table 5). Nevertheless, a few reports show potential for biomarker discovery and accurate prediction of the disease (Lawton et al., 2014; Blasco et al., 2013; Rozen et al., 2005). As evident in most other metabolomics reports in neurodegenerative disorders, much more needs to be done to ascertain biological and clinical validity of putative biomarkers.

**Table 5** A Summary of Metabolomics Studies in Amyotrophic Lateral Sclerosis

| Organism | Sample Tissue/ Fluid | Platform | Findings | References |
|---|---|---|---|---|
| Human | Plasma | LC-mass spec. | Metabolic profiles of control subjects, motor neuron disease patients taking Riluzole, and motor neuron disease patients not taking Riluzole could all be distinguished | Rozen et al. (2005) |
| Human | Serum | NMR | ALS patients had increased glutamate, beta-hydroxybutyrate, acetate, acetone, and formate, and decreased glutamine, histidine and *N*-acetyl derivatives | Kumar et al. (2010) |
| Human | CSF | NMR | Diminished acetate concentrations in ALS. Increased acetone, pyruvate, and ascorbate | Blasco et al. (2010) |
| Human | CSF | LC-mass spec. | Identified metabolic signature predictive of ALS with 80% accuracy | Blasco et al. (2013) |
| Human | CSF | GC-mass spec. | Reduced glutamine and glutamate in ALS, particularly familial ALS with *SOD1* mutation. Differences in metabolomic signatures in ALS with and without *SOD1* mutation were observed | Wuolikainen, Moritz, Marklund, Antti, & Andersen (2011) |

ALS, amyotrophic lateral sclerosis; CSF, cerebral spinal fluid; LC, liquid chromatography; GC, gas chromatography; NMR, nuclear magnetic resonance; SOD1, superoxide dismutase-1.

## 4. SUMMARY

All neurodegenerative disorders show heterogeneity in pathology and clinical presentation. They may overlap. They can co-occur (Shaw, Korecka, Clark, Lee, & Trojanowski, 2007). These challenges make finding a valuable metabolic biomarker for any given neurodegenerative disease more difficult, but also more crucial. To ensure validity, standardization of protocols is necessary. This starts from the selected clinical cohort, as possible comorbidities and heterogeneity of patients can substantially hamper data interpretation. Acquisition of the data as well as data analysis needs to be reproducible across sites and technologies. Once this is achieved, large cohorts need to be assessed and this can be accomplished only through multicenter studies. Cross-sectional data needs to be correlated with other clinical data, and longitudinal studies are essential to ascertain the feasibility of the putative biomarkers. Regardless of the road ahead the field of metabolomics holds a promise of significant, meaningful, and valuable discoveries.

## ACKNOWLEDGMENTS

This work was supported by the BCM Medical Scientist Training Program (H. C. M.); and the Dana Foundation, McKnight Endowment for Science, and Nancy Chang Award for Excellence (M. M.-S.).

The work is also partially supported by P30HD024064 Intellectual and Developmental Disabilities Research Grant from the Eunice Kennedy Shriver National Institute of Child Health and Human Development.

*Conflict of Interest:* Authors declare no conflicts of interest.

## REFERENCES

Aasly, J., Garseth, M., Sonnewald, U., Zwart, J. A., White, L. R., & Unsgard, G. (1997). Cerebrospinal fluid lactate and glutamine are reduced in multiple sclerosis. *Acta Neurologica Scandinavica, 95*(1), 9–12.

Allen, G. I., & Maletic-Savatic, M. (2011). Sparse non-negative generalized PCA with applications to metabolomics. *Bioinformatics, 27*(21), 3029–3035. http://dx.doi.org/10.1093/bioinformatics/btr522.

Allen, G. I., Peterson, C., Vannucci, M., & Maletić-Savatić, M. (2013). Regularized partial least squares with an application to NMR spectroscopy. *Statistical Analysis and Data Mining, 6*(4), 302–314.

Alonso Vilatela, M. E., López-López, M., & Yescas-Gómez, P. (2012). Genetics of Alzheimer's disease. *Archives of Medical Research, 43*, 622–631.

Alzheimer's Disease International. (2010). The global economic impact of dementia. *World Alzheimer Report*, 1–50.

Amara, A. W., & Standaert, D. G. (2013). Metabolomics and the search for biomarkers in Parkinson's disease. *Movement Disorders: Official Journal of the Movement Disorder Society, 28*(12), 1620–1621.

Andreasson, U., Vanmechelen, E., Shaw, L. M., Zetterberg, H., & Vanderstichele, H. (2012). Analytical aspects of molecular Alzheimer's disease biomarkers. *Biomarkers in Medicine, 6*, 377–389.

Ascherio, A., LeWitt, P. A., Xu, K., Eberly, S., Watts, A., Matson, W. R., et al., Parkinson Study Group DATATOP Investigators. (2009). Urate as a predictor of the rate of clinical decline in Parkinson disease. *Archives of Neurology, 66*(12), 1460–1468.

Astarita, G., Jung, K. M., Vasilevko, V., Dipatrizio, N. V., Martin, S. K., Cribbs, D. H., et al. (2011). Elevated stearoyl-CoA desaturase in brains of patients with Alzheimer's disease. *PloS One, 6*(10), e24777. http://dx.doi.org/10.1371/journal.pone.0024777.

Beach, T. G., Monsell, S. E., Phillips, L. E., & Kukull, W. (2012). Accuracy of the clinical diagnosis of Alzheimer disease at National Institute on Aging Alzheimer Disease Centers, 2005–2010. *Journal of Neuropathology and Experimental Neurology, 71*(4), 266–273. http://dx.doi.org/10.1097/NEN.0b013e31824b211b.

Blasco, H., Corcia, P., Pradat, P. F., Bocca, C., Gordon, P. H., Veyrat-Durebex, C., et al. (2013). Metabolomics in cerebrospinal fluid of patients with amyotrophic lateral

sclerosis: An untargeted approach via high-resolution mass spectrometry. *Journal of Proteome Research*, *12*(8), 3746–3754. http://dx.doi.org/10.1021/pr400376e.
Blasco, H., Corcia, P., Moreau, C., Veau, S., Fournier, C., Vourc'h, P., et al. (2010). 1H-NMR-based metabolomic profiling of CSF in early amyotrophic lateral sclerosis. *PLoS One*, *5*(10), e13223.
Bogdanov, M., Matson, W. R., Wang, L., Matson, T., Saunders-Pullman, R., Bressman, S. S., et al. (2008). Metabolomic profiling to develop blood biomarkers for Parkinson's disease. *Brain: A Journal of Neurology*, *131*(Pt 2), 389–396.
Castro-Perez, J., Roddy, T. P., Nibbering, N. M., Shah, V., McLaren, D. G., Previs, S., et al. (2011). Localization of fatty acyl and double bond positions in phosphatidylcholines using a dual stage CID fragmentation coupled with ion mobility mass spectrometry. *Journal of the American Society for Mass Spectrometry*, *22*, 1552–1567.
Chan, R. B., Oliveira, T. G., Cortes, E. P., Honig, L. S., Duff, K. E., Small, S. A., et al. (2012). Comparative lipidomic analysis of mouse and human brain with Alzheimer disease. *Journal of Biological Chemistry*, *287*(4), 2678–2880. http://dx.doi.org/10.1074/jbc.M111.274142.
Cloarec, O., Dumas, M. E., Craig, A., Barton, R. H., Trygg, J., Hudson, J., et al. (2005). Statistical total correlation spectroscopy: An exploratory approach for latent biomarker identification from metabolic 1H NMR data sets. *Analytical Chemistry*, *77*(5), 1282–1289. http://dx.doi.org/10.1021/ac048630x.
Coen, M., Holmes, E., Lindon, J. C., & Nicholson, J. K. (2008). NMR-based metabolic profiling and metabonomic approaches to problems in molecular toxicology. *Chemical Research in Toxicology*, *21*(1), 9–27. http://dx.doi.org/10.1021/tx700335d.
Compston, A., & Coles, A. (2008). Multiple sclerosis. *Lancet*, *372*(9648), 1502–1517.
Cudjoe, E., Bojko, B., de Lannoy, I., Saldivia, V., & Pawliszyn, J. (2013). Solid-phase microextraction: A complementary in vivo sampling method to microdialysis. *Angewandte Chemie International Edition in English*, *52*(46), 12124–12126. http://dx.doi.org/10.1002/anie.201304538.
Cunnane, S., Nugent, S., Roy, M., Courchesne-Loyer, A., Croteau, E., Tremblay, S., et al. (2011). Brain fuel metabolism, aging, and Alzheimer's disease. *Nutrition (Burbank, Los Angeles County, Calif.)*, *27*, 3–20.
Czech, C., Berndt, P., Busch, K., Schmitz, O., Wiemer, J., Most, V., et al. (2012). Metabolite profiling of Alzheimer's disease cerebrospinal fluid. *PloS One*, 7(2), e31501. http://dx.doi.org/10.1371/journal.pone.0031501.
de Graaf, R. A. (2007). *In vivo NMR spectroscopy: Principles and techniques*. Chichester: Wiley.
Di Carlo, M., Giacomazza, D., & San Biagio, P. L. (2012). Alzheimer's disease: Biological aspects, therapeutic perspectives and diagnostic tools. *Journal of Physics. Condensed Matter*, *24*, 244102.
Dunn, W. B., Bailey, N. J., & Johnson, H. E. (2005). Measuring the metabolome: Current analytical technologies. *Analyst*, *130*(5), 606–625. http://dx.doi.org/10.1039/b418288j.
Ebbels, T. M. D., & Cavill, R. (2009). Bioinformatic methods in NMR-based metabolic profiling. *Progress in Nuclear Magnetic Resonance Spectroscopy*, *55*(4), 361–374. http://dx.doi.org/10.1016/j.pnmrs.2009.07.003.
Elias-Sonnenschein, L. S., Bertram, L., & Visser, P. J. (2012). Relationship between genetic risk factors and markers for Alzheimer's disease pathology. *Biomarkers in Medicine*, *6*, 477–495.
Fagan, A. M., & Perrin, R. J. (2012). Upcoming candidate cerebrospinal fluid biomarkers of Alzheimer's disease. *Biomarkers in Medicine*, *6*, 455–476.
Fiehn, O. (2002). Metabolomics—The link between genotypes and phenotypes. *Plant Molecular Biology*, *48*(1–2), 155–171.
Funayama, M., Li, Y., Tomiyama, H., Yoshino, H., Imamichi, Y., Yamamoto, M., et al. (2007). Leucine-rich repeat kinase 2 among the Japanese population. The

G2385R (c.7153G>A) variant was reported as a risk factor for sporadic Parkinson. *Neuroreport, 18*, 273–275.
German, J. B., Hammock, B. D., & Watkins, S. M. (2005). Metabolomics: Building on a century of biochemistry to guide human health. *Metabolomics, 1*, 3–9.
Gika, H. G., Theodoridis, G. A., Plumb, R. S., & Wilson, I. D. (2014). Current practice of liquid chromatography-mass spectrometry in metabolomics and metabonomics. *Journal of Pharmaceutical and Biomedical Analysis, 87*, 12–25. http://dx.doi.org/10.1016/j.jpba.2013.06.032.
Glazko, G. V., & Emmert-Streib, F. (2009). Unite and conquer: Univariate and multivariate approaches for finding differentially expressed gene sets. *Bioinformatics, 25*(18), 2348–2354. http://dx.doi.org/10.1093/bioinformatics/btp406.
Goodacre, R., Vaidyanathan, S., Dunn, W. B., Harrigan, G. G., & Kell, D. B. (2004). Metabolomics by numbers: Acquiring and understanding global metabolite data. *Trends in Biotechnology, 22*(5), 245–252. http://dx.doi.org/10.1016/j.tibtech.2004.03.007.
Graham, S. F., Chevallier, O. P., Roberts, D., Holscher, C., Elliott, C. T., & Green, B. D. (2013). Investigation of the human brain metabolome to identify potential markers for early diagnosis and therapeutic targets of Alzheimer's disease. *Analytical Chemistry, 85*(3), 1803–1811. http://dx.doi.org/10.1021/ac303163f.
Greenberg, N., Grassano, A., Thambisetty, M., Lovestone, S., & Legido-Quigley, C. (2009). A proposed metabolic strategy for monitoring disease progression in Alzheimer's disease. *Electrophoresis, 30*(7), 1235–1239. http://dx.doi.org/10.1002/elps.200800589.
Grimm, M. O., Grösgen, S., Riemenschneider, M., Tanila, H., Grimm, H. S., & Hartmann, T. (2011). From brain to food: Analysis of phosphatidylcholines, lysophosphatidylcholines and phosphatidylcholine-plasmalogens derivates in Alzheimer's disease human post mortem brains and mice model via mass spectrometry. *Journal of Chromatography. A, 1218*(42), 7713–7722. http://dx.doi.org/10.1016/j.chroma.2011.07.073.
Haas, R. H., Nasirian, F., Nakano, K., Ward, D., Pay, M., Hill, R., et al. (1995). Low platelet mitochondrial complex I and complex II/III activity in early untreated Parkinson's disease. *Annals of Neurology, 37*, 714–722.
Hampel, H., Lista, S., & Khachaturian, Z. S. (2012). Development of biomarkers to chart all Alzheimer's disease stages: The royal road to cutting the therapeutic Gordian knot. *Alzheimers Dement, 8*, 312–336.
Han, J., Datla, R., Chan, S., & Borchers, C. H. (2009). Mass spectrometry-based technologies for high-throughput metabolomics. *Bioanalysis, 1*(9), 1665–1684. http://dx.doi.org/10.4155/bio.09.158.
Han, X., Rozen, S., Boyle, S. H., Hellegers, C., Cheng, H., Burke, J. R., et al. (2011). Metabolomics in early Alzheimer's disease: Identification of altered plasma sphingolipidome using shotgun lipidomics. *PloS One, 6*(7), e21643. http://dx.doi.org/10.1371/journal.pone.0021643.
Hauser, M. A., Li, Y.-J., Takeuchi, S., Walters, R., Noureddine, M., Maready, M., et al. (2003). Genomic convergence: Identifying candidate genes for Parkinson's disease by combining serial analysis of gene expression and genetic linkage. *Human Molecular Genetics, 12*, 671–677.
Hejazi, L., Wong, J. W., Cheng, D., Proschogo, N., Ebrahimi, D., Garner, B., et al. (2011). Mass and relative elution time profiling: Two-dimensional analysis of sphingolipids in Alzheimer's disease brains. *Biochemical Journal, 438*(1), 165–175. http://dx.doi.org/10.1042/BJ20110566.
Hollywood, K., Brison, D. R., & Goodacre, R. (2006). Metabolomics: Current technologies and future trends. *Proteomics, 6*(17), 4716–4723. http://dx.doi.org/10.1002/pmic.200600106.
Ibanez, C., Simo, C., Martin-Alvarez, P. J., Kivipelto, M., Winblad, B., Cedazo-Minguez, A., et al. (2012). Toward a predictive model of Alzheimer's disease progression using capillary

electrophoresis-mass spectrometry metabolomics. *Analytical Chemistry, 84*(20), 8532–8540. http://dx.doi.org/10.1021/ac301243k.

Iwasaki, Y., Ikeda, K., Shiojima, T., & Kinoshita, M. (1992). Increased plasma concentrations of aspartate, glutamate and glycine in Parkinson's disease. *Neuroscience Letters, 145*, 175–177.

Jack, C., Jr., Knopman, D., Jagust, W., Shaw, L., Aisen, P., Weiner, M., et al. (2010). Hypothetical model of dynamic biomarkers of the Alzheimer's pathological cascade. *Lancet Neurology, 9*, 119–128.

Jankovic, J. (2003). Pathophysiology and clinical assessment of parkinsonian symptoms and signs. In R. Pahwa, K. Lyons, & W. C. Koller (Eds.), *Handbook of Parkinson's disease* (3rd ed., pp. 71–98). New York: Informa, Health Care.

Jimenez-Jimenez, F. J., Molina, J. A., Vargas, C., Gomez, P., Navarro, J. A., Benito-Leon, J., et al. (1996). Neurotransmitter amino acids in CSF of patients with Parkinson's disease. *Journal of Neurological Sciences, 15*, 39–44.

Jove, M., Portero-Otin, M., Naudi, A., Ferrer, I., & Pamplona, R. (2014). Metabolomics of human brain aging and age-related neurodegenerative diseases. *Journal of Neuropathology and Experimental Neurology, 73*(7), 640–657. http://dx.doi.org/10.1097/NEN.0000000000000091.

Kaddurah-Daouk, R., Rozen, S., Matson, W., Han, X., Hulette, C. M., Burke, J. R., et al. (2011). Metabolomic changes in autopsy-confirmed Alzheimer's disease. *Alzheimers & Dementia*, 7, 309–317.

Kaddurah-Daouk, R., Zhu, H., Sharma, S., Bogdanov, M., Rozen, S. G., Matson, W., et al., Pharmacometabolomics Research Network. (2013). Alterations in metabolic pathways and networks in Alzheimer's disease. *Translational Psychiatry, 3*, e244.

Kiernan, M. C., Vucic, S., Cheah, B. C., Turner, M. R., Eisen, A., Hardiman, O., et al. (2011). Amyotrophic lateral sclerosis. *Lancet, 377*(9769), 942–955.

Kline, A. (2012). Apolipoprotein E, amyloid-ß clearance and therapeutic opportunities in Alzheimer's disease. *Alzheimer's Research & Therapy, 4*, 32.

Kumar, A., Bala, L., Kalita, J., Misra, U. K., Singh, R. L., Khetrapal, C. L., et al. (2010). Metabolomic analysis of serum by (1)H NMR spectroscopy in amyotrophic lateral sclerosis. *Clinica Chimica Acta; International Journal of Clinical Chemistry, 411*(7-8), 563–567.

Kumar, K. K., Goodwin, C. R., Uhouse, M. A., Bornhorst, J., Schwerdtle, T., Aschner, M., et al. (2015). Untargeted metabolic profiling identifies interactions between Huntington's disease and neuronal manganese status. *Metallomics*, 7(2), 363–370.

Lawton, K. A., Brown, M. V., Alexander, D., Li, Z., Wulff, J. E., Lawson, R., et al. (2014). Plasma metabolomic biomarker panel to distinguish patients with amyotrophic lateral sclerosis from disease mimics. *Amyotrophic Lateral Sclerosis and Frontotemporal Degeneration, 15*(5–6), 362–370.

LeWitt, P. (2012). Recent advances in CSF biomarkers for Parkinson's disease. *Parkinsonism & Related Disorders, 18*(Suppl. 1), S49–S51. http://dx.doi.org/10.1016/S1353-8020(11)70017-7.

Lewitt, P. A., Li, J., Lu, M., Beach, T. G., Adler, C. H., Guo, L., & Arizona Parkinson's Disease Consortium. (2013). 3-hydroxykynurenine and other Parkinson's disease biomarkers discovered by metabolomic analysis. *Movement Disorders: Official Journal of the Movement Disorder Society, 28*(12), 1653–1660.

LeWitt, P., Schultz, L., Auinger, P., Lu, M., & Parkinson Study Group, D. I. (2011). CSF xanthine, homovanillic acid, and their ratio as biomarkers of Parkinson's disease. *Brain Research, 1408*, 88–97. http://dx.doi.org/10.1016/j.brainres.2011.06.057.

Li, N. J., Liu, W. T., Li, W., Liu, S. Q., Chen, X. H., Bi, K. S., et al. (2010). Plasma metabolic profiling of Alzheimer's disease by liquid chromatography/mass spectrometry. *Clinical Biochemistry, 43*(12), 992–997. http://dx.doi.org/10.1016/j.clinbiochem.2010.04.072.

Liu, C. C., Kanekiyo, T., Xu, H., & Bu, G. (2013). Apolipoprotein E and Alzheimer disease: Risk, mechanisms, and therapy. *Nature Reviews Neurology, 9*, 106–118.

Lutz, N. W., Viola, A., Malikova, I., Confort-Gouny, S., Audoin, B., Ranjeva, J. P., et al. (2007). Inflammatory multiple-sclerosis plaques generate characteristic metabolic profiles in cerebrospinal fluid. *PloS One*, *2*(7), e595. http://dx.doi.org/10.1371/journal.pone.0000595.

Lynch, J., Peeling, J., Auty, A., & Sutherland, G. R. (1993). Nuclear magnetic resonance study of cerebrospinal fluid from patients with multiple sclerosis. *The Canadian Journal of Neurological Sciences. Le Journal Canadien des Sciences Neurologiques*, *20*(3), 194–198.

Ma, L. H., Li, Y., Djurić, P. M., & Maletić-Savatić, M. (2011). Systems biology approach to imaging of neural stem cells. *Methods in Molecular Biology*, *711*, 421–434.

Maletic-Savatic, M., Vingara, L. K., Manganas, L. N., Li, Y., Zhang, S., Sierra, A., et al. (2008). Metabolomics of neural progenitor cells: A novel approach to biomarker discovery. *Cold Spring Harbor Symposia on Quantitative Biology*, *73*, 389–401. http://dx.doi.org/10.1101/sqb.2008.73.021.

Mally, J., Szalai, G., & Stone, T. W. (1997). Changes in the concentration of amino acids in serum and cerebrospinal fluid of patients with Parkinson's disease. *Journal of Neurological Sciences*, *151*, 159–162.

Mangalam, A., Poisson, L., Nemutlu, E., Datta, I., Denic, A., Dzeja, P., et al. (2013). Profile of circulatory metabolites in a relapsing-remitting animal model of multiple sclerosis using global metabolomics. *Journal of Clinical & Cellular Immunology*, *4*, 150.

Manganas, L., & Maletic-Savatic, M. (2005). Stem cell therapy for CNS demyelinating diseases. *Current Neurology and Neuroscience Report*, *5*(3), 225–231.

Mapstone, M., Cheema, A. K., Fiandaca, M. S., Zhong, X., Mhyre, T. R., MacArthur, L. H., et al. (2014). Plasma phospholipids identify antecedent memory impairment in older adults. *Nature Medicine*, *20*(4), 415–418. http://dx.doi.org/10.1038/nm.3466.

Marjanska, M., Curran, G. L., Wengenack, T. M., Henry, P. G., Bliss, R. L., Poduslo, J. F., et al. (2005). Monitoring disease progression in transgenic mouse models of Alzheimer's disease with proton magnetic resonance spectroscopy. *Proceedings of the National Academy of Sciences of the United States of America*, *102*(33), 11906–11910.

Mason, S., & Barker, R. A. (2015). Progress in Huntington's disease: The search for markers of disease onset and progression. *Journal of Neurology*. [Epub ahead of print].

Metz, T. (2011). *Metabolic profiling: Methods and protocols*. New York: Springer Verlag.

Mishur, R. J., & Rea, S. L. (2012). Applications of mass spectrometry to metabolomics and metabonomics: Detection of biomarkers of aging and of age-related diseases. *Mass Spectrometry Reviews*, *31*, 70–95.

Myint, K. T., Aoshima, K., Tanaka, S., Nakamura, T., & Oda, Y. (2009). Quantitative profiling of polar cationic metabolites in human cerebrospinal fluid by reversed-phase nanoliquid chromatography/mass spectrometry. *Analytical Chemistry*, *81*(3), 1121–1129. http://dx.doi.org/10.1021/ac802259r.

Nevedomskaya, E., Ramautar, R., Derks, R., Westbroek, I., Zondag, G., van der Pluijm, I., et al. (2010). CE-MS for metabolic profiling of volume-limited urine samples: Application to accelerated aging TTD mice. *Journal of Proteome Research*, *9*, 4869–4874.

Nicoli, F., Vion-Dury, J., Confort-Gouny, S., Maillet, S., Gastaut, J. L., & Cozzone, P. J. (1996). Cerebrospinal fluid metabolic profiles in multiple sclerosis and degenerative dementias obtained by high resolution proton magnetic resonance spectroscopy. *Comptes Rendus de l'Académie des Sciences Série III*, *319*(7), 623–631.

Noga, M. J., Dane, A., Shi, S., Attali, A., van Aken, H., Suidgeest, E., et al. (2012). Metabolomics of cerebrospinal fluid reveals changes in the central nervous system metabolism in a rat model of multiple sclerosis. *Metabolomics*, *8*(2), 253–263.

Oresic, M., Hyotylainen, T., Herukka, S. K., Sysi-Aho, M., Mattila, I., Seppanan-Laakso, T., et al. (2011). Metabolome in progression to Alzheimer's disease. *Translational Psychiatry*, *1*, e57. http://dx.doi.org/10.1038/tp.2011.55.

Paisán-Ruíz, C., Jain, S., Evans, E. W., Gilks, W. P., Simón, J., Brug, M., et al. (2004). Cloning of the gene containing mutations that cause PARK8-linked Parkinson's disease. *Neuron*, *18*, 575–577.
Penn, A. M., Roberts, T., Hodder, J., Allen, P. S., Zhu, G., & Martin, W. R. (1995). Generalized mitochondrial dysfunction in Parkinson's disease detected by magnetic resonance spectroscopy of muscle. *Neurology*, *45*, 2097–2099.
Peterson, C., Vannucci, M., Karakas, C., Choi, W., Ma, L., & Maletic-Savatic, M. (2013). Inferring metabolic networks using the Bayesian adaptive graphical lasso with informative priors. *Statistics and Its Interface*, *6*(4), 547–558. http://dx.doi.org/10.4310/SII.2013.v6.n4.a12.
Pieragostino, D., D'Alessandro, M., di Ioia, M., Rossi, C., Zucchelli, M., Urbani, A., et al. (2015). An integrated metabolomics approach for the research of new cerebrospinal fluid biomarkers of multiple sclerosis. *Molecular BioSystems*, *11*(6), 1563–1572.
Pringsheim, T., Jette, N., Frolkis, A., & Steeves, T. D. (2014). The prevalence of Parkinson's disease: A systematic review and meta-analysis. *Movement Disorders*, *29*(13), 1583–1590.
Ramos, L. (2012). Critical overview of selected contemporary sample preparation techniques. *Journal of Chromatography A*, *1221*, 84–98. http://dx.doi.org/10.1016/j.chroma.2011.11.011.
Regenold, W. T., Phatak, P., Makley, M. J., Stone, R. D., & Kling, M. A. (2008). Cerebrospinal fluid evidence of increased extra-mitochondrial glucose metabolism implicates mitochondrial dysfunction in multiple sclerosis disease progression. *Journal of Neurological Sciences*, *275*(1–2), 106–112. http://dx.doi.org/10.1016/j.jns.2008.07.032.
Reinke, S. N., Broadhurst, D. L., Sykes, B. D., Baker, G. B., Catz, I., Warren, K. G., et al. (2014). Metabolomic profiling in multiple sclerosis: Insights into biomarkers and pathogenesis. *Multiple Sclerosis (Houndmills, Basingstoke, England)*, *20*(10), 1396–1400.
Richards, S. E., Dumas, M.-E., Fonville, J. M., Ebbels, T. M. D., Holmes, E., & Nicholson, J. K. (2010). Intra- and inter-omic fusion of metabolic profiling data in a systems biology framework. *Chemometrics and Intelligent Laboratory Systems*, *104*(1), 121–131. http://dx.doi.org/10.1016/j.chemolab.2010.07.006.
Roede, J. R., Uppal, K., Park, Y., Lee, K., Tran, V., Walker, D., et al. (2013). Serum metabolomics of slow vs. rapid motor progression Parkinson's disease: A pilot study. *PLoS One*, *8*(10), e77629.
Rozen, S., Cudkowicz, M. E., Bogdanov, M., Matson, W. R., Kristal, B. S., Beecher, C., et al. (2005). Metabolomic analysis and signatures in motor neuron disease. *Metabolomics*, *1*(2), 101–108. http://dx.doi.org/10.1007/s11306-005-4810-1.
Salek, R. M., Xia, J., Innes, A., Sweatman, B. C., Adalbert, R., Randle, S., et al. (2010). A metabolomic study of the CRND8 transgenic mouse model of Alzheimer's disease. *Neurochemistry International*, *56*(8), 937–947.
Sato, Y., Suzuki, I., Nakamura, T., Bernier, F., Aoshima, K., & Oda, Y. (2012). Identification of a new plasma biomarker of Alzheimer's disease using metabolomics technology. *Journal of Lipid Research*, *53*(3), 567–576. http://dx.doi.org/10.1194/jlr.M022376.
Scherzer, C. R., Eklund, A. C., Morse, L. J., Liao, Z., Locascio, J. J., Fefer, D., et al. (2007). Molecular markers of early Parkinson's disease based on gene expression in blood. *Proceedings of the National Academy of Sciences of the United States of America*, *104*, 955–960.
Shaw, L. M., Korecka, M., Clark, C. M., Lee, V. M., & Trojanowski, J. Q. (2007). Biomarkers of neurodegeneration for diagnosis and monitoring therapeutics. *Nature Reviews. Drug Discovery*, *6*(4), 295–303. http://dx.doi.org/10.1038/nrd2176.
Simone, I. L., Federico, F., Trojano, M., Tortorella, C., Liguori, M., Giannini, P., et al. (1996). High resolution proton MR spectroscopy of cerebrospinal fluid in MS patients. Comparison with biochemical changes in demyelinating plaques. *Journal of Neurological Sciences*, *144*(1–2), 182–190.

Sinclair, A. J., Viant, M. R., Ball, A. K., Burdon, M. A., Walker, E. A., Stewart, P. M., et al. (2010). NMR-based metabolomic analysis of cerebrospinal fluid and serum in neurological diseases–a diagnostic tool? *NMR in Biomedicine*, *23*(2), 123–132.

Small, G., Mazziotta, J., Collins, M., Baxter, L., Phelps, M., Mandelkern, M., et al. (1995). Apolipoprotein E type 4 allele and cerebral glucose metabolism in relatives at risk for familial Alzheimer disease. *JAMA: The journal of the American Medical Association*, *273*(12), 942–947.

Sowell, R. A., Koeniger, S. L., Valentine, S. J., Moon, M. H., & Clemmer, D. E. (2004). Nanoflow LC/IMS-MS and LC/IMS-CID/MS of protein mixtures. *Journal of the American Society for Mass Spectrometry*, *15*, 1341–1353.

Takeuchi, K., Ohishi, M., Ota, S., et al. (2013). Metabolic profiling to identify potential serum biomarkers for gastric ulceration induced by nonsteroid anti-inflammatory drugs. *Journal of Proteome Research*, *12*, 1399–1407.

Trushina, E., Dutta, T., Persson, X. M., Mielke, M. M., & Petersen, R. C. (2013). Identification of altered metabolic pathways in plasma and CSF in mild cognitive impairment and Alzheimer's disease using metabolomics. *PloS One*, *8*(5), e63644. http://dx.doi.org/10.1371/journal.pone.0063644.

Trushina, E., Nemutlu, E., Zhang, S., Christensen, T., Camp, J., Mesa, J., et al. (2012). Defects in mitochondrial dynamics and metabolomic signatures of evolving energetic stress in mouse models of familial Alzheimer's disease. *PLoS One*, 7(2), e32737.

Trushina, E., & Mielke, M. M. (2014). Recent advances in the application of metabolomics to Alzheimer's Disease. *Biochimica et Biophysica Acta*, *1842*(8), 1232–1239. http://dx.doi.org/10.1016/j.bbadis.2013.06.014.

Tsang, T. M., Woodman, B., McLoughlin, G. A., Griffin, J. L., Tabrizi, S. J., Bates, G. P., et al. (2006). Metabolic characterization of the R6/2 transgenic mouse model of Huntington's disease by high-resolution MAS 1H NMR spectroscopy. *Journal of Proteome Research*, *5*(3), 483–492.

Ulrich, E. L., Akutsu, H., Doreleijers, J. F., Harano, Y., Ioannidis, Y. E., Lin, J., et al. (2008). BioMagResBank. *Nucleic Acids Research*, *36*(Database issue), D402–D408. http://dx.doi.org/10.1093/nar/gkm957.

Underwood, B. R., Broadhurst, D., Dunn, W. B., Ellis, D. I., Michell, A. W., Vacher, C., et al. (2006). Huntington disease patients and transgenic mice have similar pro-catabolic serum metabolite profiles. *Brain: A Journal of Neurology*, *129*, 877–886.

Verwaest, K. A., Vu, T. N., Laukens, K., Clemens, L. E., Nguyen, H. P., Van Gasse, B., et al. (2011). (1)H NMR based metabolomics of CSF and blood serum: A metabolic profile for a transgenic rat model of Huntington disease. *Biochimica et Biophysica Acta*, *1812*(11), 1371–1379.

Vingara, L. K., Yu, H. J., Wagshul, M. E., Serafin, D., Christodoulou, C., Pelczer, I., et al. (2013). Metabolomic approach to human brain spectroscopy identifies associations between clinical features and the frontal lobe metabolome in multiple sclerosis. *NeuroImage*, *82*, 586–594. http://dx.doi.org/10.1016/j.neuroimage.2013.05.125.

Walker, F. O. (2007). Huntington's disease. *Lancet*, *369*(9557), 218–228.

Weckwerth, W., & Morgenthal, K. (2005). Metabolomics: From pattern recognition to biological interpretation. *Drug Discovery Today*, *10*(22), 1551–1558. http://dx.doi.org/10.1016/S1359-6446(05)03609-3.

Weljie, A. M., Newton, J., Mercier, P., Carlson, E., & Slupsky, C. M. (2006). Targeted profiling: Quantitative analysis of 1H NMR metabolomics data. *Analytical Chemistry*, *78*(13), 4430–4442. http://dx.doi.org/10.1021/ac060209g.

Wishart, D. S. (2007). Current progress in computational metabolomics. *Briefings in Bioinformatics*, *8*(5), 279–293. http://dx.doi.org/10.1093/bib/bbm030.

Wishart, D. S., Tzur, D., Knox, C., Eisner, R., Guo, A. C., Young, N., et al. (2007). HMDB: The Human Metabolome Database. *Nucleic Acids Research*, *35*(Database issue), D521–D526. http://dx.doi.org/10.1093/nar/gkl923.

Wuolikainen, A., Moritz, T., Marklund, S. L., Antti, H., & Andersen, P. M. (2011). Disease-related changes in the cerebrospinal fluid metabolome in amyotrophic lateral sclerosis detected by GC/TOFMS. *PLoS One*, *6*(4), e17947.

Yin, P., & Xu, G. (2014). Current state-of-the-art of nontargeted metabolomics based on liquid chromatography-mass spectrometry with special emphasis in clinical applications. *Journal of Chromatography A*, *1374C*, 1–13. http://dx.doi.org/10.1016/j.chroma.2014.11.050.

Zilka, N., & Novak, M. (2006). The tangled story of Alois Alzheimer. *Bratislavské Lekárske Listy*, *107*, 343–345.

Zinnel, N. F., Pai, P. J., & Russell, D. H. (2012). Ion mobility-mass spectrometry (IM-MS) for top-down proteomics: Increased dynamic range affords increased sequence coverage. *Analytical Chemistry*, *84*, 3390–3397.

CHAPTER THREE

# Parkinson's Disease: *In Vivo* Brain Metabolomics by MRS

**Mario Rango**[1]

Department of Neurological Sciences and Excellence Center for advanced MR studies, IRCCS Ca' Granda-Ospedale Maggiore Policlinico Foundation, University of Milan, Milano, Italy

[1]Corresponding author: e-mail address: mariocristia@yahoo.it

## Contents

1. Proton MRS 82
2. 1H MRS: Compounds Detectable *In Vivo* 82
3. Phosphorus MRS 83
4. Mitochondrial Dysfunction 89
5. Other Findings 89
6. High Magnetic Field 90
7. Parkinson's Disease and Solvent Exposure 90
8. Conclusions 91
References 91

## Abstract

*In vivo* brain metabolomics in Parkinson's disease is still in its infancy. This chapter will review brain metabolomics in the human brain as studied noninvasively by magnetic resonance spectroscopy. Although preliminary, the results shed some light on the pathophysiology of Parkinson's disease.

Opposite to classical biochemical approaches that focus on single metabolites and single metabolic reactions and their kinetic properties, metabolomics collects quantitative data on a broad series of metabolites to gain an overall picture of metabolism (Kristal et al., 2007a, 2007b).

Magnetic resonance spectroscopy (MRS) is particularly useful in providing maps of biochemical pathways or networks, which serve as crucial inputs for quantitative flux analysis (Dauner, Bailey, & Sauer, 2001; de Graaf et al., 2000).

We will focus on proton and phosphorus MRS.

*International Review of Neurobiology*, Volume 122
ISSN 0074-7742
http://dx.doi.org/10.1016/bs.irn.2015.05.007

## 1. PROTON MRS

Two methods of proton MRS are available: single voxel and multi-voxel, with or without spectroscopic imaging. Single-voxel proton MRS provides a rapid biochemical profile of a localized volume within a region.

Spectroscopic imaging provides biochemical information about multiple volumes focalized on a particular region of interest that allows the mapping of metabolic tissue distribution. The data obtained are treated by computer and superimposed on the image illustrating the distribution of such metabolites within a certain area.

Two localization methods are commonly used in clinical proton MRS: point-resolved spectroscopy and stimulated echo acquisition mode. Protons are stimulated within the volume of interest with minimal stimulation outside of this volume (Atlas, 2009).

Mostly important is the choice of echo time. With short echo times (less than 30 ms), the magnetic resonance spectrum detects larger numbers of metabolites, but peak superimposition will occur causing difficulty in spectroscopic curve interpretation.

By using long echo times (more than 135 ms), smaller numbers of metabolites are detected, but with better definition of peaks.

*In vivo* proton MRS allows the presence of certain metabolites in brain tissue to be detected if the minimum concentrations are between 0.5 and 1.0 mM (Atlas, 2009).

The spectrum represents radiofrequency signals emitted from the proton nuclei of the different metabolites into the region of interest. Specific metabolites always appear at the same frequencies, expressed as parts per million, and are represented on the horizontal axis of the graph. The vertical axis shows the heights of the metabolite peaks, represented on an arbitrary intensity scale.

The study of proton MRS can be either qualitative or quantitative. Qualitative study results in graphs of metabolites from a given region of the brain.

Quantitative study measures the real concentration of metabolites, which is proportional to the area under the peak, or the relationship of their rates with each other, through height measurement of the peaks.

## 2. 1H MRS: COMPOUNDS DETECTABLE *IN VIVO*

1H MRS visualizes signals from nonexchangeable protons, carbon bound, with the highest information density in the spectral region from 1 to 5 ppm.

The metabolites detected by 1H MRS are *N*-acetylaspartate (NAA), an amino acid which, in adults, is present in neurons and is an expression of neuronal integrity, choline-containing compounds (including metabolites involved in phospholipid membrane synthesis), creatine (including phosphocreatine (PCr)), and lactate as an indicator of anaerobic glycolysis. Several other compounds and neurotransmitters can be also studied, such as glutamate, glutamine, gaba, and myoinositol (Atlas, 2009).

Several studies have shown a reduction of NAA in conditions in which neuronal or axonal loss is known to occur.

Most MRS studies have used metabolite ratios to quantify changes in individual compounds. The peak of creatine/PCr has been used because these two compounds are in chemical equilibrium and their total amount would be expected to remain constant even in disease states.

## 3. PHOSPHORUS MRS

Clinical scanners can be modified to collect brain MRS data from metabolites containing the 31Phosphorous nucleus (31P-MRS) including PCr, ATP, phosphomonoesters (mainly phosphorylethanolamine and phosphorylcholine) that are precursors for membrane phospholipid synthesis, phosphodiesters that are breakdown products of membrane phospholipids, and inorganic phosphate. These measurements provide insight into the status of high-energy phosphates (HEP) and membrane turnover. The resonance frequency of inorganic phosphate is sensitive to the intracellular pH. Therefore, measures of the resonance frequency of inorganic phosphate can be used to estimate the pH of the intracellular compartment in brain tissue. The variable obtained by the sum of PCr and ATP (PCr + ATP) is a marker of mitochondrial energetics functioning (Erecińska & Silver, 1989; Rango, Bozzali, Prelle, Scarlato, & Bresolin, 2001).

Parkinson's disease (PD) is a sporadic condition of uncertain etiology (Daroff & Bradley, 2012). Several lines of evidence suggest that a defect in oxidative phosphorylation contributes to its pathogenesis. For instance, 1-methyl-4-phenyl-1,2,3,6-tetrahydropyridine, a neurotoxin that blocks complex I (NADH-ubiquinone oxidoreductase) of the mitochondrial electron transport chain (Langston & Ballard, 1983) resembles in humans the hallmarks of PD (Javitch, D'Amato, Strittmatter, & Snyder, 1985). Reduction in complex I activity has been reported in PD tissues (Benecke, Strümper, & Weiss, 1993; Haas et al., 1995; Krige, Carroll, Cooper, Marsden, & Schapira, 1992; Mizuno et al., 1989; Schapira et al., 1989, 1998; Swerdlow et al., 1996).

Experimental and postmortem studies have implicated oxidative damage (Beal, 1995; Cassarino et al., 1997) in PD pathogenesis, although the source of this damage has not been clear. Candidates for production of reactive oxygen species are mainly dopamine metabolism and dysfunction of mitochondria (Beal, 1995; Cassarino et al., 1997). These studies suggest that disrupted mitochondrial complex I activity and oxidative stress participate in the killing of dopaminergic neurons in PD. In turn, normal mitochondrial activity may be affected by environmental chemicals (both natural and synthetic) (Berenguer, Soulage, Perrin, Pequignot, & Abraini, 2003; Chan, Nutt, & Holford, 2004) and by mitochondrial DNA and nuclear genes polymorphisms and mutations (Bandmann, Sweeney, Daniel, Marsden, & Wood, 1997; Cooper, Mann, Krige, & Schapira, 1992; Ikebe, Tanaka, & Ozawa, 1995; Shoffner et al., 1993), which are all implicated in PD pathogenesis.

Inactivation of parkin and synuclein overexpression can cause mitochondrial dysfunction (Beal, 2004; Palacino et al., 2004). The recent discovery of PINK1, a putative mitochondrial protein kinase that is implied in some cases of PD (Valente et al., 2004), has opened new avenues of investigation into both basic mitochondrial biology and neurodegenerative disease. Finally, neuroleptic medications used to treat psychiatric and other disorders can induce Parkinsonism in humans.

Burkhardt, Kelly, Lim, Filley, and Parker (1993) studied the effects of representative compounds from several classes of neuroleptic drugs and found that they tend to be very potent inhibitors of rat brain complex I activity.

Although the magnitude of the complex I defect in PD is unclear (range 16–71%, in published studies), even small perturbations of the electron transport chain may carry pathogenic significance (Parker, Boyson, & Parks, 1989; Shoffner, Watts, Juncos, Torroni, & Wallace, 1991), since the effects of bioenergetic processes on cellular metabolism are protean.

The main mitochondrial function is to maintain adequate concentration of HEP in the cells, most of the HEP being produced by oxidative phosphorylation (Brady, Siegel, Wayne Albers, & Price, 2011; Chance et al., 1986; Erecińska & Silver, 1989; Siesjo, 1978). Rango et al. have developed a system to study brain energetics and mitochondrial function in the human brain by observing HEP in the brain visual areas by 31P-MRS during very short activation with a spatial resolution better than 10 mL (Rango, Castelli, & Scarlato, 1997; Rango et al., 2001).

They applied the technique to the study of idiopathic PD as well as normal subjects (Rango, Bonifati, & Bresolin, 2006). In normal subjects, HEPs remained unchanged during activation, but rose significantly (by 16%) during recovery. The intracellular brain pH increased during visual activation with a slow return to rest values. In PD patients, HEPs were within the normal range at rest and did not change during activation, but fell significantly (by 36%) in the recovery period; pH did not reveal a homogeneous pattern with a wide spread of values. They have shown that energy unbalance under increased oxidative metabolism requirements discloses a mitochondrial dysfunction already present in the brain of patients with PD even in the absence of overt clinical manifestations, as in the visual cortex.

PET studies have shown that glucose metabolism in the visual cortex at rest is decreased in PD patients (Bohnen, Minoshima, Giordani, Frey, & Kuhl, 1999; Eberling, Richardson, Reed, Wolfe, & Jagust, 1994). This finding may be explained either by damage/loss of neurons, which however is not usually found given normal NAA content (Birken & Oldendorf, 1989; Rango et al., 1995), or rather by diminished energetics requirement from reduced nigrostriatal outflow and visual areas functional deafferentation (Bohnen et al., 1999; Eberling et al., 1994). Under the latter condition, which is characterized by a mitochondrial metabolic state 4 (Chance et al., 1986), increased, rather than normal, PCr and PCr/ATP content would be expected in the visual cortex. In this light, the finding of normal PCr/ATP content (Rango et al., 2006) is, paradoxically, suggestive of impaired energetics and their study of brain energetics under increased requirement, which is functional activation and recovery, has shown that this is, indeed, the case.

In normal subjects, there is a postactivation increase of HEPs that lasts long after stimulation has ceased (Rango et al., 2001). This finding is in line with findings from other authors (Madsen, Linde, Hasselbalch, Paulson, & Lassen, 1998) who have reported an increase of glucose oxidation during the postactivation phase, as compared with rest and activated conditions. Although part of increased glucose oxidation is likely to provide energy to restore rest conditions (i.e., intracellular and extracellular $Na^+/K^+$ gradients, neurotransmitter synthesis, etc.) (Erecińska & Silver, 1989; Siesjo, 1978), increased glucose oxidation is in excess of actual energy requirement. Conversely, in patients with mitochondrial disease without clinical CNS involvement as well as in PD patients, there is a postactivation decrease of HEPs, suggesting that oxidative phosphorylation/mitochondrial impairment is present in brain of PD patients even in the absence of clinical involvement.

Findings in PD patients (Rango et al., 2006) overlap with findings in patients with mitochondrial diseases without clinical CNS involvement. At rest, Rango et al. (2006) found no difference between HEP content in normal subjects and in PD patients. The HEP content remained unchanged during activation in PD patients, as in normal subjects, but it decreased in the postactivation period. This means that the brain of PD patients cannot cope with increased oxidative requirements such as those of the postactivation period that eventually lead to energy imbalance. Conversely, activation causes no energy failure because during this period additional energy demands are low and primarily sustained by an increase of anaerobic glycolysis that does not rely on mitochondria (Fox, Raichle, Mintun, & Dence, 1988).

In conclusion, the mitochondrial oxidative phosphorylation is impaired in the brain of PD patients, even in areas not directly involved such as the visual cortex. The heterogeneity of the physicochemical environment found, as expressed by the wide SD of the pH, indicates that the degree of brain involvement may vary in severity among patients.

The exact role of oxidative phosphorylation/mitochondrial impairment in PD remains unclear. It has been recently hypothesized that aging and various degenerative disorders may share a common pathogenesis involving mitochondrial defects and energy failure (Müller-Höcker, 1992; Wallace, 1992). However, the effect of repeated energy failure in the human brain is currently unknown. The current findings suggest that whereas stimulation "prepares" the normal brain for increased energy requirements, the brain of patients with PD may be most vulnerable to repeat activation. Although initial clinical CNS involvement in patients with PD points mainly to the basal ganglia, with time some of them may develop additional clinical features, which suggest involvement of other brain regions. Although the mitochondrial dysfunction that we detected in the visual cortex is somewhat silent since it has no major clinical expression, repeated energy failure from repeat neuronal activation may eventually lead to neuronal dysfunction. In fact, it has been recently reported that with progression of disease, there is a longitudinal deterioration of color discrimination and contrast sensitivity in PD as well in patients with mitochondrial myopathies (Diederich, Raman, Leurgans, & Goetz, 2002).

Although the reason for mitochondrial impairment remains unclear, oxidative damage from dopamine metabolism does not appear to be the main cause of mitochondrial impairment in PD patients since the visual cortex is barely, if not at all, implied in such metabolism (Daroff & Bradley, 2012).

Rather, its adjunctive effect may enhance mitochondrial impairment and suffering of substantia nigra neurons.

In PD, the genes *PARK2, DJ1,* and *PINK1* are all linked to either oxidative stress or mitochondrial dysfunction but differently from idiopathic PD.

Rango et al. reported of a study of a subject with *PINK1* PD and a group of idiopathic PD subjects in whom brain mitochondrial function was assessed by 31P functional MRS (Rango et al., 2001, 2006) at rest, during brain activation, and after brain activation in the patient and 10 age-matched healthy females, and 10 age- and UPDRS-matched females with idiopathic PD. Visual cortex pH in the patient at rest was alkaline (7.20; normal range at rest: 6.78–7.14); it was 7.18 during light stimulation and 7.16 during recovery. In the idiopathic Parkinson group, mean pH was $6.93 \pm 0.10$ SD at rest, $7.01 \pm 0.11$ SD during light stimulation, and $6.97 \pm 0.09$ SD during recovery.

In the *PINK1* patient, mitochondrial function at rest was already depressed as assessed by the reduction of PCr + ATP (PCr + βATP, arbitrary units) content (Rango et al., 2006) below the normal range (6.28; normal range: 9.82–15.31). Activation further reduced PCr + βATP (5.13; normal range: 9.91–15.47), and PCr + βATP recovered partially (to 7.31) during recovery without reaching the normal recovery range (12.12–16.93). In contrast, the mean PCr + βATP content in idiopathic Parkinson patients was normal at rest ($12.10 \pm 1.98$ SD) and under activation ($12.14 \pm 2.02$ SD), and decreased during the recovery period ($8.17 \pm 1.66$ SD). In healthy subjects, the PCr + βATP content remained unchanged from rest ($11.99 \pm 1.64$ SD) during activation ($12.19 \pm 1.87$ SD), and increased during the recovery period ($14.23 \pm 1.32$ SD).

Proton MRS spectral profiles were normal in the PINK1 patient, except for an increase of the myoinositol peak above the upper limit of the normal range in all the three studied areas (visual cortex: +22%; right centrum semiovale: +24%; right lenticular nucleus: +21%) compared with healthy subjects. No increase of myoinositol was observed in idiopathic PD patients, instead. Lactate was undetectable in all subjects.

In conclusion, the *PINK1* neurochemical/metabolic phenotype is clearly distinguishable from idiopathic PD. In fact, the physicochemical environment is perturbed at rest in *PINK1*, as shown by abnormally alkaline intracellular pH. In parallel, the reported patient exhibited mitochondrial energy failure in rest conditions that was aggravated during brain activation and persisted during recovery. By contrast, mitochondrial energy failure is apparent in typical PD only during recovery (i.e., during maximal respiratory chain activity) (Rango et al., 2006). These findings suggest that the mitochondrial machinery is more heavily affected in *PINK1* than in idiopathic PD. Indeed, *PINK1* mutation involves several steps at the mitochondrial level (e.g., fission, fusion, and mitophagy), as well as others with several different effects on the respiratory chain (Heeman et al., 2011); *in vitro* studies have shown that reduced cellular ATP content is further reduced during periods of increased cellular demand (Heeman et al., 2011), while mitochondrial defect in idiopathic PD appears to be more limited and mostly confined to respiratory chain complex I (Rango et al., 2006).

Although there is mitochondrial energy failure in *PINK1*, glycolysis is not activated to compensate—as shown by normal PET-FDG glucose metabolic rates. The excess of substrate not entering the respiratory chain does not accumulate as lactate, as shown by normal lactate content, but is very likely converted into myoinositol, as suggested by the increase of myoinositol in all of the brain areas studied (Cilia et al., 2007; Rango et al., 2008). Indeed, glycolysis is a source of myoinositol, which derives from the conversion of glucose-6-phosphate (Rango et al., 2008). This is not the case in idiopathic PD, in which cortical glucose metabolism is depressed but the respiratory chain works enough to maintain normal high-energy phosphate content at rest and during activation (Borghammer et al., 2010).

Holshouser et al. (1995) performed a large multicenter 1H MRS study of 151 patients with PD. Spectra were collected from the basal ganglia with 80–90% of the volume localized to the striatum. No significant reduction in the NAA/creatine ratio was observed in the PD group. A decrease in the NAA/choline ratio was present in the older PD patients suggesting a slight decrease in NAA or, alternatively, increased levels of choline and creatine in this subgroup. In a 1H MRS study of five PD patients by Clarke, Lowry, and Horsman (1997), absolute quantification of metabolites showed no significant difference in the concentration of metabolites, including NAA, choline, and creatine.

Concentration of glutamine or glutamate in the basal ganglia was normal. Davie, Pirtosek, et al. (1995) and Davie, Wenning, et al. (1995) carried out 1H MRS localized to the lentiform nucleus in patients with asymmetrical, levodopa-responsive PD, and patients with clinically probable MSA, who were subdivided into striatonigral and olivopontocerebellar atrophy variants. No significant differences were observed between the PD patients and controls. Instead, the MSA patients showed a reduction in the absolute levels of NAA and in the NAA/creatine ratio in the lentiform nucleus. This was most striking in the striatonigral patients. Lemmens et al. showed that the reduction in the NAA/creatine ratio observed in five clinically probable

MSA patients was present in both putamen. The same authors showed no significant difference in the NAA/creatine ratio in a group of PD patients. There was, however, a significant reduction of NAA/choline ratios in drug-naive PD patients compared with a treated group and a control group.

## 4. MITOCHONDRIAL DYSFUNCTION

None of the studies has demonstrated elevated lactate levels in the basal ganglia in PD. Bowen et al. performed 1H MRS on a large volume of brain (27 mL) centered on the occipital lobe in 14 patients with PD. The authors demonstrated a significant group increase in lactate in the PD patients in particular in a subgroup of four Parkinsonian patients with dementia. However, the authors also found elevated lactate levels in several controls. The detection of lactate by 1H MRS in healthy controls is well established. It must be borne in mind that lactate levels may be increased by functional stimulation. This has been demonstrated both in the occipital cortex and in the basal ganglia. The presence of cognitive impairment in patients diagnosed as PD raises the possibility of an alternative diagnosis, such as Lewy body dementia. A study in patients with suspected vascular ischemic Parkinsonism did not show an elevated lactate signal in the striatum. A study by Davie, Pirtosek, et al. (1995) and Davie, Wenning, et al. (1995) in three former professional boxers with Parkinsonism unresponsive to levodopa showed significantly reduced concentrations of NAA in the lentiform nucleus but no evidence of lactate production.

## 5. OTHER FINDINGS

Federico et al. found, in five patients with progressive supranuclear paralysis (PSP), a significant reduction of NAA/creatine and NAA/choline ratios in the lentiform nucleus compared with eight patients with PD and nine age-matched controls. Again, no significant abnormalities were observed in the PD patients. A study by Davie, Pirtosek, et al. (1995) and Davie, Wenning, et al. (1995) in a group of nine patients with PSP showed an absolute reduction in the concentration of NAA in the lentiform nucleus.

Tedeschi et al. (1997) showed no specific differences from controls in any of the regions studied in PD patients.

O'Neill et al. investigated 10 patients with PD and 13 age-matched, healthy control with magnetic resonance imaging and 1H MRS of the substantia nigra, basal ganglia, and cerebral cortex. Compared to controls, the

PD patients had approximately 24% lower creatine content in the region of the substantia nigra and smaller volumes of the putamen (11%), globus pallidus (16%), and prefrontal cortex (6%). No other significant between-group differences were found in nine regions examined.

## 6. HIGH MAGNETIC FIELD

Significant NAA/creatine reductions have been shown in the pontine base both of patients with cerebellar variant of MSA and of patients with MSA with predominant Parkinsonism (MSA-P), while putaminal NAA/creatine was reduced only in the patients with MSA-P. Eight of the 11 MSA-P patients (as opposed to none of the PD or control group subjects) were classified correctly by combining individual NAA/creatine reductions in the pontine base and in the putamen. The combined assessment of NAA/creatine in the pontine base and putamen may be effective in differentiating MSA-P from PD (on the basis of high specificity of reduced NAA/creatine in the pontine base and in the putamen in patients with MSA-P).

## 7. PARKINSON'S DISEASE AND SOLVENT EXPOSURE

Some patients with PD have a history of chronic exposure to hydrocarbon solvents. Chronic exposure to hydrocarbon solvents is a risk factor for more severe forms of PD with earlier onset of symptoms and reduced response to dopaminergic therapy. A correlation between disease severity and degree of exposure has previously been shown. However, in previous MRS studies, past exposure to solvents has not usually been among patient inclusion criteria. Rango et al. studied seven PD patients with solvent exposure (two with low-degree exposure and five with high-degree exposure), 10 unexposed PD patients matched for sex, age, and Hoehn and Yahr scale (=3 in the "on" phase), and 10 unexposed PD patients matched for sex, age, and levodopa daily intake instead of disease severity (these patients were Hoehn and Yahr scale = 3.5 in the "on" phase). The purpose of the study was to assess neuronal degeneration in the striatum of exposed versus unexposed PD patients. The authors investigated whether neuronal damage/loss was detectable in the lentiform nucleus measuring NAA levels by 1H MRS. Multiple single-voxel MRS water-suppressed spectra were also obtained from the white matter and the occipital lobe. They found that NAA was normal in the lentiform nucleus of patients with low exposure as well as in patients with no exposure, whereas it was decreased in PD patients with high exposure. White matter and occipital lobe NAA content were normal both in exposed and in unexposed PD patients. The clinical expression is more severe in PD patients with a high degree of previous solvent exposure because of the associated postsynaptic damage to the nigrostriatal pathway.

## 8. CONCLUSIONS

*In vivo* brain metabolomics is still in its infancy. However, many useful informations have come out from spectroscopic studies. Likely, in the next years, MRS will elucidate several other aspects of brain metabolomics in PD.

## REFERENCES


Atlas, S. W. (2009). *Magnetic resonance imaging of the brain and spine: Vol. 1*. Philadelphia, PA, USA: Lippincott.

Bandmann, O., Sweeney, M. G., Daniel, S. E., Marsden, C. D., & Wood, N. W. (1997). Mitochondrial DNA polymorphisms in pathologically proven Parkinson's disease. *Journal of Neurology, 244*(4), 262–265.

Beal, M. F. (1995). Metabolic disorders and neurotoxicology. *Current Opinion in Neurology, 8*(6), 467–468, Review.

Beal, M. F. (2004). Mitochondrial dysfunction and oxidative damage in Alzheimer's and Parkinson's diseases and coenzyme Q10 as a potential treatment. *Journal of Bioenergetics and Biomembranes, 36*(4), 381–386.

Benecke, R., Strümper, P., & Weiss, H. (1993). Electron transfer complexes I and IV of platelets are abnormal in Parkinson's disease but normal in Parkinson-plus syndromes. *Brain, 116*(Pt. 6), 1451–1463.

Berenguer, P., Soulage, C., Perrin, D., Pequignot, J. M., & Abraini, J. H. (2003). Behavioral and neurochemical effects induced by subchronic exposure to 40 ppm toluene in rats. *Pharmacology, Biochemistry and Behavior, 74*(4), 997–1003.

Birken, D. L., 1, & Oldendorf, W. H. (1989). N-acetyl-L-aspartic acid: A literature review of a compound prominent in 1H-NMR spectroscopic studies of brain. *Neuroscience and Biobehavioral Reviews, 13*(1), 23–31, Spring.

Bohnen, N. I., Minoshima, S., Giordani, B., Frey, K. A., & Kuhl, D. E. (1999). Motor correlates of occipital glucose hypometabolism in Parkinson's disease without dementia. *Neurology, 52*(3), 541–546.

Borghammer, P., Chakravarty, M., Jonsdottir, K. Y., Sato, N., Matsuda, H., Ito, K., et al. (2010). Cortical hypometabolism and hypoperfusion in Parkinson's disease is extensive: Probably even at early disease stages. *Brain Structure & Function, 214*(4), 303–317. http://dx.doi.org/10.1007/s00429-010-0246-0, Review.

Brady, S., Siegel, G., Wayne Albers, R., & Price, D. (2011). *Basic neurochemistry: Principles of molecular, cellular, and medical neurobiology* (8th ed.).

Burkhardt, C., Kelly, J. P., Lim, Y. H., Filley, C. M., & Parker, W. D., Jr. (1993). Neuroleptic medications inhibit complex I of the electron transport chain. *Annals of Neurology, 33*(5), 512–517.

Cassarino, D. S., Fall, C. P., Swerdlow, R. H., Smith, T. S., Halvorsen, E. M., Miller, S. W., et al. (1997). Elevated reactive oxygen species and antioxidant enzyme activities in animal and cellular models of Parkinson's disease. *Biochimica et Biophysica Acta, 1362*(1), 77–86.

Chan, P. L., Nutt, J. G., & Holford, N. H. (2004). Modeling the short- and long-duration responses to exogenous levodopa and to endogenous levodopa production in Parkinson's disease. *Journal of Pharmacokinetics and Pharmacodynamics*, *31*(3), 243–268.
Chance, B., Leigh, J. S., Jr., Kent, J., McCully, K., Nioka, S., Clark, B. J., et al. (1986). Multiple controls of oxidative metabolism in living tissues as studied by phosphorus magnetic resonance. *Proceedings of the National Academy of Sciences of the United States of America*, *83*(24), 9458–9462.
Cilia, R., Righini, A., Marotta, G., Benti, R., Marconi, R., Isaias, I. U., et al. (2007). Clinical and imaging characterization of a patient with idiopathic progressive ataxia and palatal tremor. *European Journal of Neurology*, *14*(8), 944–946.
Clarke, C. E., Lowry, M., & Horsman, A. (1997). Unchanged basal ganglia N-acetylaspartate and glutamate in idiopathic Parkinson's disease measured by proton magnetic resonance spectroscopy. *Movement Disorders*, *12*(3), 297–301.
Cooper, J. M., Mann, V. M., Krige, D., & Schapira, A. H. (1992). Human mitochondrial complex I dysfunction. *Biochimica et Biophysica Acta*, *1101*(2), 198–203, Review.
Daroff, R. B., & Bradley, W. G. (2012). *Bradley's neurology in clinical practice* (6th ed.). R. B. Daroff, et al. (Eds.). Philadelphia, PA: Elsevier/Saunders.
Dauner, M., Bailey, J. E., & Sauer, U. (2001). Metabolic flux analysis with a comprehensive isotopomer model in Bacillus subtilis. *Biotechnology and Bioengineering*, *76*(2), 144–156.
Davie, C. A., Pirtosek, Z., Barker, G. J., Kingsley, D. P., Miller, P. H., & Lees, A. J. (1995). Magnetic resonance spectroscopic study of parkinsonism related to boxing. *Journal of Neurology, Neurosurgery and Psychiatry*, *58*(6), 688–691.
Davie, C. A., Wenning, G. K., Barker, G. J., Tofts, P. S., Kendall, B. E., Quinn, N., et al. (1995). Differentiation of multiple system atrophy from idiopathic Parkinson's disease using proton magnetic resonance spectroscopy. *Annals of Neurology*, *37*(2), 204–210.
de Graaf, A. A., Mahle, M., Möllney, M., Wiechert, W., Stahmann, P., & Sahm, H. (2000). Determination of full 13C isotopomer distributions for metabolic flux analysis using heteronuclear spin echo difference NMR spectroscopy. *Journal of Biotechnology*, *77*(1), 25–35.
Diederich, N. J., Raman, R., Leurgans, S., & Goetz, C. G. (2002). Progressive worsening of spatial and chromatic processing deficits in Parkinson disease. *Archives of Neurology*, *59*(8), 1249–1252.
Eberling, J. L., Richardson, B. C., Reed, B. R., Wolfe, N., & Jagust, W. J. (1994). Cortical glucose metabolism in Parkinson's disease without dementia. *Neurobiology of Aging*, *15*(3), 329–335.
Erecińska, M., 1, & Silver, I. A. (1989). ATP and brain function. *Journal of Cerebral Blood Flow and Metabolism*, *9*(1), 2–19.
Fox, P. T., Raichle, M. E., Mintun, M. A., & Dence, C. (1988). Nonoxidative glucose consumption during focal physiologic neural activity. *Science*, *241*(4864), 462–464.
Haas, R. H., Nasirian, F., Nakano, K., Ward, D., Pay, M., Hill, R., et al. (1995). Low platelet mitochondrial complex I and complex II/III activity in early untreated Parkinson's disease. *Annals of Neurology*, *37*(6), 714–722.
Heeman, B., Van den Haute, C., Aelvoet, S. A., Valsecchi, F., Rodenburg, R. J., Reumers, V., et al. (2011). Depletion of PINK1 affects mitochondrial metabolism, calcium homeostasis and energy maintenance. *Journal of Cell Science*, *124*(Pt. 7), 1115–1125. http://dx.doi.org/10.1242/jcs.078303.
Holshouser, B. A., 1, Komu, M., Möller, H. E., Zijlmans, J., Kolem, H., Hinshaw, D. B., Jr., et al. (1995). Localized proton NMR spectroscopy in the striatum of patients with idiopathic Parkinson's disease: A multicenter pilot study. *Magnetic Resonance in Medicine*, *33*(5), 589–594.

Ikebe, S., Tanaka, M., & Ozawa, T. (1995). Point mutations of mitochondrial genome in Parkinson's disease. *Brain Research Molecular Brain Research*, *28*(2), 281–295.

Javitch, J. A., D'Amato, R. J., Strittmatter, S. M., & Snyder, S. H. (1985). Parkinsonism-inducing neurotoxin, N-methyl-4-phenyl-1,2,3,6-tetrahydropyridine: Uptake of the metabolite N-methyl-4-phenylpyridine by dopamine neurons explains selective toxicity. *Proceedings of the National Academy of Sciences of the United States of America*, *82*(7), 2173–2177.

Krige, D., Carroll, M. T., Cooper, J. M., Marsden, C. D., & Schapira, A. H. (1992). Platelet mitochondrial function in Parkinson's disease. The Royal Kings and Queens Parkinson Disease Research Group. *Annals of Neurology*, *32*(6), 782–788.

Kristal, B. S., Shurubor, Y. I., Kaddurah-Daouk, R., & Matson, W. R. (2007a). Metabolomics in the study of aging and caloric restriction. *Methods in Molecular Biology (Clifton, N. J.)*, *371*, 393–409. Review.

Kristal, B. S., Shurubor, Y. I., Kaddurah-Daouk, R., & Matson, W. R. (2007b). High-performance liquid chromatography separations coupled with coulometric electrode array detectors: a unique approach to metabolomics. *Methods in Molecular Biology (Clifton, N. J.)*, *358*, 159–174.

Langston, J. W., & Ballard, P. A., Jr. (1983). Parkinson's disease in a chemist working with 1-methyl-4-phenyl-1,2,5,6-tetrahydropyridine. *The New England Journal of Medicine*, *309*(5), 310, No abstract available.

Madsen, P. L., Linde, R., Hasselbalch, S. G., Paulson, O. B., & Lassen, N. A. (1998). Activation-induced resetting of cerebral oxygen and glucose uptake in the rat. *Journal of Cerebral Blood Flow and Metabolism*, *18*(7), 742–748.

Mizuno, Y., Ohta, S., Tanaka, M., Takamiya, S., Suzuki, K., Sato, T., et al. (1989). Deficiencies in complex I subunits of the respiratory chain in Parkinson's disease. *Biochemical and Biophysical Research Communications*, *163*(3), 1450–1455.

Müller-Höcker, J. (1992). Mitochondria and ageing. *Brain Pathology*, *2*(2), 149–158, Review.

Palacino, J. J., 1, Sagi, D., Goldberg, M. S., Krauss, S., Motz, C., Wacker, M., et al. (2004). Mitochondrial dysfunction and oxidative damage in parkin-deficient mice. *The Journal of Biological Chemistry*, *279*(18), 18614–18622.

Parker, W. D., Jr., Boyson, S. J., & Parks, J. K. (1989). Abnormalities of the electron transport chain in idiopathic Parkinson's disease. *Annals of Neurology*, *26*(6), 719–723.

Rango, M., Bonifati, C., & Bresolin, N. (2006). Parkinson's disease and brain mitochondrial dysfunction: A functional phosphorus magnetic resonance spectroscopy study. *Journal of Cerebral Blood Flow and Metabolism*, *26*(2), 283–290.

Rango, M., Bozzali, M., Prelle, A., Scarlato, G., & Bresolin, N. (2001). Brain activation in normal subjects and in patients affected by mitochondrial disease without clinical central nervous system involvement: A phosphorus magnetic resonance spectroscopy study. *Journal of Cerebral Blood Flow and Metabolism*, *21*(1), 85–91.

Rango, M., Castelli, A., & Scarlato, G. (1997). Energetics of 3.5 s neural activation in humans: A 31P MR spectroscopy study. *Magnetic Resonance in Medicine*, *38*(6), 878–883.

Rango, M., Cogiamanian, F., Marceglia, S., Barberis, B., Arighi, A., Biondetti, P., et al. (2008). Myoinositol content in the human brain is modified by transcranial direct current stimulation in a matter of minutes: A 1H-MRS study. *Magnetic Resonance in Medicine*, *60*(4), 782–789. http://dx.doi.org/10.1002/mrm.21709.

Rango, M., Spagnoli, D., Tomei, G., Bamonti, F., Scarlato, G., & Zetta, L. (1995). Central nervous system trans-synaptic effects of acute axonal injury: A 1H magnetic resonance spectroscopy study. *Magnetic Resonance in Medicine*, *33*(5), 595–600.

Schapira, A. H., Cooper, J. M., Dexter, D., Jenner, P., Clark, J. B., & Marsden, C. D. (1989). Mitochondrial complex I deficiency in Parkinson's disease. *Lancet*, *1*(8649), 1269, No abstract available.

Schapira, A. H., Gu, M., Taanman, J. W., Tabrizi, S. J., Seaton, T., Cleeter, M., et al. (1998). Mitochondria in the etiology and pathogenesis of Parkinson's disease. *Annals of Neurology*, *44*(3 Suppl. 1), S89–S98, Review.

Shoffner, J. M., Brown, M. D., Torroni, A., Lott, M. T., Cabell, M. F., Mirra, S. S., et al. (1993). Mitochondrial DNA variants observed in Alzheimer disease and Parkinson disease patients. *Genomics*, *17*(1), 171–184.

Shoffner, J. M., Watts, R. L., Juncos, J. L., Torroni, A., & Wallace, D. C. (1991). Mitochondrial oxidative phosphorylation defects in Parkinson's disease. *Annals of Neurology*, *30*(3), 332–339.

Siesjo, B. (1978). *Brain energy metabolism*. New York: Wiley.

Swerdlow, R. H., Parks, J. K., Miller, S. W., Tuttle, J. B., Trimmer, P. A., Sheehan, J. P., et al. (1996). Origin and functional consequences of the complex I defect in Parkinson's disease. *Annals of Neurology*, *40*(4), 663–671.

Tedeschi, G., Litvan, I., Bonavita, S., Bertolino, A., Lundbom, N., Patronas, N. J., et al. (1997). Proton magnetic resonance spectroscopic imaging in progressive supranuclear palsy, Parkinson's disease and corticobasal degeneration. *Brain*, *120*(Pt. 9), 1541–1552.

Valente, E. M., Abou-Sleiman, P. M., Caputo, V., Muqit, M. M., Harvey, K., et al. (2004). Hereditary early-onset Parkinson's disease caused by mutations in PINK1. *Science*, *304*, 1158–1160.

Wallace, D. C. (1992). Mitochondrial genetics: A paradigm for aging and degenerative diseases? *Science*, *256*(5057), 628–632.

CHAPTER FOUR

# Recent Advances and Applications of Metabolomics to Investigate Neurodegenerative Diseases

**Clara Ibáñez, Alejandro Cifuentes, Carolina Simó**[1]

Laboratory of Foodomics, Institute of Food Science Research (CIAL), CSIC, Madrid, Spain

[1]Corresponding author: e-mail address: c.simo@csic.es

## Contents

1. Introduction 96
2. Metabolomics and Neurodegenerative Disorders 100
   2.1 Metabolomics of Neurological Diseases in CSF Samples 101
   2.2 Metabolomics of Neurological Diseases in Blood Samples 106
   2.3 Metabolomics of Neurological Diseases in Other Samples 116
3. Conclusions 123
References 126

## Abstract

Metabolomics is gaining an important role in the investigation of neurological pathologies such as Alzheimer's disease, Parkinson's disease, and amyotrophic lateral sclerosis which are characterized by the absence of reliable diagnostic markers. The magnitude of emotional, physical, and financial burden related to these three devastating pathologies can be deduced considering that nearly 20 million people worldwide suffer from these three pathologies.

In this chapter, an overview of the recent advances and applications of metabolomics to investigate these major neurodegenerative diseases will be presented. Metabolomics strategies are now being developed to map potential perturbations in biochemical pathways linked to neurodegeneration. Going further, there is more and more evidence supporting the concept that these pathologies can begin years or even decades before the onset of clinical symptoms, and thus, metabolomics is also increasingly being used to discover preclinical biomarkers of these neurological diseases.

*International Review of Neurobiology*, Volume 122
ISSN 0074-7742
http://dx.doi.org/10.1016/bs.irn.2015.05.015

## 1. INTRODUCTION

Degenerative diseases of the central nervous system (CNS) include a heterogeneous group of slowly progressive disorders (Waggie, Kahle, & Tolwani, 1999) among which Alzheimer's disease (AD), Parkinson's disease (PD), and amyotrophic lateral sclerosis (ALS) are the most common and most costly to society (Mayeux, 2003). AD is the most prevalent form of late-life mental failure in humans (Blennow, de Leon, & Zetterberg, 2006; Selkoe, 2001) and its incidence is expected to triple over the next 50 years (Wimo et al., 2013). PD is the second most common neurodegenerative disorder (Sharma et al., 2013) with an incidence rate over age 50 of around 15 per 100,000 individuals in the European Union (von Campenhausen et al., 2005). In fact, PD is the most common age-related movement disorder, with a prevalence of approximately 2% among people over 65 years of age (Fasano, Alberio, & Lopiano, 2008). Compared to AD and PD, ALS is less frequent, accounting with an annual incidence rate around 2 per 100,000 individuals (Kiernan et al., 2011). ALS is the most common motor neuron disease affecting upper and lower motor neurons and leading to paralysis and death within 3–5 years (Tarasiuk, Kułakowska, Drozdowski, Kornhuber, & Lewczuk, 2012). Epidemiologically, it is of particular relevance to point out that nearly 20 million people worldwide suffer the devastating effects of these three chronic pathologies (Mayeux, 2003).

Although the etiology and clinical features of the three disorders are very distinct, there are some common features. For instance AD, PD, and ALS present middle to late age of onset and bring about gradual loss of specific populations of neurons (Mayeux, 2003; Waggie et al., 1999). Also, in all three disorders there is aggregation and deposition of altered proteins. In this respect, AD, PD, and ALS neurodegenerative diseases are increasingly being recognized to have common cellular and molecular mechanisms (Ross & Poirier, 2004). Another common aspect is that these pathologies present either inherited or sporadic forms. Familial forms have been identified and different genes have been related to each of the three disorders suffered by a scarce portion of the total of patients compared to occurrence of the sporadic cases (which represent more than 90% of total cases) (Esposito et al., 2002). Unfortunately, origin and trigger factors behind the sporadic forms of AD, PD, and ALS suffered by the majority of patients are still unclear (Schon & Manfredi, 2003). The great lack of knowledge of pathophysiological processes that govern these neurodegenerative diseases entails the absence of biomarkers and reliable diagnostic tools plus the lack of effective preventive therapies or treatment to reverse the consequences of the neurodegeneration (Blasco et al., 2013; Jankovic & Stacy, 2007; Tiraboschi, Hansen, Thal, & Corey-Bloom, 2004).

Neuropsychological evaluation, clinical history examination, analyses of blood and specialized medical imaging techniques are ordinarily used to diagnose AD, PD, and ALS, while still there is no definitive test available for either of them (Blasco et al., 2013; Dubois et al., 2007; Jankovic & Stacy, 2007). Anyhow, diagnostic test vary for the three pathologies considering the different pathogenicity and dissimilar clinical features. For instance, PD manifests by a heterogeneous and broad spectrum of motor and non-motor features. Rest tremor, bradykinesia, rigidity, and loss of postural reflexes are typically suffered by PD patients. No definitive diagnostic test is useful for differentiating PD from other syndromes with similar symptomatology that are known as Parkinsonian disorders (Jankovic & Stacy, 2007). That issue is well illustrated since more than 77% of patients with Parkinsonism are diagnosed of PD (Stacy & Jankovic, 1992) but up to 25% of them are found to have lesions incompatible with PD at autopsy (Hughes, Daniel, Kilford, & Lees, 1992). The pathological hallmark of PD is degeneration of dopaminergic neurons coupled with intracytoplasmic proteinaceous inclusions known as Lewy bodies and their postmortem detection has been considered the definitive criterion of PD diagnosis (Gibb & Lees, 1988). Similarly, AD can only be definitively diagnosed by autopsy. In this latter case, detection of neurofibrillary tangles and amyloid plaques in postmortem brain tissue points out AD diagnosis (Tiraboschi et al., 2004). These formations are considered to affect neuronal function and bring about cell death (Calissano, Matrone, & Amadoro, 2009) resulting in an unspecific symptomatology that begins with cognitive deficits to remember autobiographical events specific to a time and place (Welsh, Butters, Hughes, Mohs, & Heyman, 1992) and progressing to dementia syndrome (Nestor, Scheltens, & Hodges, 2004). Interestingly, neurological features present in both AD and PD (i.e., neurofibrillary tangles, amyloid plaques, Lewy bodies) have been also found in brains from asymptomatic-aged individuals and thus it is not clear whether these formations occur with ordinary aging or reflect a presymptomatic pathological stage (Przedborski, Vila, & Jackson-Lewis, 2003). In line with PD and AD diagnosis, ALS neurodegenerative disease lacks a specific diagnosis test. The *El Escorial Criteria* are routinely used for diagnosis of ALS and include a combination of upper and lower motor neuron signs in the limbs to establish levels of diagnostic certainty (Brooks, 1994). However, poor sensitivity for those criteria has been reported mostly in the identification of early stages of ALS. Thus, there is often a long delay before the patient can be diagnosed leading to use of inappropriate therapies over the course of the disease (Traynor et al., 2000). As can be observed much effort must be paid to advance the accurate and effective diagnosis of these neurological disorders.

Going further, of particular importance is the development of effective tools to accurately identify future potential patients suffering from these pathologies. Diagnosis at preclinical stages, state that precedes the onset of the characteristic disease symptoms, is challenging and its investigation represents a high research priority. There is evidence suggesting AD (Morris, 2005), PD (Panyakaew & Bhidayasiri, 2013), and ALS (Eisen, Kiernan, Mitsumoto, & Swash, 2014) pathological processes begin years or even decades before clinical symptoms onset. A long preclinical period offers an opportunity for protective and/or preventive interventions despite accounting for a challenge in research for disease recognition through early biomarkers determination and establishment of diagnostic criteria for this prodromal phase. After preclinical phase, still some intermediate states preceding pathophysiological processes related to AD, PD, and ALS have been identified. Development and biological events associated to those preceding states are also under intense investigation due to their special relevance in the elucidation of neurodegenerative mechanisms. For instance, AD is preceded by a mild cognitive impairment (MCI) state followed by dementia. The USA National Institute of Aging and the Alzheimer's disease Association is working on the determination of the best predictor factors in the progression from normal cognition (presymptomatic or preclinical state) to MCI (Sperling et al., 2011). Annually, conversion rate from MCI to dementia is about 15% (DeCarli, 2003) and reach up to 80% in a 6-year follow-up (Petersen, 2004). Thus, many efforts are being made in the discovery of predictor markers of progression (Buerger et al., 2002; Guarch, Marcos, Salamero, & Blesa, 2004; Toledo-Morrell et al., 2004). However, until date, the lack of predictors and early biomarkers linked to AD progression represent a great clinical need. On the other hand in PD, there is a preceding state of non-motor precursor symptoms during which Lewy bodies may be found during various years before the onset of classic clinical PD (Dickson et al., 2008; Muzerengi, Contrafatto, & Chaudhuri, 2007; Panyakaew & Bhidayasiri, 2013). Even more it has even been postulated that PD could start in the perinatal period when environmental and genetic influences enable normal function that remains for decades (Le, Chen, & Jankovic, 2009). Then, as a result of neuronal attrition associated to aging, PD manifests when neuronal loss reaches up 60% which is the critical threshold for PD onset (Le et al., 2009). Likewise, ALS is known to be clinically preceded by pathological changes years before the onset. Decrease in motor unit number estimates (Aggarwal & Nicholson, 2002) and abnormalities in the performance of upper motor neuron (Vucic, Ziemann, Eisen, Hallett, & Kiernan, 2013) have been reported among the different preceding events associated to ALS. More recently, it has been stated that prior years or decades before ALS onset cells are affected leading to molecular disturbances (Eisen et al., 2014). Actually, those alterations are not sufficient to cause clinical features but the accumulation of biological abnormalities reflects a long-lasting morbid process progressing over years before the first ALS symptoms appear. In light of this information and the lengthy premonitory period for the three pathologies, the discovery of biomarkers suitable to monitor the evolution and progression from the preclinical phases is particularly challenging and may offer key information as to the origin, causes, and pathophysiology that are so far unknown.

At the same time, diagnosis of preclinical and other preceding stages entails an ethical conflict because of the potential emotional repercussion given the lack of effective strategies to stop disease progression. Thus management of these chronic pathologies on the one hand attempts to slow the progress of neurodegeneration with palliative caring, therapy, or stimulation and on the other hand relieve motor symptoms for ALS and PD. Included in the group of therapeutic approach to slow down progression, a combination of cholinesterase inhibitors with memantine is the most common strategy in moderate-to-severe AD patients (Gauthier & Molinuevo, 2013). To slow down ALS, advance riluzole is the only drug approved by the Food and Drug Administration increasing the life span of the patients with an average of 2–3 months (Miller, Mitchell, Lyon, & Moore, 2007) but its effectiveness is limited to a portion of the patients and presents a number of side effects. Besides as stated before, there are also some drugs that help controlling and relieving motor symptoms for ALS and PD. One of the most extended PD drugs is Levodopa which temporarily diminishes the motor symptoms. It is expected, in view of this information that to be diagnosed of any of these disabling illnesses is devastating for the patient and family members. The search for preventive and or therapeutic treatments at all neurodegenerative phases is imperative since up to date, no drug can reverse pathological process of these chronic illnesses.

## 2. METABOLOMICS AND NEURODEGENERATIVE DISORDERS

Given the lack of knowledge on pathophysiological processes that govern ALS, PD, and AD neurodegenerative diseases, and the absence of biomarkers, novel and non-targeted approaches are needed to deepen in the investigation of prevention, prognosis, diagnosis, and risk factor assessment related to these pathological processes. Without available treatment to reverse the neurodegenerative damage and progressive illness advance, the discovery of early and high confident biomarkers and targets for novel drug development has become a necessary matter.

Metabolomics, the newest "omic" technology, presents the ability to detect slight changes in the metabolic pathways and alteration in the homeostasis even before any phenotypical sign is detectable (Nambiar, Gupta, & Misra, 2010). Metabolomics allows the comprehensive study of the metabolites (small molecules, generally less than 1500 Da) in a biological system (cell, biofluid, tissue, or organism) at a time under given conditions (Fiehn, 2001). Metabolome study in biological samples is a powerful tool to characterize organism phenotypes and to discover biomarkers for health and disease states (Oresic, Vidal-Puig, & Hänninen, 2006). Mass spectrometry (MS) and nuclear magnetic resonance (NMR) are the two analytical platforms most predominantly used in metabolomics. NMR permits the analysis of complex mixtures of metabolites with little or no sample preparation in a rapid and non-destructive way (Zhang, Nagana-Gowda, Ye, & Raftery, 2010) and has been largely applied in metabolomics (Zhang & Powers, 2012). Although NMR spectra are very informative, low sensitivity and high data complexity limit quantitative profiling to less than100 compounds in most biological samples (Bain et al., 2009). MS has the advantage of much higher sensitivity compared with NMR. Modern MS platforms such as those that incorporate time of flight (TOF), Orbitrap, and Fourier transform ion cyclotron resonance (FT-ICR) mass analyzers offer very high mass resolution and mass accuracy. Typically, MS technique is preceded by a separation technique, such as, liquid chromatography (LC), gas chromatography (GC), or capillary electrophoresis (CE), increasing the separation power up to thousands of metabolites. A less common detector in metabolomics is electrochemical array detection (ECA) characterized to be extremely selective and sensitive. However, this technique is less informative about the metabolite content compared to NMR and MS detection. As can be seen in Tables 1–3, NMR and MS-based metabolomics platforms are predominantly applied to neurodegenerative disease investigations.

The lack of knowledge about the pathophysiology involved in neurodegeneration makes the use of "unbiased" approaches an excellent strategy for a deeper understanding of the processes involved. In this sense, "metabolic fingerprinting" approach (Fiehn, 2002) has been demonstrated as a powerful tool in the investigation of AD, ALS, and PD (Tables 1–3) revealing a number of potential biomarkers (Table 4). Similar to other pathological processes such as cancer (Armitage & Barbas, 2014), diabetes (Bain et al., 2009), or cardiovascular diseases (Senn, Hazen, & Tang, 2012), metabolomics is playing an important role in the understanding of pathological processes linked to neurological disorders and is offering unique insights into metabolic alterations as will be discussed later in this chapter. Most of research is based on cerebrospinal fluid (CSF) and blood analysis, although there are a number of studies that have examined other samples such as other tissues or urine (*vide infra*).

## 2.1 Metabolomics of Neurological Diseases in CSF Samples

CSF is a fluid produced in CNS in equilibrium with the brain and spinal cord and as an extracellular fluid it is more likely to reflect the state of health and activity of the CNS than other biofluids. CSF has become the preferred sample to study CNS (Huhmer, Biringer, Amato, Fonteh, & Harrington, 2006). Among CSF functions such as mechanical protection or transport of nutrients to CNS cells (Roche, Gabelle, & Lehman, 2008), the role of CSF as a connective tissue between the brain and the bloodstream makes CSF unique biomarker discovery. CSF is one of the preferred samples for neurological diseases study by metabolomics, which is in accordance to its potential to reflect the changes due to CNS pathological processes. Table 1 shows an overview of the CSF-based metabolomics studies linked to AD, ALS, and PD investigation. CSF protein removal is typically carried out by ultrafiltration or protein precipitation prior to metabolite profiling/fingerprinting.

### *2.1.1 CSF Metabolomics in AD*

In 2008, Jukarainen and colleagues published the first work showing non-targeted metabolomics for the investigation of AD with the aim to find out if CSF composition could reflect and anticipate a pathological state of the metabolism of the brain related to AD (Jukarainen et al., 2008). For that purpose, NMR was used to compare non symptomatic individuals with

**Table 1** CSF Metabolomics Studies of Neurological Disorders

| Disorder | Groups of Samples | Analytical Platform | References |
|---|---|---|---|
| AD | Healthy subjects with typical AD biomarkers (Aβ y tau) ($n=10$) and without typical AD biomarkers ($n=34$) | NMR | Jukarainen et al. (2008) |
| AD | AD patients ($n=79$) and control subjects ($n=51$) | GC-TOF MS LC-MS/MS | Czech et al. (2012) |
| AD | AD ($n=23$), MCI with progression to AD ($n=9$), MCI without progression to AD ($n=22$), and control ($n=19$) subjects. Validation set ($n=12$) | CE-TOF MS | Ibañez et al. (2012) |
| AD | AD ($n=21$), MCI with progression to AD ($n=12$), MCI without progression to AD ($n=21$), and control ($n=21$) subjects | UHPLC-TOF MS | Ibañez et al. (2013) |
| AD | AD ($n=40$), MCI ($n=36$), and control ($n=38$) subjects | HPLC-ECA | Kaddurah-Daouk et al. (2013) |
| AD | AD patients ($n=40$) and control subjects ($n=38$) | HPLC-ECA GC-TOF MS | Motsinger-Reif et al. (2013) |
| AD | AD ($n=15$), MCI ($n=15$), and control ($n=15$) subjects | UHPLC-TOF MS | Trushina, Dutta, Persson, Mielke, and Petersen (2013) |
| ALS | 16 ALS patients | GC-TOF MS NMR | Wuolikainen et al. (2009) |
| ALS | ALS patients ($n=78$) and control subjects ($n=110$) | GC-TOF MS | Wuolikainen, Moritz, Marklund, Antti, and Andersen (2011) |
| ALS | ALS patients ($n=16$) with six different mutations in the *SOD1* gene, and control subjects ($n=16$) | GC-TOF MS | Wuolikainen, Andersen, Moritz, Marklund, and Antti (2012) |

**Table 1** CSF Metabolomics Studies of Neurological Disorders—cont'd

| Disorder | Groups of Samples | Analytical Platform | References |
|---|---|---|---|
| ALS | ALS patients ($n=9$) and control subjects ($n=13$) | NMR | Toczylowska, Jamrozik, Liebert, and Kwiecinski (2013) |
| ALS | ALS patients ($n=66$) and control subjects ($n=128$) | UHPLC-Q/ Orbitrap MS | Blasco et al. (2013) |
| PD | PD patients ($n=48$) and control subjects ($n=57$) | UHPLC-MS/MS GC-TOF MS | Lewitt et al. (2013) |
| PD | PD patients ($n=20$) and control subjects ($n=20$) | GC-TOF MS | Trupp et al. (2014) |

and without typical protein biomarkers for AD (higher protein β-amyloid and tau concentrations). Large variations in metabolite content could be appreciated between the two groups, although creatinine was the only metabolite significantly altered: lower creatinine levels were found in individuals with typical β-amyloid and tau AD profile. With the aim to investigate early biomarkers related to AD by CE-MS, a group of MCI patients was also evaluated (Ibañez et al., 2012). Namely, CSF was extracted from 23 AD patients, 19 matched controls, and 31 MCI patients. During a 2-year follow-up period, there were 22 MCI patients who did not progress to AD, while 9 MCI patients progressed to AD. After CE-MS data processing, a total of 71 metabolites were detected. It was observed that control and MCI patients who did not progress to AD presented the most similar metabolic profiles. Considering that similarity in the statistical model, a 97% of correct classification of all samples in their correct diagnostic group was achieved. A group of 14 potential biomarkers were uncovered and validated in a group of 12 blinded samples. Interestingly, some of the metabolites such as carnitine and creatine that decreased in progression to AD were related to energy provision (Ibañez et al., 2012).

With the aim to increase CSF metabolome coverage, RP/UHPLC-MS and HILIC/UHPLC-MS were applied to detect early metabolite biomarkers of AD (Ibañez et al., 2013). Thus, subjects with no MCI/AD symptoms, MCI patients without progression to AD (in a 2-year follow-up), MCI patients with progression to AD (in a 2-year follow-up), and AD patients, were studied. With the determination of 17 potential biomarkers, a 98.7% of correct classification was achieved. Decreased levels of neuroprotective metabolite as taurine and increased levels of neurotoxic metabolites such as dopamine-quinone or methylsalsolinol were observed (Ibañez et al., 2013).

It is clear that no analytical platform is able to detect the complete set of metabolites from a certain biological sample. For this reason, metabolomics studies using multi-platforms is becoming a common strategy to increase maximum metabolome coverage. For instance, CSF from 79 AD patients and 51 age-matched controls were analyzed by GC-MS and LC-MS/MS (Czech et al., 2012). After CSF deproteinization, metabolite extract was divided into polar and no polar fractions and analyzed by GC-MS and LC-MS/MS, respectively. More than 340 metabolic species were detected, and the pair cysteine-uridine was suggested to be the best predictor for AD. A different combination of analytical platforms (LC-ECA and GC-MS) was selected to find differences in the metabolic signatures of 40 AD patients and 38 healthy subjects (Motsinger-Reif et al., 2013). From the two predictive models built for each analytical technique, GC-MS model gave lower predictive performance. On the other hand, two metabolite signals were highlighted in LC-ECA model as very good predictors of AD, although unfortunately they could not be identified. With a similar approach, LC-ECA was applied to unravel potential markers of AD progression (Kaddurah-Daouk et al., 2013), and thus, a group of subjects with MCI was also included in the study together with healthy and AD groups of patients. It was found a partial correlation between protein markers of AD and metabolites, namely, between the levels of vanillylmandelic acid and xanthine with total-tau protein, which could indicate that norepinephrine pathway and purine pathway may be involved in total-tau aggregation and pathology generation (Kaddurah-Daouk et al., 2013).

### 2.1.2 CSF Metabolomics in PD

Few reports have published non-targeted metabolite analysis if CSF in PD development. Trupp et al. (2014) developed a GC-MS method for the analysis of CSF from 20 control subjects and 20 PD patients at the time of diagnosis (Trupp et al., 2014). Among other changes, a pronounced decrease of 3-hydroxyisovaleric acid, tryptophan, and creatinine was observed in PD patients. As occurred with AD, diagnosis of PD is not definitive until postmortem analysis of the brain, and thus, postmortem CSF from PD patients and age-matched controls was also studied with the aim to determine alternative PD metabolite biomarkers (Lewitt et al., 2013). For that, three methodologies, namely, UHPLC-MS/MS optimized for basic metabolites,

UHPLC-MS/MS optimized for acidic species, and GC-TOF MS, were selected. After univariate statistical analysis to determine significant differences a multivariate analysis was used to detect the combination of top discriminating markers. A total of 19 metabolites were highlighted as potential PD biomarkers. Among them 16 compounds decreased and 3 increased in CSF samples from PD subjects. Interestingly oxidized glutathione was decreased by 40% in PD samples; in addition, marked increase in levels of 3-hydroxykynurenine in PD patients were observed. That investigation supported the hypothesis of relevant mechanisms such as excitotoxicity, neuroinflammation, or oxidant stress to be involved in PD pathogenesis (Lewitt et al., 2013).

### 2.1.3 CSF Metabolomics in ALS

CSF sample analysis in ALS is particularly important because 46% of ALS patients have blood-CSF barrier alterations (Tarasiuk et al., 2012). Thus, CSF analysis could provide insight into disease pathomechanisms.

After stability study of the effect of storage conditions of CSF samples from ALS patients, Wuolikainen and coworkers investigated in 2011 the different metabolic fingerprints of ALS patients depending on the mutated genes and also comparing familial ALS with sporadic cases (Wuolikainen et al., 2009). CSF samples from ALS patients and control subjects were subjected to metabolic extraction via methanol–water (1:9, v/v) and derivatization to be analyzed by GC-TOF MS (Wuolikainen et al., 2011). Multivariate statistical analysis was performed by means of orthogonal partial least squares discriminant analysis (OPLS-DA). As a result, fingerprints from sporadic ALS cases were found to be more heterogeneous than the familial ones and most metabolites were observed to be decreased in ALS patients. More recently, to deepen in the mechanisms of the disease and the possible metabolic alterations CSF from ALS patients with and without mutations causative of ALS and age-matched control subjects were studied (Wuolikainen et al., 2012). ALS patients with D90A mutation on superoxide dismutase (*SOD1*) gene conformed the group of subjects more differentiated compared to other mutations and to sporadic ALS cases. In part that different fingerprint was due to decreased levels of primarily amino acids in CSF from carriers of D90A mutation (Wuolikainen et al., 2012).

By using a LC-MS analytical platform, CSF samples from ALS patients and control subjects were analyzed using both positive (ESI +) and negative (ESI −) electrospray ionization modes (Blasco et al., 2013). Multivariate statistical analysis by means of OPLS-DA model was carried out and then based on the variable importance parameter (VIP) obtained for each metabolite the univariate statistical analysis was performed. 20 and 13 metabolites were selected for univariate statistical analysis for the positive and negative ion modes, respectively. As a result, four VIP metabolites were significantly decreased in ALS patients. MS/MS was applied to identify those species but unfortunately they were not identified. Toczylowska et al. (2013) used also VIP scores to select the most important metabolites (Toczylowska et al., 2013). In that study, CSF from ALS patients and age-matched controls were analyzed by NMR. In order to find potential ALS biomarkers, multivariate analysis by means of partial least square discriminant analysis (PLS-DA) and OPLS-DA methods were developed. Only those variables with the VIP > 1.0 were considered to build the statistical model. Especially elevated levels of lactate, acetate, and sum of glutamine and glutamic acid were observed in ALS patients compared to control group. Also, 90.9% of the samples could be correctly classified as control or ALS patients using the OPLS-DA statistical model. In addition, a general increase of the vast amount of metabolites was observed in ALS patients suggesting that ALS may represent a state of excessive anaerobic metabolism and excitotoxicity.

## 2.2 Metabolomics of Neurological Diseases in Blood Samples

While CSF has been the preferred sample for AD and ALS metabolomics studies, blood has been more often examined in PD investigation as can be observed in Tables 1 and 2. As stated before, CSF is more likely to reflect the changes due to CNS pathological processes. However, lumbar puncture is more expensive and invasive technique than blood extraction. Thus, minimum invasive samples such as blood are increasingly being used toward the search of biomarkers (Aftab & Waraich, 2012). Blood is a complex biological sample that includes various cellular compartments and a constantly changing environment of proteins, lipids, and other biomolecules (Thambisetty & Lovestone, 2010). Blood represents a great biomarkers source for neurological diseases with the main limitation focused on the high selectivity of blood–brain barrier that entails limited usefulness of blood biomarkers since exchanges between blood and CSF are not well elucidated yet (Irizarry, 2004). Another minor limitation of blood biomarkers in comparison with CSF biomarkers is less reproducibility within and between laboratories. Great efforts are being made to develop reproducible and useful metabolic biomarkers in blood that would be more widely available than CSF based

**Table 2** Blood-Based Metabolomics Studies of Neurological Disorders

| Disorder | Sample | Groups of Samples | Analytical Platform | References |
|---|---|---|---|---|
| AD | Plasma | AD patients ($n$ = 20), healthy subjects ($n$ = 20) | UHPLC-QqQ/MS | Li et al. (2010) |
| AD | Plasma | AD ($n$ = 15), MCI ($n$ = 15), and control ($n$ = 15) subjects | UHPLC-TOF MS | Trushina et al. (2013) |
| AD | Plasma | AD ($n$ = 57), MCI ($n$ = 58), and control ($n$ = 57) subjects | UHPLC-Q/TOF MS GC-Q/TOF MS | Wang et al. (2014) |
| AD | Postmortem plasma | AD patients ($n$ = 20) and control subjects ($n$ = 20) | HILIC-Q MS | Inoue et al. (2015) |
| AD | Serum | AD ($n$ = 37), MCI with progression to AD ($n$ = 52), MCI without progression to AD ($n$ = 91), and control ($n$ = 46) subjects | UHPLC-MS GCxGC-TOF MS | Oresic et al. (2011) |
| AD | Serum | AD ($n$ = 42), MCI ($n$ = 14), and control ($n$ = 37) subjects | CE-TOF MS | González-Domínguez, García, et al. (2014) |
| AD | Serum | AD patients ($n$ = 22), healthy subjects ($n$ = 18) | DI-ESI MS | González-Domínguez, García-Barrera, and Gómez-Ariza (2014) |
| AD | Serum | AD patients ($n$ = 30), healthy subjects ($n$ = 30) | FIA-Q/TOF MS | González-Domínguez, García-Barrera, and Gómez-Ariza (2015) |
| AD | Serum | AD patients ($n$ = 46), healthy subjects ($n$ = 36) | UHPLC-Q/TOF MS | Cui et al. (2014) |

*Continued*

**Table 2** Blood-Based Metabolomics Studies of Neurological Disorders—cont'd

| Disorder | Sample | Groups of Samples | Analytical Platform | References |
|---|---|---|---|---|
| ALS | Plasma | Two distinct cross-sectional studies. Study 1: ALS patients ($n=62$) and control subjects ($n=69$). Study 2: ALS patients ($n=99$) and control subjects ($n=48$) | [a]NA | Lawton et al. (2012) |
| ALS | Plasma | ALS patients ($n=172$), healthy controls ($n=50$), and patients with mimic neurological disease ($n=73$) | [a]NA | Lawton et al. (2014) |
| PD | Plasma | PD patients ($n=66$) and control subjects ($n=25$) | LC-ECA | Bogdanov et al. (2008) |
| PD | Plasma | Idiopathic ($n=41$) and with G2019S mutation ($n=12$) PD patients. Healthy family members with ($n=21$) and without mutation ($n=10$). Control subjects ($n=15$) | LC-ECA | Johansen et al. (2009) |
| PD | Plasma | PD patients ($n=20$) and control subjects ($n=20$) | GC-TOF MS | Trupp et al. (2014) |
| PD | Serum | PD patients ($n=23$) and control subjects ($n=23$) | GC-TOF MS | Michell et al. (2008) |
| PD | Serum | Patients with rapid ($n=39$) and slow ($n=41$) progression of PD and control subjects ($n=20$) | UHPLC-Q/Orbitrap MS | Roede et al. (2013) |

[a]NA, not available.

ones (Snyder et al., 2014). One of the challenges of the development of reproducible and widespread blood-based biomarkers is the variability derived from the subjects under study and variability derived from pre-analytical aspects such as anticoagulant choice, needle type, and storage among others (Snyder et al., 2014). Thus, established protocols for subject selection and/or metabolic content normalization, as well as for all procedures involving sample extraction and storage are imperative to overcome reproducibility issues of blood biomarkers.

Blood contains around 60–80 mg/mL protein (Porter, Haver, & Bush, 1984) which is >200 times of protein content than CSF. Thus, before metabolomics analysis sample treatment is mandatory. Although similar methods for metabolic purification are used in CSF and blood, in the latter case protein precipitation with organic solvents, is by far the most widely method used. Methanol-based solvents are preferred for protein precipitation although other organic solvents may also be used such as acetonitrile, acetone, and ethanol among others (Bruce et al., 2009).

### 2.2.1 Blood-Based Metabolomics in AD

Since biomolecule trafficking between blood and CSF are mostly undisclosed how blood can reflect CNS changes is of high interest. At this respect, CSF and plasma from AD, MCI, and control individuals was examined to directly correlate CSF and blood changes metabolic fingerprints (Trushina et al., 2013). Integrated information from CSF and plasma samples was used to select and validate reliable plasma biomarkers related to AD. Around 30% and 60% of the metabolic pathways altered in MCI and AD patients, respectively, were affected in both CSF and plasma samples from the same individuals. Therefore, certain correlation between biofluids was observed. Interestingly, the number of affected pathways in MCI and AD individuals was larger in plasma suggesting possible alterations in organs other than brain associated with AD. Moreover, increased levels of beta-alanine, aspartate and asparagine, alanine, L-cysteine, L-methionine, and methionine-cysteine-glutamate were observed in CSF and plasma of AD patients. In addition, it was observed that the number of pathways affected by the pathology was also correlated with disease progression from control to MCI and to AD states (Trushina et al., 2013). Biomarkers of progression were also investigated in plasma from AD, MCI, and control individuals by UHPLC-Q/TOF MS and GC-Q/TOF MS (Wang et al., 2014). Metabolites with the VIP > 1 in OPLS-DA and a $p$ value <0.05 in the student's $t$-test were considered significantly altered between groups of samples.

AD and control subjects could be discriminated with a biomarker panel consisting of six plasma metabolites (arachidonic acid, *N,N*-dimethylglycine, thymine, glutamine, glutamic acid, and cytidine). In addition, MCI and control individuals could be differentiated with another group of five plasma metabolites (thymine, arachidonic acid, 2-aminoadipic acid, *N,N*-dimethylglycine, and 5,8-tetradecadienoic acid). Results summarized in Fig. 1 indicated altered fatty acid metabolism, amino acid metabolism, carbohydrate metabolism, and TCA cycle linked to energy metabolism and oxidative stress. Also linked to energy metabolism and oxidative stress, a panel of polar biomarkers has been recently found in serum from AD, MCI, and control individuals (González-Domínguez, García, et al., 2014). After dilution and ultrafiltration, serum was analyzed by CE-MS. Significant increase of choline, creatinine, asymmetric dimethyl-arginine, homocysteine-cysteine disulfide, phenylalanyl-phenylalanine, together with a significant decrease of asparagine, methionine, histidine, carnitine, acetyl-spermidine, and different acyl carnitines were observed from control to MCI and to AD (González-Domínguez, García, et al., 2014). However as stated before MCI does not necessarily progress to AD and thus, to uncover biomarkers of progression to AD, a prospective study is compulsory. In this line plasma from control, MCI with and without progression to AD (in a 1–4-year follow-up) and AD diagnosed subjects were examined in the search of biomarkers of progression (Oresic et al., 2011). Samples were analyzed by two different analytical platforms, namely, GCxGC-MS and UHPLC-MS, and 683 metabolites including 139 lipids and 544 polar compounds were detected. Most relevant remarks observed were an alteration of pentose phosphate pathway when the two MCI groups (with and without progression to AD) were compared accompanied by a global trend toward decreased lipid levels in AD patients (Oresic et al., 2011).

Nonetheless, an intense research in AD investigation is focused on the evaluation and comparison of AD fingerprints with age-matched controls which could be potentially useful for diagnosis or even to unravel new targets for therapy. Thus, plasma from control subjects and AD patients was evaluated by means of UHPLC-MS in the positive and negative ionization modes (Li et al., 2010). AD and control metabolic fingerprints could be differentiated through a PCA statistical analysis. Metabolic alterations indicated a decrease on lysophosphatidyl choline related to lecithin metabolism in AD group. A C18 column was suitable to separate molecules with low to medium polarity and thus to appreciate differences on those hydrophobic species (lysophosphatidyl-cholines) (Li et al., 2010). However, polar fraction

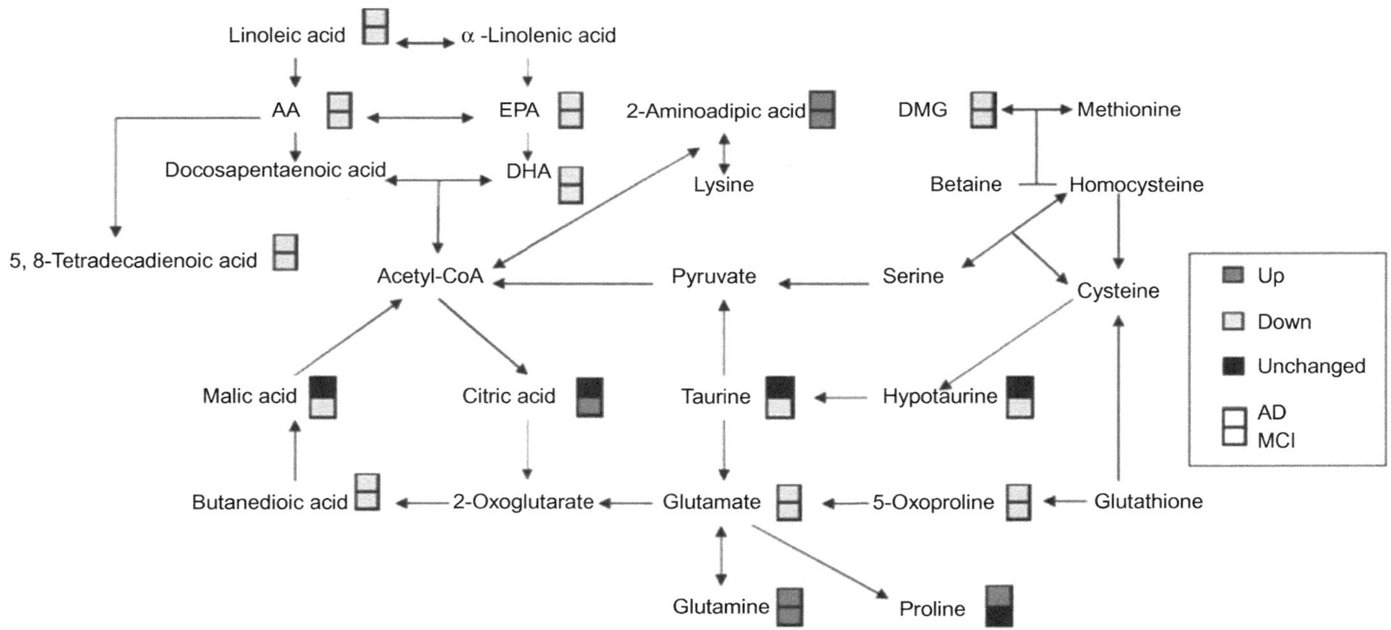


**Figure 1** Altered metabolic pathways in AD and MCI. *Reprinted with permission from Wang et al. (2014).*

can be also of importance in the search of blood biomarkers. For instance, plasma contains about 90% water and thus it is expected that many endogenous metabolites are polar molecules. Focusing in that polar fraction a UHPLC-MS method in the HILIC mode was developed (Inoue et al., 2015). For that purpose, seven different chromatographic columns were tested of which two columns were selected as the most suitable for plasma metabolic fingerprinting of postmortem plasma from AD patients and controls. Statistical multivariate analysis was applied to both of the analytical columns and the two resultant statistical models were able to differentiate AD and control groups (as can be seen in Fig. 2).

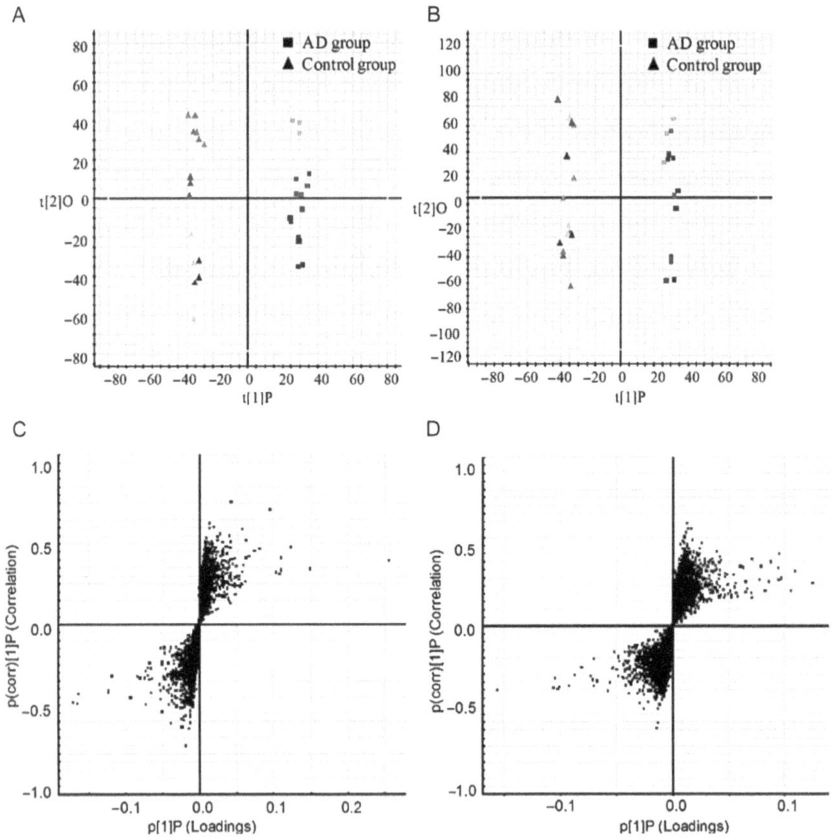


**Figure 2** OPLS-DA from two columns between AD and control groups using HILIC/MS. (A) OPLS-DA score plot using HILIC/MS with a TSK-Amide 80, (B) OPLS-DA score plot using HILIC/MS with a TSKgel-NH2, (C) S-plot using HILIC/MS with a TSK-Amide 80, (D) S-plot using HILIC/MS with a TSKgel-NH2. *Reprinted with permission from Inoue et al. (2015).*

Although CE, LC, or GC are typically coupled to MS for metabolomics studies, direct infusion has also been used to evaluate serum metabolic fingerprints from AD patients and control subjects (González-Domínguez, García-Barrera, & Gómez-Ariza, 2014). Metabolite extraction was performed via protein precipitation with methanol to obtain the polar metabolic extract and a second step of chloroform-methanol (50%) addition enabled the extraction of the most lipophilic compounds adsorbed to protein precipitate from first methanol extraction. Both extracts were analyzed in the positive and negative ion modes. After a PLS-DA statistical analysis, altered levels of plasmalogens and free fatty acids as well as perturbation on phospholipid content, including phosphatidylcholines and lysophosphatidylcholines were observed in AD samples. With those results, authors stated the great potential of direct infusion ESI MS for the study of AD in a high-throughput manner (González-Domínguez, García-Barrera, & Gómez-Ariza, 2014).

In addition to ESI, atmospheric pressure chemical ionization and atmospheric pressure photo-ionization (APPI) are other ionization techniques more suitable for less polar fraction of the metabolome than ESI. Among the three ionization techniques, APPI is the most suitable for less polar compounds and is by far the least used in metabolomics until date. Recently, APPI technique was applied in the investigation of AD biomarkers (González-Domínguez, García-Barrera, & Gómez-Ariza, 2015). Namely, a flow injection analysis (FIA)-APPI-Q/TOF MS method was developed for the analysis of serum samples from AD patients and age-matched controls. Two PLS-DA models for positive and negative APPI ionization modes were built. Most remarkable results observed in that study were altered levels of primary fatty acid amides and major neurotransmitters. Moreover increased serum levels of ceramides, diacylglycerols, and free fatty acids made the authors suggest a possible cellular membrane destabilization linked to AD (González-Domínguez, García-Barrera, & Gómez-Ariza, 2015).

### 2.2.2 Blood-Based Metabolomics in PD

Correlation of metabolic content in different biofluids linked to PD could be very useful for pathophysiological mechanisms knowledge and represents an unexplored research area. In this sense, CSF and plasma samples from PD patients and age-matched controls were evaluated via GC-MS analysis (Trupp et al., 2014). Increased levels of several amino acids, pyroglutamate and 2-oxoisocaproate and decreased levels in C16–C18 saturated and unsaturated fatty acids were observed in PD patients as compared to control subjects. CSF samples reflected an overall diminished concentration of metabolites compared to blood, particularly marked in 3-hydroxyisovaleric acid, tryptophan, and creatinine levels. The authors stated that more biomarkers must be included in the statistical model to build a sufficiently robust method (Trupp et al., 2014).

As stated before, discovery and research of biomarkers for PD diagnosis, prognosis, and to monitor disease progression are compulsory since no effective diagnostic tools are available. The extent of nigrostriatal degeneration determined by neuroimaging techniques is considered one of the most well-defined diagnostic markers of PD (Wang, Hoekstra, Zuo, Cook, & Zhang, 2012). Metabolomics could shed light on biomolecules and pathways altered linked to disease onset and progression. Even metabolic events associated with known familial PD forms are still not explored. *LRRK2* gene has been identified as the most clinical relevant genetic factor in PD development (Schiesling, Kieper, Seidel, & Kruger, 2008). However, there are *LRRK2* mutation carriers who do not develop PD. Until date, it is not possible to predict carriers who will eventually develop PD or to assess probability of pathology onset. Going further, *LRRK2* PD patients are indistinguishable from idiopathic PD from a clinical point of view. To investigate this intriguing topic, Johansen et al. (2009) evaluated the plasma metabolic fingerprints from 12 PD patients and 21 healthy relatives, all of them carriers of G2019S mutation in *LRRK2* gene, and compared them with those metabolic fingerprints obtained from idiopathic PD patients and healthy subjects without mutation in *LRRK2* gene (Johansen et al., 2009). Samples were analyzed via LC-ECA and all four groups of samples were compared through multivariate statistical analysis. Good discrimination between all groups was achieved although unfortunately the majority of the metabolites could not be identified. Uric acid levels were observed to be lower in PD patients (both idiopathic and *LRRK2*) compared to controls (18% decrease, $p < 0.01$). Moreover, in view of the results authors suggest a potential role of the purine pathway in the pathogenesis of PD (Johansen et al., 2009). The same research group, following a similar analytical approach, compared plasma samples from idiopathic PD patients and age-matched controls in order to uncover PD biomarkers useful for diagnosis and prognosis of patients (Bogdanov et al., 2008), finding also uric acid significantly reduced in PD patients. Moreover, increased levels in glutathione were observed linked to PD suggesting that oxidative damage could have an important role in the pathophysiological mechanisms of the disease.

PD patients suffer from a very heterogeneous progression of motor degeneration and that variability hampers PD biomarker discovery. In order to find out the biochemical processes responsible for progression velocity and potentially useful biomarkers for PD prognosis, Roede et al. (2013) evaluated 100 serum samples (Roede et al., 2013). Serum was obtained from 39 and 41 PD patients with rapid and slow progression, respectively, as well as 20 control subjects. PD patients were classified into slow and rapid progressing phenotypes according to annual increase in Unified Parkinson's Disease Rating Scale motor score. After UHPLC-Orbitrap MS analysis, statistical analysis including PCA and OPLS-DA was carried out. As a result of the discriminant analysis, 152 compounds were found to be the most responsible of the separation between slow and rapid progressing phenotypes. Then, topological comparison of the metabolic networks in slow and rapid PD phenotypes was performed using the module preservation function "Weighted Gene co-expression Network Analysis" (WGCNA) package in R. Results from WGCNA together with preservation of the evaluated modules are shown in Fig. 3. Most of modules were preserved although subtle differences were observed suggesting that the differences among both phenotypes are due to small perturbations in the metabolic network structure caused by differential expression of few key metabolites. For instance, $N^8$-acetylspermidine was highlighted as crucial metabolite and thus quantified in all samples showing increased levels in rapid progressors (14.7 nM) compared to slow progressors (12.3 nM) and healthy controls (10.9 nM). Most of the metabolites could not be identified via database matches. Data from high-resolution MS from those unknowns showed matches with numerous phytochemicals, suggesting dietary ingredients might protect against disease development (Roede et al., 2013).

### 2.2.3 Blood-Based Metabolomics in ALS

Only one research group has focused on the research of biomarkers linked to ALS in peripheral blood applying non-targeted metabolomics approach. In the first published work, evaluation of plasma from two cross-sectional studies (study 1 and study 2) was performed. 62 and 69 ALS patients were recruited in study 1 and 2, respectively; in addition to 69 and 48 plasma samples from control subjects in study 1 and 2, respectively (Lawton et al., 2012). Altered levels in 23 metabolites were found in the two study populations and were linked to neuronal change, hypermetabolism, oxidative damage, mitochondrial dysfunction, and possible hepatic dysfunction in PD patients. More recently, with the aim to differentiate ALS from other disease mimics

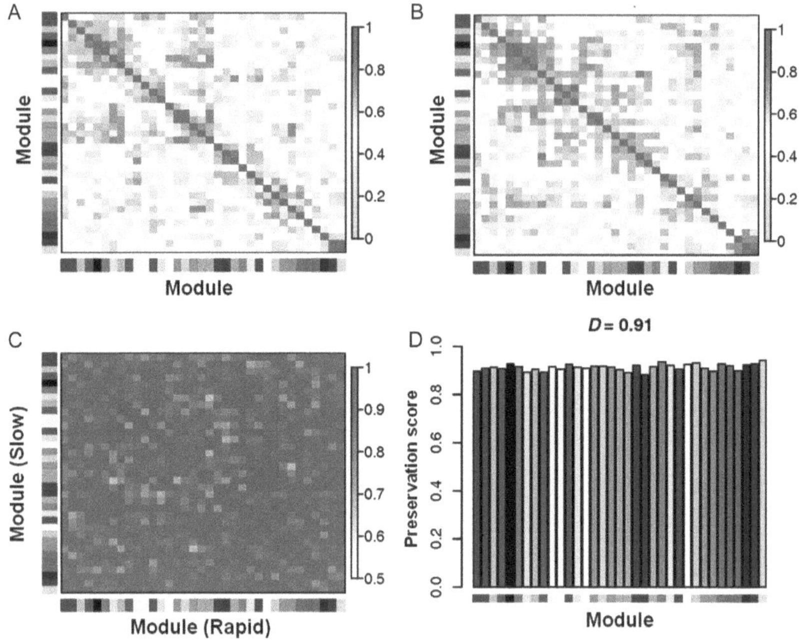


**Figure 3** Summary plot of consensus eigengene networks and their differential analysis comparing slow versus rapid progression PD. The eigengene networks in the two sets, slow (A) and rapid (B) are shown as heatmaps. In the heatmaps, red (dark gray in the print version) denotes high adjacency (positive correlation) and green (light gray in the print version) denotes low adjacency (negative correlation). The Preservation heatmap (C) shows the preservation network, defined as one minus the absolute difference of the eigengene networks in the two datasets. The barplot (D) shows the mean preservation of adjacency for each of the eigengenes to all other eigengenes; in other words, the barplot depicts the column means of the preservation heatmap. *Reprinted with permission from Roede et al. (2013).*

plasma from ALS patients, healthy controls, and patients with mimic neurological diseases was collected and analyzed (Lawton et al., 2014). Considering for statistical analysis exclusively metabolites present in at least 50% of samples, a method to discriminate the different conditions was built with the selection of 32 metabolites. Classification was achieved with 58% sensitivity and 90% specificity.

## 2.3 Metabolomics of Neurological Diseases in Other Samples

Urine and tissue samples have also been evaluated in the search of biomarkers of neurodegenerative diseases as can be seen in Table 3. Human

**Table 3** Other Samples Analyzed in Metabolomics Studies of Neurological Disorders

| Disorder | Sample | Groups of samples | Analytical Platform | References |
|---|---|---|---|---|
| AD | Urine | AD patients ($n=46$), healthy subjects ($n=36$) | UHPLC-Q/TOF MS | Cui et al. (2014) |
| AD | Rat urine | Control ($n=4$) and transgenic APP/tau rats at three life-time points: 4 ($n=4$), 10 ($n=4$), and 15 ($n=3$) months | NMR | Fukuhara et al. (2013) |
| AD | Mice urine | APP/PS1 transgenic mice ($n=10$) and wild type ($n=10$) | DI-ESI MS | González-Domínguez, García-Barrera, Vitorica, and Gómez-Ariza (2014) |
| AD | Mice urine | TgCRND8 ($n=12$) and wild-type ($n=12$) mice. Samples collected at three different ages, namely, 15–17 weeks, 25–28 weeks, and 30–31 weeks | LC-FT-ICR MS | Peng et al. (2014) |
| AD | Postmortem mice brain | 8 brain regions from young mice TgCRND8 ($n=5$) and control young mice ($n=4$), and aged mice TgCRND8 ($n=3$) and control old mice ($n=5$) | NMR | Salek et al. (2010) |
| AD | Postmortem human brain | AD patients ($n=15$) and control subjects ($n=15$). Validation set ($n=60$) | UHPLC-Q/TOF MS | Graham et al. (2013) |
| AD | Postmortem mice brain | 5 brain regions extracted at 1, 3, 6, and 11 month of age from single-transgenic Tg2576 mouse model and control | NMR | Lalande et al. (2014) |

*Continued*

**Table 3** Other Samples Analyzed in Metabolomics Studies of Neurological Disorders—cont'd

| Disorder | Sample | Groups of samples | Analytical Platform | References |
|---|---|---|---|---|
| AD | Postmortem human brain | AD patients ($n=15$) and control subjects ($n=15$) | NMR | Graham, Hölscher, and Green (2014) |
| AD | Postmortem mice brain | 5 brain regions from APP/PS1 transgenic mice ($n=30$) and wild type ($n=30$) | GC-IT/Q MS UHPLC-Q/TOF MS | González-Domínguez, Castilla-Quintero, García-Barrera, and Gómez-Ariza (2014) |
| AD | Postmortem mice brain | 4 brain regions from APP/PS1 transgenic mice ($n=30$) and wild type ($n=30$) | DI-ESI MS | González-Domínguez, García-Barrera, Vitorica, and Gómez-Ariza (2015) |
| AD, ALS | Postmortem human brain | 19 frontal cortex extracts from AD ($n=8$) and ALS ($n=11$) patients | NMR | Botosoa et al. (2012) |
| PD | Urine | PD patients ($n=23$) and control subjects ($n=23$) | GC-TOF MS | Michell, Mosedale, Grainger, and Barker (2008) |
| PD | Postmortem mice brain | Mesencephalon of MPTP-induced PD mice with ($n=10$) and without ($n=10$) administration of herbal extract and control mice ($n=10$) | UHPLC-Q/TOF MS | Li et al. (2013) |
| PD | Postmortem goldfish brain | MPTP-induced PD goldfish ($n=19$) and control goldfish ($n=19$) | NMR | Lu et al. (2014) |

MPTP: 1-methyl-4-phenyl-1,2,3,6-tetrahydropyridin.

urine represents a minimum invasive sample and is easy to obtain. Moreover, it presents low content on interfering molecules, such as proteins. Thus, minimum sample treatment is generally required (i.e., filtration, centrifugation, dilution). Optimization of sample treatment and data normalization of urine samples has been recently developed for direct infusion MS to prevent ion suppression problems (González-Domínguez, García-Barrera, Vitorica, et al., 2014). Most suitable sample treatment was observed to be a simple 10 fold-dilution of urine samples. However, urine is characterized by high complexity and heterogeneity among individuals. Moreover as an end-product of the body it is easily affected by diet and environmental factors that act as confounding factors increasing intra- and interindividual variability. Complexity and heterogeneity makes human urine particularly difficult to understand and interpret (Bouatra et al., 2013). For those reasons, the two published works that evaluate biomarkers linked to neurodegeneration in human urine also includes other sample obtained from the same subjects under study (Cui et al., 2014; Michell et al., 2008). In the first study, evaluation of the metabolic fingerprints of plasma and urine samples from PD patients and control subjects was carried out by GC-MS (Michell et al., 2008). To minimize variability among samples all individuals under study were females in initial stages of the disease. First, PCA was used for extreme outliers removal. Metabolomic data from urine samples, from serum samples and taking into account both (urine and serum) were used to build three different PLS-DA models. However, only subtle differences were detected and none of the metabolites highlighted in the three methods of classification was significantly different between PD and control groups in univariate analysis (Michell et al., 2008). On the contrary, identification of significant biomarkers linked to AD in urine was possible via LC-MS and LC-MS/MS methods (Cui et al., 2014). In order to determine metabolic pathways altered in AD, serum and urine from AD patients and age-matched controls were analyzed by LC-MS. Potential biomarkers were determined by multivariate analysis and then submitted to confirmation applying tandem MS. Potential biomarkers unraveled were palmitic amide, lysophosphatidylcholine (LysoPC, 18:0), LysoPC(18:2), L-glutamine, and 5-L-glutamylglycine. Following that non-targeted approach, most remarkable facts observed linked to AD were alteration in amino acid and phospholipid metabolism and dysregulated palmitic amide (Cui et al., 2014).

A number of investigations linked to neurodegenerative diseases have been performed in animals mostly based on rodent models (see Table 3). Among neurodegenerative diseases, most studies using animal models are focus on AD research. Mice models to investigate AD usually include human mutations in amyloid precursor protein (APP) and tau. For instance, the TgCRND8 transgenic mouse express human double-mutant APP (Chishti et al., 2001) and the APP/PS1 model express mutant APP and presenilin protein (PS) (Mucke et al., 2000) have been analyzed through metabolomics. Unlike AD, animal models for metabolomics of ALS and PD are not yet well-established. The few animal based studies published on PD metabolomics use animal models treated with dopaminergic neuronal damage substances (i.e., 1-methyl-4-phenyl-1,2,3,6-tetrahydropyridine, MPTP) to represent PD pathology (Li et al., 2013; Lu et al., 2014).

The use of urine from animal models (normally rodents) present clear advantages such as less heterogeneity, total control of environmental and dietary factors, and thus easier interpretation over human urine metabolomics studies. However, a limited volume of urine can be collected from rodents impeding the use of several analytical platforms. In order to obtain the maximum metabolomics information by using only one analytical platform, Peng et al. (2014) optimized a method based on differential isotope labeling LC-MS. That analytical approach was able to detect and quantify more than 950 metabolites in mice urine. In that work, 12 TgCRND8 transgenic and 12 wild-type mice were compared at 3 different time points. Namely, urine samples were collected at 15–17 weeks, 25–28 weeks, and 30–31 weeks to represent different stages of disease development. Increased levels ($p < 0.01$) of methionine and desaminotyrosine while decreased levels of 5-hydroxyindoleacetic acid and $N^1$-acetylspermidine were observed in transgenic mice urine (Peng et al., 2014). Moreover, different metabolic content was detected depending on the time of collection that represented different stages of AD development. Because urine is a noninvasive sample animals can be monitored during disease progression. In this sense, urine NMR fingerprints from four control mice and four transgenic APP/tau mice were evaluated at three different time points to represent AD progression states, namely, prior to onset (at 4 months), early-middle progress (at 10 months) and last period of AD (at 15 months) (Fukuhara et al., 2013). Multivariate statistical analysis by means of PCA and OPLS-DA showed a clear discrimination between non-transgenic versus transgenic mice even at onset time point (4 months). At 15 months, increased levels of citrate and urea and decreased levels of 2-oxoglutarate, dimethylamine, trimethylamine, trigonelline, and 1-methylnicotinamide were observed in transgenic mice. Interestingly, 3-hydroxykynurenine, homogentisate, and tyrosine were only differentially expressed in transgenic mice prior to the onset of dementia (4 months) and then at 10 and 15 months presented no significant differences. Thus, these biomarkers closely related to oxidative stress could provide an early indication of AD risk (Fukuhara et al., 2013).

Depending on neurodegenerative disorder, different brain areas are expected to be affected and thus biomarkers will be found with more probability there. PD affects neurons from the substantia nigra located in the mesencephalon, in the mid-brain region of the brain. ALS affects motor cortex, brainstem, and spinal cord leading to atrophy of motor neurons and muscles. In AD, especially damaged areas are cerebral cortex, certain subcortical regions, and the hippocampus and cerebral atrophy occurs in temporoparietal location. As can be deduced from AD complexity, the majority of metabolomics studies cover the analysis of several brain regions (Botosoa et al., 2012; González-Domínguez, Castilla-Quintero, et al., 2014; González-Domínguez, García-Barrera, Vitorica, et al., 2015; Lalande et al., 2014; Salek et al., 2010). For instance, metabolic fingerprints of eight different brain regions of TgCRND8 mice (five young and three aged mice) and control mice (four young and five aged mice) were obtained by NMR (Salek et al., 2010). After uni- and multivariate statistical analysis, altered levels of metabolites were observed to be dependent on the brain area. Thus, decreased levels of taurine were observed in transgenic mice except for hippocampus. Also increased levels of glycine for all brain regions except for midbrain were also shown. Some common to all brain areas alterations such as increase in lactate, aspartate, leucine, and valine and decrease in *N*-acetyl-L-aspartate, glutamate, glutamine among others were observed in transgenic mice compared to controls. It was also observed that age was linked to the severity of hippocampus and cortical regions affection (Salek et al., 2010).

More recently, metabolic fingerprinting of postmortem human brain tissue from 15 AD patients and 15 control subjects were compared. From the total ions detected by UHPLC-MS in both positive and negative ionization mode, 39 and 37 metabolic signals were found to be significantly different among control and AD tissue in the positive and negative ion modes, respectively. Based on both ionization modes datasets, two predictive models of sample discrimination were built with a predictive accuracy of 91–97% (Graham et al., 2013).

ALS and AD have been also compared in a NMR-based metabolomics study of postmortem frontal cortex extracts from 9 AD and 11 ALS subjects (Botosoa et al., 2012). The brain location was chosen based on the fact that although the initial brain areas affected in AD and ALS are different, they both reach frontal cortex at their end stage. After OPLS-DA statistical method, increased levels of alanine, acetate, glutamate, and glutamine and decreased levels of lactate and creatine were observed in AD compared to ALS (Fig. 4). On the other hand higher concentrations of lactate, *N*-acetyl-aspartate, creatine, choline, and myo-inositol were found in ALS brain (Botosoa et al., 2012).

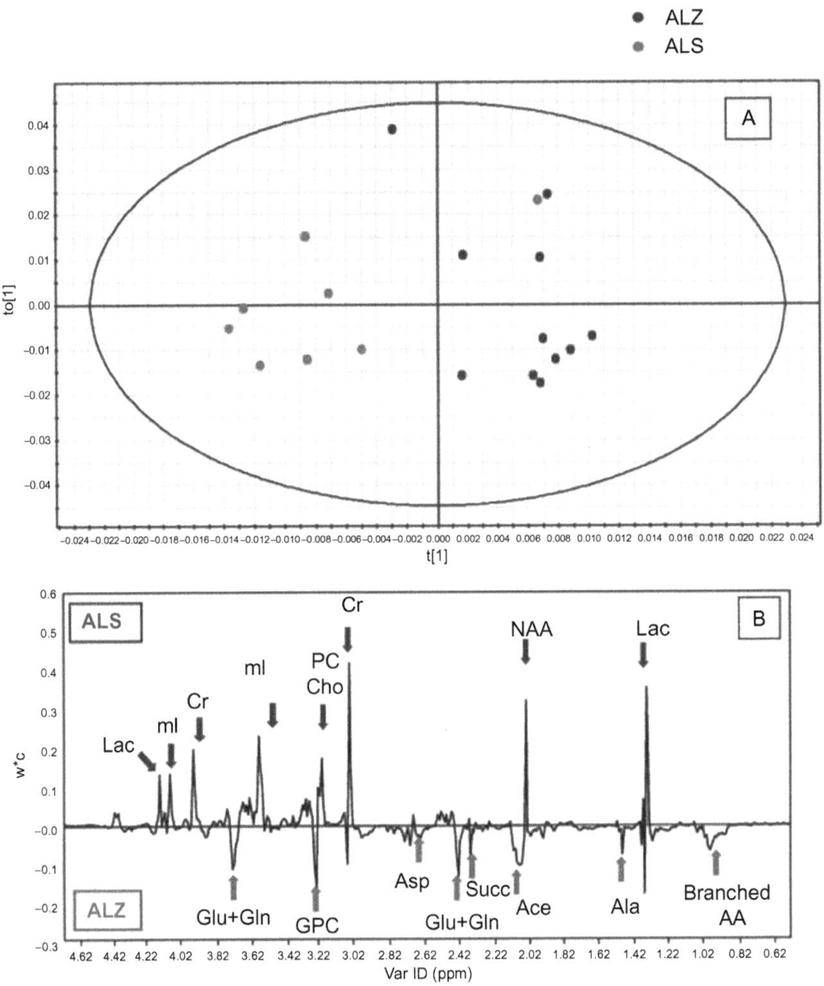


**Figure 4** (A) Orthogonal partial least square (OPLS) score plot showing the separation of patients suffering from Alzheimer's disease (ALZ, red (light gray in the print version) circles) and patients suffering from amyotrophic lateral sclerosis (ALS, blue (dark gray in the print version) circles). Horizontal axis: first orthogonal component containing variation orthogonal to group separation. Vertical axis: predictive component containing all information responsible for group separation. (B) OPLS loading plot showing buckets (assigned to the metabolites) responsible for the discrimination observed in the corresponding score plot. *Reprinted with permission from Botosoa et al. (2012).*

As stated before, PD animal models for metabolomics studies are not yet well established and little research has been developed until date. Recently, goldfish treated with the dopaminergic neuronal damage substance MPTP was used as animal model to represent PD pathology in a metabolomics study (Lu et al., 2014). Metabolic fingerprints of brain tissue from 19 PD induced and 19 control goldfish were obtained via NMR and multivariate statistical analysis. As a result, a number of metabolites were observed to be significantly increased (i.e., myo-inositol, 18:2 fatty acid, total fatty acids, etc.) and decreased (i.e., *N*-acetylaspartate, phosphocreatine, phosphocholine, etc.) and involved in oxidative stress, energy failure, neuronal cell injury and death, pathways known to be altered in PD (Lu et al., 2014).

Another metabolomics non-targeted approach has been developed using the same toxic agent (Li et al., 2013). In that later case, the aim was to deepen in the possible neuroprotective effect of a plant extract (*Acanthopanax senticosus*, AS) when administered with MPTP toxic substance. For that purpose, among the 20 mice treated with MPTP, 10 were also fed with AS extract. A control group of 10 mice without neither MPTP nor plant extract administration, was included in this study. Mesencephalon from all mice was analyzed by LC-MS and data was subsequently submitted to OPLS-DA multivariate analysis. Interestingly, it was observed that metabolic alteration induced by MPTP (similar to PD pathology) was restored after extract administration except for the levels of Cer(d18:0/18:0), LysoPC(20:4 (5Z,8Z,11Z,14Z)), and morphiceptin. The authors could link extract administration with metabolic pathways restoration, thereby potentially opening new strategies for PD treatment (Li et al., 2013).

## 3. CONCLUSIONS

In this chapter, an overview of non-targeted metabolomics strategies in the advance of AD, PD, and ALS investigations has been presented. Different biological matrixes have been investigated for the research of these pathologies. CSF and blood (plasma or serum) are by far the most predominant samples employed for metabolomics of neurodegenerative diseases. Urine has been used in a lesser extent although its minimally invasive collection could stand for an advantageous source of biomarkers.

Most of the presented studies aim to further understanding of the origin, cause, and pathophysiology of AD, PD, and ALS. From the works presented in this chapter, relevant information (summarized in Table 4) has been extracted about, e.g., amino acid metabolism, energy metabolism, and oxidative stress and their role in disease through several metabolomics

**Table 4** Summary of Some Relevant Metabolic Variations Discussed in This Chapter Related to AD, PD, and ALS

| Scope of the Study | Metabolite Variations | Sample | References |
|---|---|---|---|
| **Increased levels of** | | | |
| PD biomarkers identification | Glutathione | Plasma | Bogdanov et al. (2008) |
| AD biomarkers identification | Glycine, lactate, aspartate, leucine, and valine | Brain | Salek et al. (2010) |
| AD biomarkers identification | Beta-alanine, aspartate and asparagine, alanine, L-cysteine, L-methionine, methionine-cysteine-glutamate | CSF | Czech et al. (2012) |
| Identification of oxidative stress biomarkers in AD | Citrate, urea | Urine | Fukuhara et al. (2013) |
| Progression to AD | Methylsalsolinol, dopamine, quinone | CSF | Ibañez et al. (2013) |
| Alteration of metabolic networks in AD | Vanillylmandelic acid, xanthine | CSF | Kaddurah-Daouk et al. (2013) |
| PD biomarkers identification | 3-Hydroxykynurenine | CSF | Lewitt et al. (2013) |
| Biomarkers of rapid PD progressors | $N^8$-acetylspermidine | Serum | Roede et al. (2013) |
| ALS biomarkers identification | Lactate, acetate, sum of glutamine and glutamic acid | CSF | Toczylowska et al. (2013) |
| Progression to AD | Glutamine, 2-aminoadipic acid, proline | CSF and plasma | Trushina et al. (2013) |
| Progression to AD | Choline, creatinine, asymmetric dimethyl-arginine, homocysteine-cysteine disulfide, phenylalanyl-phenylalanine | Serum | González-Domínguez, García, et al. (2014) |
| PD biomarkers identification | Myo-inositol, 18:2 fatty acid, total fatty acids | Brain | Lu et al. (2014) |

**Table 4** Summary of Some Relevant Metabolic Variations Discussed in This Chapter Related to AD, PD, and ALS—cont'd

| Scope of the Study | Metabolite Variations | Sample | References |
|---|---|---|---|
| Progression to AD | Methionine, desaminotyrosine | Urine | Peng et al. (2014) |
| PD biomarkers identification | Amino acids, pyroglutamate, 2-oxoisocaproate | CSF and plasma | Trupp et al. (2014) |
| AD biomarkers identification | Ceramides, diacylglycerols, and free fatty acids | Serum | González-Domínguez, García-Barrera, and Gómez-Ariza (2015) |
| **Decreased levels of** | | | |
| PD biomarkers identification | Uric acid | Plasma | Bogdanov et al. (2008) |
| Identification of early AD biomarkers | Creatinine | CSF | Jukarainen et al. (2008) |
| PD biomarkers identification | Uric acid | Plasma | Johansen et al. (2009) |
| AD biomarkers identification | Lysophosphatidyl choline | Plasma | Li et al. (2010) |
| AD biomarkers identification | Taurine, *N*-acetyl-L-aspartate, glutamate, glutamine | Brain | Salek et al. (2010) |
| Progression to AD | Lipidic molecules | Serum | Oresic et al. (2011) |
| AD biomarkers identification | Uridine | CSF | Czech et al. (2012) |
| Progression to AD | Carnitine | CSF | Ibáñez et al. (2012) |
| Identification of oxidative stress biomarkers in AD | 2-Oxoglutarate, dimethylamine, trimethylamine, trigonelline, and 1-methylnicotinamide | Urine | Fukuhara et al. (2013) |
| Progression to AD | Creatine, taurine | CSF | Ibañez et al. (2013) |
| PD biomarkers identification | Oxidized glutathione | CSF | Lewitt et al. (2013) |

*Continued*

**Table 4** Summary of Some Relevant Metabolic Variations Discussed in This Chapter Related to AD, PD, and ALS—cont'd

| Scope of the Study | Metabolite Variations | Sample | References |
|---|---|---|---|
| Progression to AD | Linoleic acid, butedioic acid, arachidonic acid, glutamic acid, oxoproline, methionine, *N*,*N*-dimethylglycine | CSF and plasma | Trushina et al. (2013) |
| Progression to AD | Asparagine, methionine, histidine, carnitine, acetyl-spermidine and different acyl carnitines | Serum | González-Domínguez, García, et al. (2014) |
| PD biomarkers identification | *N*-acetylaspartate, phosphocreatine, phosphocholine | Brain | Lu et al. (2014) |
| Progression to AD | 5-Hydroxyindoleacetic acid, $N^1$-acetylspermidine | Urine | Peng et al. (2014) |
| PD patients | 3-Hydroxyisovaleric acid, tryptophan, creatinine, C16–C18 saturated and unsaturated fatty acids | CSF and plasma | Trupp et al. (2014) |

investigation; therefore, important consideration must be given to these results for future investigations. Moreover, the lengthy premonitory period for the three pathologies emphasizes the need to continue the search for early disease biomarkers.

In summary, although metabolomics offers unique insights into metabolic alterations of neurodegeneration associated with AD, PD, and ALS, much more work still needs to be done. For instance, it seems mandatory to validate the biomarkers and disturbed metabolic pathways revealed in the presented works by increasing the cohort of individuals under study.

## REFERENCES

Aftab, M. F., & Waraich, R. S. (2012). A review of biochemical markers for early diagnosis of Alzheimer's disease. *American Journal of Neuroscience*, *3*, 54–62.

Aggarwal, A., & Nicholson, G. (2002). Detection of preclinical motor neurone loss in SOD1 mutation carriers using motor unit number estimation. *Journal of Neurology, Neurosurgery and Psychiatry*, *73*, 199–201.

Armitage, E. G., & Barbas, C. (2014). Metabolomics in cancer biomarker discovery: Current trends and future perspectives. *Journal of Pharmaceutical and Biomedical Analysis*, *87*, 1–11.

Bain, J. R., Stevens, R. D., Wenner, B. R., Ilkayeva, O., Muoio, D. M., & Newgard, C. B. (2009). Metabolomics applied to diabetes research: Moving from information to knowledge. *Diabetes*, *58*, 2429–2443.

Blasco, H., Corcia, P., Pradat, P. F., Bocca, C., Gordon, P. H., Veyrat-Durebex, C., et al. (2013). Metabolomics in cerebrospinal fluid of patients with amyotrophic lateral sclerosis: An untargeted approach via high-resolution mass spectrometry. *Journal of Proteome Research*, *12*, 3746–3754.

Blennow, K., de Leon, M. J., & Zetterberg, H. (2006). Alzheimer's disease. *Lancet*, *368*, 387–403.

Bogdanov, M., Matson, W. R., Wang, L., Matson, T., Saunders-Pullman, R., Bressman, S. S., et al. (2008). Metabolomic profiling to develop blood biomarkers for Parkinson's disease. *Brain*, *131*, 389–396.

Botosoa, E. P., Zhu, M., Marbeuf-Gueye, C., Triba, M. N., Dutheil, F., Duyckäerts, C., et al. (2012). NMR metabolomic of frontal cortex extracts: First study comparing two neurodegenerative diseases, Alzheimer disease and amyotrophic lateral sclerosis. *IRBM*, *33*, 281–286.

Bouatra, S., Aziat, F., Mandal, R., Guo, A. C., Wilson, M. R., Knox, C., et al. (2013). The human urine metabolome. *PLoS One*, *8*, e73076.

Brooks, B. R. (1994). El Escorial world federation of neurology criteria for the diagnosis of amyotrophic lateral sclerosis. Subcommittee on motor neuron diseases/amyotrophic lateral sclerosis of the world federation of neurology research group on neuromuscular diseases and the El Escorial "clinical limits of amyotrophic lateral sclerosis" workshop contributors. *Journal of the Neurological Sciences*, *124*, 96–107.

Bruce, S. J., Tavazzi, I., Parisod, V., Rezzi, S., Kochhar, S., & Guy, P. A. (2009). Investigation of human blood plasma sample preparation for performing metabolomics using ultrahigh performance liquid chromatography/mass spectrometry. *Analytical Chemistry*, *81*, 3285–3296.

Buerger, K., Teipel, S. J., Zinkoiwski, R., Blennow, K., Arai, H., Engel, R., et al. (2002). CSF tau protein phosphorylated at threonine 231 correlates with cognitive decline in MCI subjects. *Neurology*, *59*, 627–629.

Calissano, P., Matrone, C., & Amadoro, G. (2009). Apoptosis and in vitro Alzheimer disease neuronal models. *Communicative & Integrative Biology*, *2*, 163–169.

Chishti, M. A., Yang, D. S., Janus, C., Phinney, A. L., Horne, P., Pearson, J., et al. (2001). Early-onset amyloid deposition and cognitive deficits in transgenic mice expressing a double mutant form of amyloid precursor protein 695. *The Journal of Biological Chemistry*, *276*, 21562–21570.

Cui, Y., Liu, X., Wang, M., Liu, L., Sun, X., Ma, L., et al. (2014). Lysophosphatidylcholine and amide as metabolites for detecting Alzheimer disease using ultrahigh-performance liquid chromatography-quadrupole time-of-flight mass spectrometry-based metabonomics. *Journal of Neuropathology and Experimental Neurology*, *73*, 954–963.

Czech, C., Berndt, P., Busch, K., Schmitz, O., Wiemer, J., Most, V., et al. (2012). Metabolite profiling of Alzheimer's disease cerebrospinal fluid. *PLoS One*, *7*, e31501.

DeCarli, C. (2003). Mild cognitive impairment: Prevalence, prognosis, aetiology, and treatment. *Lancet Neurology*, *2*, 15–21.

Dickson, D. W., Fujishiro, H., DelleDonne, A., Menke, J., Ahmed, Z., Klos, K. J., et al. (2008). Evidence that incidental lewy body disease is pre-symptomatic Parkinson's disease. *Acta Neuropathologica*, *115*, 437–444.

Dubois, B., Feldman, H. H., Jacova, C., Dekosky, S. T., Barberger-Gateau, P., Cummings, J., et al. (2007). Research criteria for the diagnosis of Alzheimer's disease: Revising the NINCDS-ADRDA criteria. *Lancet Neurology*, *6*, 734–746.

Eisen, A., Kiernan, M., Mitsumoto, H., & Swash, M. (2014). Amyotrophic lateral sclerosis: A long preclinical period? *Journal of Neurology, Neurosurgery and Psychiatry*, *85*, 1232–1238.

Esposito, E., Rotilio, D., Di Matteo, V., Di Giulio, C., Cacchio, M., & Algeri, S. (2002). A review of specific dietary antioxidants and the effects on biochemical mechanisms related to neurodegenerative processes. *Neurobiology of Aging*, *23*, 719–735.

Fasano, M., Alberio, T., & Lopiano, L. (2008). Peripheral biomarkers of Parkinson's disease as early reporters of central neurodegeneration. *Biomarkers in Medicine*, *2*, 465–478.

Fiehn, O. (2001). Combining genomics, metabolome analysis, and biochemical modelling to understand metabolic networks. *Comparative and Functional Genomics*, *2*, 155–168.

Fiehn, O. (2002). Metabolomics: The link between genotypes and phenotypes. *Plant Molecular Biology*, *48*, 155–171.

Fukuhara, K., Ohno, A., Ota, Y., Senoo, Y., Maekawa, K., Okuda, H., et al. (2013). NMR-based metabolomics of urine in a mouse model of Alzheimer's disease: Identification of oxidative stress biomarkers. *Journal of Clinical Biochemistry and Nutrition*, *52*, 133–138.

Gauthier, S., & Molinuevo, J. L. (2013). Benefits of combined cholinesterase inhibitor and memantine treatment in moderate-severe Alzheimer's disease. *Alzheimers Dement*, *9*, 326–331.

Gibb, W. R., & Lees, A. J. (1988). The relevance of the lewy body to the pathogenesis of idiopathic Parkinson's disease. *Journal of Neurology, Neurosurgery and Psychiatry*, *51*, 745–752.

González-Domínguez, R., Castilla-Quintero, R., García-Barrera, T., & Gómez-Ariza, J. L. (2014). Development of a metabolomic approach based on urine samples and direct infusion mass spectrometry. *Analytical Biochemistry*, *465C*, 20–27.

González-Domínguez, R., García, A., García-Barrera, T., Barbas, C., & Gómez-Ariza, J. L. (2014). Metabolomic profiling of serum in the progression of Alzheimer's disease by capillary electrophoresis-mass spectrometry. *Electrophoresis*, *35*, 3321–3330.

González-Domínguez, R., García-Barrera, T., & Gómez-Ariza, J. L. (2014). Combination of metabolomic and phospholipid-profiling approaches for the study of Alzheimer's disease. *Journal of Proteomics*, *104*, 37–47.

González-Domínguez, R., García-Barrera, T., & Gómez-Ariza, J. L. (2015). Application of a novel metabolomic approach based on atmospheric pressure photoionization mass spectrometry using flow injection analysis for the study of Alzheimer's disease. *Talanta*, *131*, 480–489.

González-Domínguez, R., García-Barrera, T., Vitorica, J., & Gómez-Ariza, J. L. (2014). Region-specific metabolic alterations in the brain of the APP/PS1 transgenic mice of Alzheimer's disease. *Biochimica et Biophysica Acta*, *1842*, 2395–2402.

González-Domínguez, R., García-Barrera, T., Vitorica, J., & Gómez-Ariza, J. L. (2015). Metabolomic screening of regional brain alterations in the APP/PS1 transgenic model of Alzheimer's disease by direct infusion mass spectrometry. *Journal of Pharmaceutical and Biomedical Analysis*, *102*, 425–435.

Graham, S. F., Chevallier, O. P., Roberts, D., Hölscher, C., Elliott, C. T., & Green, B. D. (2013). Investigation of the human brain metabolome to identify potential markers for early diagnosis and therapeutic targets of Alzheimer's disease. *Analytical Chemistry*, *85*, 1803–1811.

Graham, S. F., Hölscher, C., & Green, B. D. (2014). Metabolic signatures of human Alzheimer's disease (AD): 1H NMR analysis of the polar metabolome of post-mortem brain tissue. *Metabolomics*, *10*, 744–753.

Guarch, J., Marcos, T., Salamero, M., & Blesa, R. (2004). Neuropsychological markers of dementia in patients with memory complaints. *International Journal of Geriatric Psychiatry*, *19*, 352–358.

Hughes, A. J., Daniel, S. E., Kilford, L., & Lees, A. J. (1992). Accuracy of clinical diagnosis of idiopathic Parkinson's disease: A clinico-pathological study of 100 cases. *Journal of Neurology, Neurosurgery and Psychiatry*, *55*, 181–184.

Huhmer, A. F., Biringer, R. G., Amato, H., Fonteh, A. N., & Harrington, M. G. (2006). Protein analysis in human cerebrospinal fluid: Physiological aspects, current progress and future challenges. *Disease Markers*, *22*, 3–26.

Ibañez, C., Simo, C., Barupal, D. K., Fiehn, O., Kivipelto, M., Cedazo-Mínguez, A., et al. (2013). A new metabolomic workflow for early detection of Alzheimer's disease. *Journal of Chromatography A*, *1302*, 65–71.

Ibañez, C., Simo, C., Martín-Álvarez, P. J., Kivipelto, M., Winblad, B., Cedazo-Mínguez, A., et al. (2012). Toward a predictive model of Alzheimer's disease progression using capillary electrophoresis-mass spectrometry metabolomics. *Analytical Chemistry*, *84*, 8532–8540.

Inoue, K., Tsuchiya, H., Takayama, T., Akatsu, H., Hashizume, Y., Yamamoto, T., et al. (2015). Blood-based diagnosis of Alzheimer's disease using fingerprinting metabolomics based on hydrophilic interaction liquid chromatography with mass spectrometry and multivariate statistical analysis. *Journal of Chromatography B: Analytical Technologies in the Biomedical and Life Sciences*, *974*, 24–34.

Irizarry, M. C. (2004). Biomarkers of Alzheimer disease in plasma. *NeuroRx*, *1*, 226–234.

Jankovic, J., & Stacy, M. (2007). Medical management of levodopa-associated motor complications in patients with Parkinson's disease. *CNS Drugs*, *21*, 677–692.

Johansen, K. K., Wang, L., Aasly, J. O., White, L. R., Matson, W. R., Henchcliffe, C., et al. (2009). Metabolomic profiling in LRRK2-related Parkinson's disease. *PLoS One*, *4*, e7551.

Jukarainen, N. M., Korhonen, S. P., Laakso, M. P., Korolainen, M. A., Niemitz, M., Soininen, P. P., et al. (2008). Quantification of 1 H NMR spectra of human cerebrospinal fluid: A protocol based on constrained total-line-shape analysis. *Metabolomics*, *4*, 150–160.

Kaddurah-Daouk, R., Zhu, H., Sharma, S., Bogdanov, M., Rozen, S. G., Matson, W., et al. (2013). Alterations in metabolic pathways and networks in Alzheimer's disease. *Translational Psychiatry*, *3*, e244.

Kiernan, M. C., Vucic, S., Cheah, B. C., Turner, M. R., Eisen, A., Hardiman, O., et al. (2011). Amyotrophic lateral sclerosis. *Lancet*, *377*, 942–955.

Lalande, J., Halley, H., Balayssac, S., Gilard, V., Déjean, S., Martino, R., et al. (2014). 1H NMR metabolomic signatures in five brain regions of the AβPPswe Tg2576 mouse model of Alzheimer's disease at four ages. *Journal of Alzheimer's Disease*, *39*, 121–143.

Lawton, K. A., Brown, M. V., Alexander, D., Li, Z., Wulff, J. E., Lawson, R., et al. (2014). Plasma metabolomic biomarker panel to distinguish patients with amyotrophic lateral sclerosis from disease mimics. *Amyotrophic Lateral Sclerosis & Frontotemporal Degeneration*, *15*, 362–370.

Lawton, K. A., Cudkowicz, M. E., Brown, M. V., Alexander, D., Caffrey, R., Wulff, J. E., et al. (2012). Biochemical alterations associated with ALS. *Amyotrophic Lateral Sclerosis*, *13*, 110–118.

Le, W., Chen, S., & Jankovic, J. (2009). Etiopathogenesis of Parkinson disease: A new beginning. *The Neuroscientist*, *15*, 28–35.

Lewitt, P. A., Li, J., Lu, M., Beach, T. G., Adler, C. H., & Guo, L. (2013). Arizona Parkinson's disease consortium. 3-hydroxykynurenine and other Parkinson's disease biomarkers discovered by metabolomic analysis. *Movement Disorders*, *28*, 1653–1660.

Li, N. J., Liu, W. T., Li, W., Li, S. Q., Chen, X. H., Bi, K. S., et al. (2010). Plasma metabolic profiling of Alzheimer's disease by liquid chromatography/mass spectrometry. *Clinical Biochemistry*, *43*, 992–997.

Li, X. Z., Zhang, S. N., Lu, F., Liu, C. F., Wang, Y., Bai, Y., et al. (2013). Cerebral metabonomics study on Parkinson's disease mice treated with extract of Acanthopanax senticosus harms. *Phytomedicine*, *20*, 1219–1229.

Lu, Z., Wang, J., Li, M., Liu, Q., Wei, D., Yang, M., et al. (2014). 1H NMR-based metabolomics study on a goldfish model of Parkinson's disease induced by 1-methyl-4-phenyl-1,2,3,6-tetrahydropyridine (MPTP). *Chemico-Biological Interactions, 223C*, 18–26.

Mayeux, R. (2003). Epidemiology of neurodegeneration. *Annual Review of Neuroscience, 26*, 81–104.

Michell, A. W., Mosedale, D., Grainger, D. J., & Barker, R. A. (2008). Metabolomic analysis of urine and serum in Parkinson's disease. *Metabolomics, 4*, 191–201.

Miller, R. G., Mitchell, J. D., Lyon, M., & Moore, D. H. (2007). Riluzole for amyotrophic lateral sclerosis (ALS)/motor neuron disease (MND). *Cochrane Database of Systematic Reviews, 24*, CD001447.

Morris, J. C. (2005). Early-stage and preclinical Alzheimer disease. *Alzheimer Disease and Associated Disorders, 19*, 163–165.

Motsinger-Reif, A. A., Zhu, H., Kling, M. A., Matson, W., Sharma, S., Fiehn, O., et al. (2013). Comparing metabolomic and pathologic biomarkers alone and in combination for discriminating Alzheimer's disease from normal cognitive aging. *Acta Neuropathologica Communications, 1*, 28.

Mucke, L., Masliah, E., Yu, G. Q., Mallory, M., Rockenstein, E. M., Tatsuno, G., et al. (2000). High-level neuronal expression of abeta 1–42 in wild-type human amyloid protein precursor transgenic mice: Synaptotoxicity without plaque formation. *The Journal of Neuroscience, 20*, 4050–4058.

Muzerengi, S., Contrafatto, D., & Chaudhuri, K. R. (2007). Non-motor symptoms: Identification and management. *Parkinsonism & Related Disorders, 13*, S450–S456.

Nambiar, P. R., Gupta, R. R., & Misra, V. (2010). An "omics" based survey of human colon cancer. *Mutation Research, 693*, 3–18.

Nestor, P. J., Scheltens, P., & Hodges, J. R. (2004). Advances in the early detection of Alzheimer's disease. *Nature Medicine, 10*, S34–S41.

Oresic, M., Hyötyläinen, T., Herukka, S. K., Sysi-Aho, M., Mattila, I., Seppänan-Laakso, T., et al. (2011). Metabolome in progression to Alzheimer's disease. *Translational Psychiatry, 1*, e57.

Oresic, M., Vidal-Puig, A., & Hänninen, V. (2006). Metabolomic approaches to phenotype characterization and applications to complex diseases. *Expert Review of Molecular Diagnostics, 6*, 575–585.

Panyakaew, P., & Bhidayasiri, R. (2013). The spectrum of preclinical gait disorders in early Parkinson's disease: Subclinical gait abnormalities and compensatory mechanisms revealed with dual tasking. *Journal of Neural Transmission, 120*, 1665–1672.

Peng, J., Guo, K., Xia, J., Zhou, J., Yang, J., Westaway, D., et al. (2014). Development of isotope labeling liquid chromatography mass spectrometry for mouse urine metabolomics: Quantitative metabolomic study of transgenic mice related to Alzheimer's disease. *Journal of Proteome Research, 13*, 4457–4469.

Petersen, R. C. (2004). Mild cognitive impairment as a diagnostic entity. *Journal of Internal Medicine, 256*, 183–194.

Porter, W. H., Haver, V. M., & Bush, B. A. (1984). Effect of protein concentration on the determination of digoxin in serum by fluorescence polarization immunoassay. *Clinical Chemistry, 30*, 1826–1829.

Przedborski, S., Vila, M., & Jackson-Lewis, V. (2003). Series introduction: Neurodegeneration: What is it and where are we? *The Journal of Clinical Investigation, 111*, 3–10.

Roche, S., Gabelle, A., & Lehman, S. (2008). Clinical proteomics of the cerebrospinal fluid: Towards the discovery of new biomarkers. *Proteomics Clinical Applications, 2*, 428–436.

Roede, J. R., Uppal, K., Park, Y., Lee, K., Tran, V., Walker, D., et al. (2013). Serum metabolomics of slow vs. rapid motor progression Parkinson's disease: A pilot study. *PLoS One, 8*, e77629.

Ross, C. A., & Poirier, M. A. (2004). Protein aggregation and neurodegenerative disease. *Nature Medicine*, *10*, S10–S17.

Salek, R. M., Xia, J., Innes, A., Sweatman, B. C., Adalbert, R., Randle, S., et al. (2010). A metabolomic study of the CRND8 transgenic mouse model of Alzheimer's disease. *Neurochemistry International*, *56*, 937–947.

Schiesling, C., Kieper, N., Seidel, K., & Kruger, R. (2008). Review: Familial Parkinson's disease-genetics, clinical phenotype and neuropathology in relation to the common sporadic form of the disease. *Neuropathology and Applied Neurobiology*, *34*, 255–271.

Schon, E. A., & Manfredi, G. (2003). Neuronal degeneration and mitochondrial dysfunction. *The Journal of Clinical Investigation*, *111*, 303–312.

Selkoe, D. J. (2001). Alzheimer's disease: Genes, proteins, and therapy. *Physiological Reviews*, *81*, 741–766.

Senn, T., Hazen, S. L., & Tang, W. H. (2012). Translating metabolomics to cardiovascular biomarkers. *Progress in Cardiovascular Diseases*, *55*, 70–76.

Sharma, S., Moon, C. S., Khogali, A., Haidous, A., Chabenne, A., Ojo, C., et al. (2013). Biomarkers in Parkinson's disease (recent update). *Neurochemistry International*, *63*, 201–229.

Snyder, H. M., Carrillo, M. C., Grodstein, F., Henriksen, K., Jeromin, A., Lovestone, S., et al. (2014). Developing novel blood-based biomarkers for Alzheimer's disease. *Alzheimers Dement*, *10*, 109–114.

Sperling, R. A., Aisen, P. S., Beckett, L. A., Bennett, D. A., Craft, S., Fagan, A. M., et al. (2011). Toward defining the preclinical stages of Alzheimer's disease: Recommendations from the national institute on aging-Alzheimer's association workgroups on diagnostic guidelines for Alzheimer's disease. *Alzheimers Dement*, *7*, 280–292.

Stacy, M., & Jankovic, J. (1992). Differential diagnosis of Parkinson's disease and the parkinsonism plus syndromes. *Neurologic Clinics*, *10*, 341–359.

Tarasiuk, J., Kułakowska, A., Drozdowski, W., Kornhuber, J., & Lewczuk, P. (2012). CSF markers in amyotrophic lateral sclerosis. *Journal of Neural Transmission*, *119*, 747–757.

Thambisetty, M., & Lovestone, S. (2010). Blood-based biomarkers of Alzheimer's disease: Challenging but feasible. *Biomarkers in Medicine*, *4*, 65–79.

Tiraboschi, P., Hansen, L. A., Thal, L. J., & Corey-Bloom, J. (2004). The importance of neuritic plaques and tangles to the development and evolution of AD. *Neurology*, *62*, 1984–1989.

Toczylowska, B., Jamrozik, Z., Liebert, A., & Kwiecinski, H. (2013). NMR-based metabonomics of cerebrospinal fluid applied to amyotrophic lateral sclerosis. *Biocybernetics and Biomedical Engineering*, *33*, 21–32.

Toledo-Morrell, L., Stoub, T. R., Bulgakova, M., Wilson, R. S., Bennett, D. A., Leurgans, S., et al. (2004). MRI-derived entorhinal volume is a good predictor of conversion from MCI to AD. *Neurobiology of Aging*, *25*, 1197–1203.

Traynor, B. J., Codd, M. B., Corr, B., Forde, C., Frost, E., & Hardiman, O. (2000). Clinical features of amyotrophic lateral sclerosis according to the El Escorial and Airlie house diagnostic criteria. *Archives of Neurology*, *57*, 1171–1176.

Trupp, M., Jonsson, P., Ohrfelt, A., Zetterberg, H., Obudulu, O., Malm, L., et al. (2014). Metabolite and peptide levels in plasma and CSF differentiating healthy controls from patients with newly diagnosed Parkinson's disease. *Journal of Parasitic Diseases*, *4*, 549–560.

Trushina, E., Dutta, T., Persson, X. M., Mielke, M. M., & Petersen, R. C. (2013). Identification of altered metabolic pathways in plasma and CSF in mild cognitive impairment and Alzheimer's disease using metabolomics. *PLoS One*, *8*, e63644.

von Campenhausen, S., Bornschein, B., Wick, R., Bötzel, K., Sampaio, C., Poewe, W., et al. (2005). Prevalence and incidence of Parkinson's disease in Europe. *European Neuropsychopharmacology*, *15*, 473–490.

Vucic, S., Ziemann, U., Eisen, A., Hallett, M., & Kiernan, M. C. (2013). Transcranial magnetic stimulation and amyotrophic lateral sclerosis: Pathophysiological insights. *Journal of Neurology, Neurosurgery and Psychiatry*, *84*, 1161–1170.

Waggie, K. S., Kahle, P. J., & Tolwani, R. J. (1999). Neurons and mechanisms of neuronal death in neurodegenerative diseases: A brief review. *Laboratory Animal Science*, *49*, 358–362.

Wang, J., Hoekstra, J. G., Zuo, C., Cook, T. J., & Zhang, J. (2012). Biomarkers of Parkinson's disease: Current status and future. *Drug Discovery Today*, *18*, 155–162.

Wang, G., Zhou, Y., Huang, F. J., Tang, H. D., Xu, X. H., Liu, J. J., et al. (2014). Plasma metabolite profiles of Alzheimer's disease and mild cognitive impairment. *Journal of Proteome Research*, *13*, 2649–2958.

Welsh, K. A., Butters, N., Hughes, J. P., Mohs, R. C., & Heyman, A. (1992). Detection and staging of dementia in Alzheimer's disease. *Archives of Neurology*, *49*, 448–452.

Wimo, A., Reed, C. C., Dodel, R., Belger, M., Jones, R. W., Happich, M., et al. (2013). The GERAS study: A prospective observational study of costs and resource use in community dwellers with Alzheimer's disease in three European countries—Study design and baseline findings. *Journal of Alzheimer's Disease*, *36*, 385–399.

Wuolikainen, A., Andersen, P. M., Moritz, T., Marklund, S. L., & Antti, H. (2012). ALS patients with mutations in the SOD1 gene have an unique metabolomic profile in the cerebrospinal fluid compared with ALS patients without mutations. *Molecular Genetics and Metabolism*, *105*, 472–478.

Wuolikainen, A., Hedenström, M., Moritz, T., Marklund, S. L., Antti, H., & Andersen, P. M. (2009). Optimization of procedures for collecting and storing of CSF for studying the metabolome in ALS. *Amyotrophic Lateral Sclerosis*, *10*, 229–236.

Wuolikainen, A., Moritz, T., Marklund, S. L., Antti, H., & Andersen, P. M. (2011). Disease-related changes in the cerebrospinal fluid metabolome in amyotrophic lateral sclerosis detected by GC/TOFMS. *PLoS One*, *6*, e17947.

Zhang, S., Nagana-Gowda, G. A., Ye, T., & Raftery, D. (2010). Advances in NMR-based biofluid analysis and metabolite profiling. *Analyst*, *135*, 1490–1498.

Zhang, B., & Powers, R. (2012). Analysis of bacterial biofilms using NMR-based metabolomics. *Future Medicinal Chemistry*, *4*, 1273–1306.

CHAPTER FIVE

# Lipidomics of Human Brain Aging and Alzheimer's Disease Pathology

**Alba Naudí*, Rosanna Cabré*, Mariona Jové*, Victoria Ayala*, Hugo Gonzalo*, Manuel Portero-Otín*, Isidre Ferrer[†,‡], Reinald Pamplona*[,1]**

*Department of Experimental Medicine, University of Lleida-Biomedical Research Institute of Lleida, Lleida, Spain
[†]Institute of Neuropathology, Bellvitge University Hospital, University of Barcelona, Biomedical Research Institute of Bellvitge, L'Hospitalet de Llobregat, Barcelona, Spain
[‡]Center for Biomedical Research on Neurodegenerative Diseases (CIBERNED), ISCIII, Madrid, Spain
[1]Corresponding author: e-mail address: reinald.pamplona@mex.udl.cat

## Contents

1. Introduction 134
2. Lipidomics of Human Brain 136
   2.1 Definition of Lipid and Classification 136
   2.2 Analytical Methods to Study Brain Lipidome 139
   2.3 Lipids in the Human Brain 143
   2.4 Functional Properties of Lipids in Human Brain 153
3. Lipidomics of Human Brain Aging 163
4. Lipidomics of Alzheimer's Disease Pathology 168
   4.1 Evidence for Disturbance of Human Brain Lipid Content in AD Pathology 170
   4.2 Docosahexaenoic Acid and Alzheimer's Disease Pathology: An Allostatic Adaption 176
5. Summary and Future Prospects 177

Acknowledgments 178
References 178

## Abstract

Lipids stimulated and favored the evolution of the brain. Adult human brain contains a large amount of lipids, and the largest diversity of lipid classes and lipid molecular species. Lipidomics is defined as "the full characterization of lipid molecular species and of their biological roles with respect to expression of proteins involved in lipid metabolism and function, including gene regulation." Therefore, the study of brain lipidomics can help to unravel the diversity and to disclose the specificity of these lipid traits and its alterations in neural (neurons and glial) cells, groups of neural cells, brain, and fluids such as cerebrospinal fluid and plasma, thus helping to uncover potential biomarkers of

*International Review of Neurobiology*, Volume 122
ISSN 0074-7742
http://dx.doi.org/10.1016/bs.irn.2015.05.008

human brain aging and Alzheimer disease. This review will discuss the lipid composition of the adult human brain. We first consider a brief approach to lipid definition, classification, and tools for analysis from the new point of view that has emerged with lipidomics, and then turn to the lipid profiles in human brain and how lipids affect brain function. Finally, we focus on the current status of lipidomics findings in human brain aging and Alzheimer's disease pathology. Neurolipidomics will increase knowledge about physiological and pathological functions of brain cells and will place the concept of selective neuronal vulnerability in a lipid context.

## 1. INTRODUCTION

The natural history of lipids is closely related with the evolution of life. The appearance of lipids was a driving force for the evolution of life and multicellularity. As a result, all living organisms (including the three domains of life: archaea, bacteria, and eukaryotes) have lipid membranes. The early evolution of lipid biosynthesis and the importance of lipid membranes are discussed by Lombard, López-García, and Moreira (2012). As Hulbert, Kelly, and Abbott (2014) note, just as DNA has been described as an "eternal molecule," so lipid membranes could be considered an "eternal structure" as such membranes are the products of pre-existing membranes. Neural cells (neurons and glial cells) are not an exception. Indeed, lipids stimulated and favored the evolution of the brain (Broadhurst et al., 2002; Crawford et al., 2013).

Among the tissues of the human body, nervous tissue is one of the richest in lipid content. It is well established that lipids account for about 10–12% of the fresh weight and half the dry matter of the brain (Sastry, 1985). Apart from their quantitative importance, the lipids of the nervous system show a great deal of structural and functional diversity. Beginning with the classic discoveries of the neurochemist J.L.W. Thudichum (Thudichum, 1884) at the turn of the twentieth century, a large body of knowledge on the biochemistry and physiology of lipids of the nervous tissue has been accumulated. Thus, all lipid classes are represented in neural cells, similarly to other cell types, and the wide spectra of lipid molecular species is an expression of the different needs and functions ascribed to them. In addition, the demonstration that lipids have broad information-carrying roles in the nervous system, the ability of profiling large-scale changes in lipid composition, and determining topographical distribution of individual lipid species in neural cells has boosted a renewed interest in this particular cell component.

Human brain performs a wide range of motor, sensory, regulatory, behavioral, and cognitive functions which are dependent on the complex organization of groups of neuronal populations composed, in turn, of a diversity of neural cells. Furthermore, neurons differ morphologically in size, number of dendrites, complexity of the dendritic tree, number and type of synapses, axonal length, and degree of axonal myelination, among other cellular and subcellular traits. Additionally, from a physiological point of view, neuronal diversity is meaningfully expressed by the chemical specificity that confers the neurotransmitters used for chemical transmission and neuromodulation, as well as by their electrical properties. This structural and functional diversity is also true for non-neuronal cells. In this context, it is postulated that this morphological and functional diversity among neural cells is also projected and achieved through the expression of particular lipid profiles.

Specific regions of the brain exhibit differential vulnerabilities to aging and age-related neurodegenerative diseases such as Alzheimer's disease (AD), with aging being the main risk factor (Jové, Portero-Otín, Naudí, Ferrer, & Pamplona, 2014; Mattson & Magnus, 2006). A central question is why some individuals' age with their cognitive function relatively preserved whereas others decline and develop AD pathology. Early studies suggested that neuronal loss was an integral feature of the aging brain. With the appearance of stereological neuronal quantification, however, it became clear that neuronal cell number is largely preserved in the neocortex and hippocampus of the aging human brain, declining only in the setting of AD. In this context, we postulated that lipid-derived adaptive mechanisms have evolved to preserve neurons and cognitive function across an entire lifespan. Therefore, specific lipidomic profiles and lipidomic signatures may be useful to improve understanding of mechanistic processes of the corresponding physiological process (brain aging) and disease (AD) and to identify potentially specific lipid markers.

This review will discuss the lipid composition of the adult human brain. We first consider a brief approach to the lipid definition, classification, and tools for analysis from the new point of view emerging with lipidomics, and then turn to the lipid profiles in human brain and how lipids affect brain function. However, the effects of development and maturation of human brain, the observations from experimental animals, the dietary influences, and drug effects on lipid metabolism and lipid composition are not covered. Finally, we focus on the current status of lipidomics findings in human brain aging and AD pathology.

# 2. LIPIDOMICS OF HUMAN BRAIN

## 2.1 Definition of Lipid and Classification

Lipids are a diverse and ubiquitous group of compounds which have key roles in cellular physiology and pathology. The diversity in lipid function is reflected by an enormous variation in the structures of lipid molecules. Contrasting the case of genes and proteins, which are primarily composed of linear combinations of 4 nucleic acids and 20 amino acids, respectively, lipid structures are more complex due to the number of different biochemical transformations which occur during their biosynthesis (Fahy, Cotter, Sud, & Subramaniam, 2011). Lipids exhibit notable structural diversity, determined by factors such as variable chain length, and biochemical transformations such as oxidations, reductions, substitutions, ring-forming transformations, as well as modification with sugar residues and other functional groups of different biosynthetic origin. There are no reliable estimates of the number of discrete lipid compounds in nature, due to the technical challenges of elucidating chemical structures, but based on acyl/alkyl chain and sugar permutations for glycerolipids, glycerophospholipids, and sphingolipids, the number of lipid molecular species can be estimated around 200,000 (Yetukuri, Ekroos, Vidal-Puig, & Oresic, 2008). This number is actually exceeded by the list of known natural products, most of which are of either prenol or polyketide origin (Buckingham, 2010). In this scenario, it is only fair to point out the work of the Lipid Metabolites and Pathways Strategy (LIPID MAPS) consortium that is actively involved in an integrated approach for the detection, quantitation, and pathway reconstruction of lipids and related genes and proteins at a systems-biology level (Fahy et al., 2011; Subramaniam et al., 2011). In any case, this extreme structural complexity is unlikely to be expressed in brain lipid composition in light of available evidence, probably due to a molecular selection process during evolution of specific lipid species according to neural cell structural and functional needs.

The concept "lipid" has been defined as any group of organic compounds that are insoluble in water but soluble in organic solvents (Smith, 2000). Currently, lipids are defined in chemical terms as small hydrophobic or amphiphilic molecules that originate either entirely or in part from two distinct types of building blocks: ketoacyl and isoprene groups (Fahy et al., 2005, 2009, 2011) (Fig. 1A). Regarding lipid classification, some approaches separate lipids into "simple" and "complex" groups, with simple lipids being

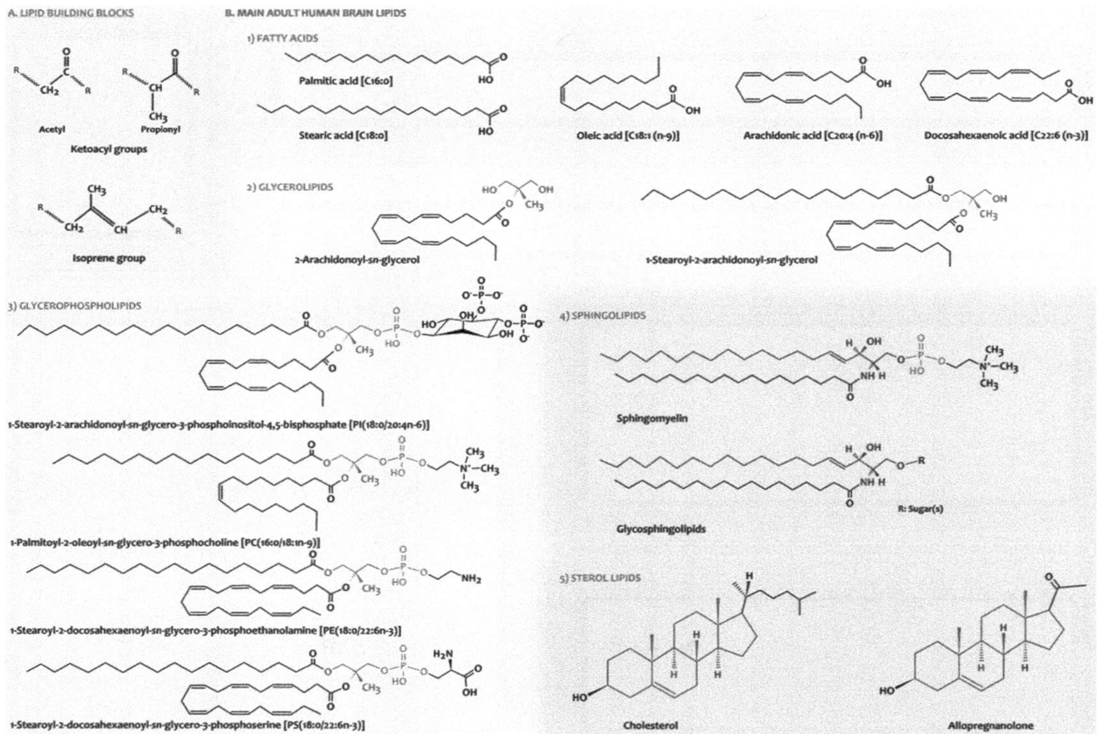


**Figure 1** See legend on next page.

those that yield at most two types of distinct entities upon hydrolysis (e.g., acylglycerols: fatty acids, and glycerol) and complex lipids (e.g., glycerophospholipids: fatty acids, glycerol, and headgroup) those yielding three or more products upon hydrolysis (see Cyberlipid Center Website, n.d.; Lipid Library Website, n.d.). Additionally, the LipidBank (Lipid Bank Website, n.d.) database in Japan defines a third major group called "derived" lipids (alcohols and fatty acids derived by hydrolyzing the simple lipids) which includes 26 top-level categories in their classification scheme, covering a wide variety of animal and plant sources. In 2005, the International Lipid Classification and Nomenclature Committee on the initiative of the LIPID MAPS Consortium developed and established a comprehensive classification system for lipids based on well-defined chemical and biochemical principles and using a framework designed to be extensible, flexible, scalable, and compatible with modern informatics technology (for more details about lipid classification and nomenclature, lipid structures, and bioinformatic tools for lipidomic analysis, see Fahy et al., 2011, 2005, 2009; Subramaniam et al., 2011). The nomenclature adopted by the LIPID MAPS consortium carefully follows existing IUPAC–IUBMB (the International Union of Pure and Applied Chemists and the International Union of Biochemistry and Molecular Biology) guidelines.

Based on this classification system, lipids have been divided into eight categories: fatty acyls (FA); glycerolipids (GL); glycerophospholipids (GP);

**Figure 1** (A) Lipid building blocks: ketoacyl groups and isoprene groups. (B) Main adult human brain lipids: (1) fatty acids (FA) contain a carboxylic group attached to an aliphatic chain. Saturated fatty acids (SFA) do not contain double bonds, whereas monounsaturated (MUFA) and polyunsaturated (PUFA) fatty acids contain one or more *cis*-double bonds. There are two types of PUFAs: omega-6 (e.g., arachidonic acid, 20:4n-6) and omega-3 (e.g., docosahexaenoic acid, 22:6n-3), which are named according to the position of the first double bond in the carbon chain, starting from the methyl end of the molecule. Fatty acids shown represent around 80–90% of total fatty acid profile of human brain (Naudí et al., 2012, 2013a, 2013b); (2) glycerolipids (GL) are fatty acid esters of glycerol and in human brain mostly comprise mono- and diacylglycerols; (3) glycerophospholipids contain phosphoric acid in ester form with a glycerolipid. They are subdivided into distinct classes based on the nature of the head group linked to the phosphate at the *sn*-3 position of the glycerol backbone. Phosphatidylcholine (PC), phosphatidylethanolamine (PE), phosphatidylserine (PS), and phosphatidylinositols (PI) are the main phospholipids present in human brain (Sastry, 1985); (4) sphingolipids contain a common sphingoid base moiety. They are acylated to form ceramides, which are modified to generate phosphosphingolipids (e.g., sphingomyelin) and glycosphingolipids; and (5) sterol lipids contain a fused four-ring core and comprise cholesterol and its steroid derivatives. *Adapted with permission from Piomelli, Astarita, and Rapaka (2007).*

sphingolipids (SP); saccharolipids (SL) and polyketides (PK) (derived from condensation of ketoacyl subunits); sterol (ST); and prenol lipids (PR) (derived from condensation of isoprene subunits). Figure 1B shows the structure of the main lipid molecular species present in adult human brain. Each category is further divided into classes, subclasses, and, in the case of some subclasses of prenol lipids, 4th-level classes. Each lipid species is assigned a unique 12- or 14-character identifier (LIPID MAPS ID or "LM ID") based on this classification scheme. The format of the LM ID contains the classification information, provides a systematic means of assigning a unique identification to each lipid molecule, and allows for the addition of large numbers of new categories, classes, and subclasses in the future (Fahy et al., 2011).

## 2.2 Analytical Methods to Study Brain Lipidome

Systems biology has revolutionized the meaning of the concept of molecular profiling in neurosciences. By way of example, a recent study shows a comprehensive atlas of the adult human brain transcriptome (Hawrylycz et al., 2012), comprising extensive histological analysis and comprehensive microarray profiling of $\sim$900 neuroanatomically precise subdivisions. Analogously, another recent study offers the proteome profiling of the human brain, but in a more restricted number of regions (Fernandez-Irigoyen et al., 2014). Although lipid research had already become an intensive area of investigation in the 1960s, the period in which the traditional lipid and fatty acids analyses were developed, and lipid biology has gained importance in the past decade with the emergence of lipidomics as a specific-derived part of metabolomics (Han, 2007; Han & Gross, 2003, 2005; Oresic, Hänninen, & Vidal-Puig, 2008; Seppänen-Laakso & Oresic, 2009), we are still far from having a comprehensive atlas of the lipidome of the adult human brain. The term "lipidome" describes the complete lipid profile within an organism, organ, tissue, cell, organelle, subcellular membrane or microdomain (e.g., lipid rafts), and biological fluids (e.g., cerebrospinal fluid (CSF) and plasma/serum). Lipidomics can be defined as "the full characterization of lipid molecular species and of their biological roles with respect to expression of proteins involved in lipid metabolism and function, including gene regulation." Neurolipidomics (Power & Patel, 2004) is a particular subset of lipidomics specifically developed in the context of the complexity and specificity of nervous system lipids. What's more, the great diversity of lipid classes and lipid molecular species expressed in brain, e.g., in sphingolipid classes, has given rise to a subset of neurolipidomics that is termed sphingolipidome (Merrill, Sullards, Allegood, Kelly, & Wang, 2005).

Because of the huge diversity of lipids, lipidomics is a challenge in field of analytical chemistry and demands specific solutions for analysis, data handling, and lipid pathway analysis (Yetukuri et al., 2008). Figure 2 offers an overview of different stages of a typical lipidomics platform, from sample preparation to bioinformatics. For in-depth discussions and specific methods, the reader is advised to refer to recently published reviews and series of books on the topic (Brown, 2007; Brown, Henage, Preininger, Xiang, & Exton, 2007; Enriquez-Algeciras & Bhattacharya, 2013; Fahy et al., 2011; Hyötyläinen & Orešič, 2014; Ivanova, Milne, Byrne, Xiang, & Brown, 2007; Li, Yang, Bai, & Liu, 2014; Seppänen-Laakso & Oresic, 2009).

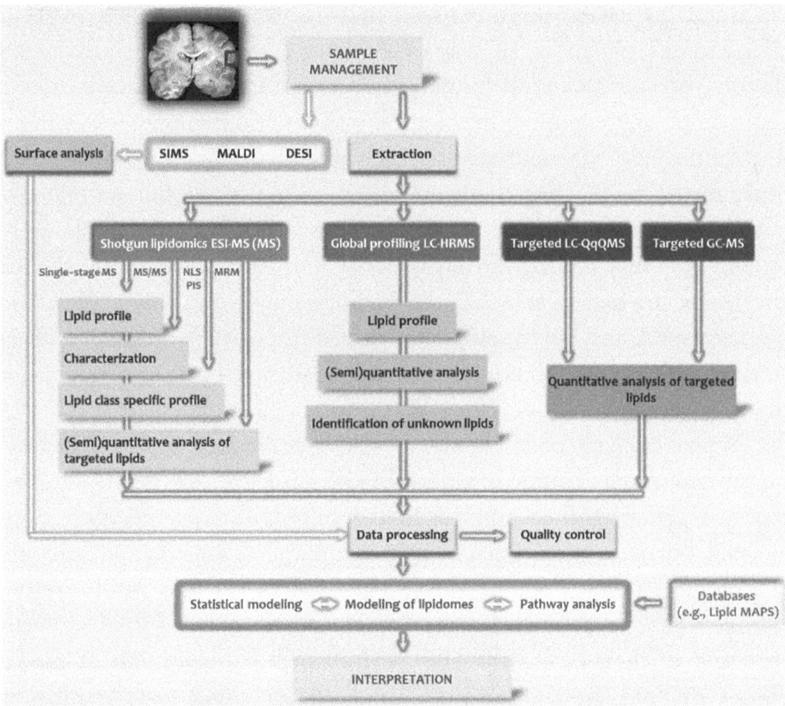


**Figure 2** Overview of different stages of a typical lipidomics platform, from sample preparation to bioinformatics. Abbreviations: DESI, desorption electrospray ionization; ESI, electrospray ionization; GC, gas chromatography; HRMS, high resolution mass spectrometry; LC, liquid chromatography; MALDI, matrix-assisted laser desorption/ionization; MRM, multiple-reaction monitoring; MS, mass spectrometry; NLS, neutral loss; PIS, precursor ion scan; QqQ, triple quadrupole; SIMS, secondary ion mass spectrometry. *Adapted with permission from Hyötyläinen and Orešič (2014).*

The first step in performing lipidomics analyses is to determine the number of lipid species to be measured. If only a defined set of metabolites are wanted to be detected, a targeted approach should be selected. However, if the aim of the experiment is whole lipidome determination, an untargeted approach should be chosen (Patti, Yanes, & Siuzdak, 2012). So, global lipidomics means mapping the entire spectrum of lipids and lipid molecular species in a biological system.

This election will also determine the extraction method to be used. Because lipids are very heterogeneous and complex molecules, a single extraction method, which is able to extract all lipid classes from a biological matrix with a good efficiency, does not exist. Therefore, a crucial step in any lipidomics analysis is the extraction of lipids and different methods have been described depending on the experiment objective (Pellegrino, Di Veroli, Valeri, Goracci, & Cruciani, 2014).

The second step in the lipidomics analyses is the detection of lipid species extracted. Mass spectrometry (MS), nuclear magnetic resonance (NMR), and other spectroscopic approaches have become powerful tools for lipid characterization. It may be termed "shotgun lipidomics" if the lipid extract is introduced directly into the mass spectrometer (Han & Gross, 2005, Schwudke et al., 2006) or hyphenated techniques such as liquid chromatography plus MS (LC-MS) when the extract is introduced into MS after chromatographic separation (Houjou, Yamatani, Imagawa, Shimizu, & Taguchi, 2005; Laaksonen et al., 2006). In addition to LC, other separation technologies that are essential/complementary tools for comprehensive analysis of lipids in complex samples are thin-layer chromatography (TLC), gas chromatography (GC), supercritical fluid chromatography (SFC), and capillary electrophoresis (CE). When these are coupled with MS, they offer a huge amount of information on lipidomics. Although there are some drawbacks to using spectroscopic approaches for lipidomics analysis, these approaches should not be ignored given their utility in visualization analysis, which is quite useful in the study of dynamic biological processes (Li et al., 2014). Furthermore, MALDI-based lipid visualization has been employed for brain analyses and can provide imaging resolution (Amoscato et al., 2014; Chen, Allegood, et al., 2008; Chen, Green, Orr, & Bazinet, 2008). Targeted lipidomics, in turn, aims to specifically detect and quantify a single lipid or multiple related lipids, e.g., oxylipids.

Though there is not a single universal technique for ionization, the most common ionization technique in untargeted lipidomics approaches is electrospray ionization (ESI), which is a soft ionization method that can be combined with several types of mass analyzers such as triple quadrupole, ion trap, time-of-flight (TOF), and Orbitrap®. ESI is most often used in positive ion mode (ESI+) for untargeted approaches, since ESI+ enables coverage of diverse classes such as major GL, GP, and SP. However, in particular when GPs are the focus, some classes such as phosphatidylinositol (PI), phosphatidylserine (PS), phosphatidic acid (PA), and free fatty acids are not suitable for ESI+ analysis, and the negative ion mode (ESI−) is advantageous. Additionally, ESI− analysis can provide information about carboxylate anions of the fatty acids in different phospholipids (Seppänen-Laakso & Oresic, 2009; Watson, 2006). Further, it may not be neglected that other ionization techniques such as chemical ionization or atmospheric pressure chemical ionization could be more sensitive to specific lipids.

Modern approaches to lipidomic analysis are dominated by MS (Want, Cravatt, & Siuzdak, 2005), usually preceded by separation by LC (Sommer, Herscovitz, Welty, & Costello, 2006) or GC (Jiye et al., 2005). New MS-based lipidomics methods allow the study of intact lipid molecular species from very small amounts of samples (Han & Gross, 2005; Schwudke et al., 2006), e.g., from cultured neural cells or (micro)regions dissected from brain. In addition, the dynamic range for analyses of lipidomes has been dramatically extended so that we are currently able to identify and quantify lipid classes only present in a very low amount (e.g., lysophospholipids, ceramide, sphingosine-1-phosphate) (Han, 2002; Han, Yang, Cheng, Fikes, & Gross, 2005) and/or achieve analysis of very low-abundant molecular species in many lipid classes that are present in medium or high total mass content (e.g., ethanolamine glycerophospholipids, cardiolipins) (Han et al., 2005; Han, Yang, Yang, Cheng, & Gross, 2006). It is expected that analysis of neurolipidomes in the near future will be a challenge of sample preparation and tissue isolation rather than an issue of the lipid analysis (Han, 2007).

Lipidomics has made rapid progress on numerous fronts over the past decade although it is yet to achieve the same level of advancement and knowledge as genomics and proteomics. The diversity of lipid species presents a challenge both from the experimental and the informatics stances. In addition to efforts to achieve technical improvement in analytical equipment, and to develop novel methods with higher sensitivity for low abundance lipids, there is also the key question of solving the need for a robust bioinformatics infrastructure for the (i) establishment of a globally accepted classification system, creation of databases of lipid structures, and lipid-related genes and proteins (in this regard, the initiative of the LIPID MAPS consortium is excellent news); (ii) efficient analysis of experimental data;

(iii) integration of experimental data and existing knowledge into metabolic and signaling pathways; and (iv) development of software for efficient search, display, and analysis of lipidomic data, among others. Although still far from providing comprehensive coverage of lipids in brain, the progress of lipidomics will provide increasing expansion into global lipidomes as well as their characterization in physiological and pathological contexts.

## 2.3 Lipids in the Human Brain

The enormous complexity of the adult human brain can be expressed with the observation that it is possible to discern around 900 neuroanatomically precise subdivisions (Hawrylycz et al., 2012). Analogous to the observation that there exists a region-specific transcriptomic profile, it may be speculated that the lipidome of each brain structure or region is different in terms of the performance of distinct functions. Although the limited available evidence seems to indicate that this is the case, currently no information is available to create a comprehensive atlas of the adult human brain lipidomes.

Adult human brain contains a large amount of lipids. The mass levels of lipids in brain are second only to the adipose tissue (Han, 2007). Furthermore, in comparison to other organs and/or systems, brain contains the largest diversity of lipid classes and lipid molecular species. For example, in addition to the presence of diverse phospholipid classes, brain also contains a large portion of sphingolipid classes. Thousands of sphingolipid molecular species are present in the sphingolipidome (Merrill et al., 2005) and the majority of these molecular species are present in brain. Cholesterol, and cholesterol metabolites, are also very important and abundant in human brain. Indeed, although the brain only accounts for 2% of the body's total weight, it contains 25% of the body's total cholesterol (Dietschy & Turley, 2001). The importance of cholesterol in the brain is also reflected by the tight regulation of its levels, which is independent of circulating cholesterol and its fluctuations (Dietschy & Turley, 2001).

Glycerophospholipids are the major phospholipid components ubiquitously found in cell membranes and, therefore, they are also found in abundance in membranes from neural cells (for review, see Sastry, 1985) (see Fig. 1B). In the human brain, phospholipids constitute around 4.5–5.4% of wet weight in whole brain and about 4.2% in the gray matter. White matter has a higher concentration of phospholipids amounting to about 7% of wet weight in humans. Phosphatidic acid, the simplest among the glycerophospholipids, and central intermediary in the biosynthetic pathways of both glycerophospholipids and neutral lipids, occurs in low concentration in brain (about 2% of total phospholipids). The predominant form of choline phosphoglycerides occurring in human brain is phosphatidylcholine (PC; 1,2-diacyl-*sn*-glycero-3-phosphocholine; 32.8%), with PC (16:0/18:1) being the major molecular species (O'Brien & Sampson, 1965a, 1965b; Rouser & Yamamoto, 1969; Rouser, Feldman, & Galli, 1965; Rouser, Galli, & Kritchevsky, 1965). The choline plasmalogen (1-alk-1′-enyl,2-acyl-*sn*-glycero-3-phosphocholine) and the alkyl analogue (1-alkyl,2-acyl-*sn*-glycero-3-phosphocholine) account for only about 2% of total choline phosphoglycerides in brain. Ethanolamine phosphoglycerides are quantitatively the major phospholipid in human brain (35.6%) (O'Brien & Sampson, 1965a, 1965b; Panganamala, Horrocks, Geer, & Cornwell, 1971) and the predominant form is the ethanolamine plasmalogen (PPE; 1-alk-1′-enyl-2-acyl-*sn*-glycero-3-phosphoethanolamine), accounting for 50–60% of the ethanolaminephosphoglyceride class of lipids in the whole human brain. The alkylacyl analogue content is relatively low (3–7% of the ethanolamine phosphoglyceride class), whereas phosphatidylethanolamine (1,2-diacyl-*sn*-glycero-3-phosphoethanolamine) makes up the remaining amount of ethanolamine phosphoglycerides. Their total fatty acid composition indicates a large content of polyunsaturates, and the positional distribution of fatty acids in ethanolamine phosphoglycerides of human brain shows that position-1 of *sn*-glycerol is occupied primarily by the palmitic acid (16:0), stearic acid (18:0), and oleic acid (18:1) groups both in the white and gray matter. Position-2 consists of the polyunsaturates and these are more numerous in the gray matter than in the white matter. The concentration of serine phosphoglycerides in human brain is about 16.6% (O'Brien & Sampson, 1965a, 1965b; Panganamala et al., 1971) of the total phospholipids. They occur as 1,2-diacyl-*sn*-glycero-3-phosphoserine (more than 90%) and also as the serine plasmalogen. Regarding the fatty acid profile, they contain mainly 18:0, 18:1, and docosahexaenoic acid (DHA, 22:6). The gray matter serine phosphoglycerides are particularly rich in 22:6. Inositol phosphoglycerides account for about 2.6% of the total phospholipids in human brain (Norton, Poduslo, & Suzuki, 1996; Rouser & Yamamoto, 1968). Phosphatidylinositol and triphosphoinositide are the major lipids with only trace amounts of diphosphoinositide. Brain contains the highest concentrations of phosphoinositides among animal tissues. The main fatty acid components of inositol phosphoglycerides are stearic (18:0) and arachidonic (20:4) acids. Finally, Kahma, Brotherus, Haltia, and Renkonen (1976) found 0.2% of phospholipids as diphosphatidylglycerol and 0.1% as bis(monoacyl glycerol) phosphate in human brain. Diphosphatidylglycerol is mainly located in brain mitochondria although small quantities are also present in nuclear and synaptosomal fraction. The main fatty acids included in this phospholipid fraction are palmitic acid (16:0), palmitoleic acid (16:1), stearic acid (18:0), oleic acid (18:1), linoleic acid (18:2), linolenic acid (18:3), and arachidonic acid (AA, 20:4). Table 1 shows the content and fatty acid composition of the main adult human brain phospholipids.

Sphingolipids are a group a complex lipids, derived from *N*-acylsphingosine (ceramide), which occur in particularly large concentrations in human brain (Maceyka & Spiegel, 2014; Sastry, 1985). Figure 3 offers a brief scheme of the sphingolipid metabolism. This group of lipids consists of sphingomyelin, cerebrosides, sulfatides, and gangliosides (see also Table 1 for sphingolipid content and fatty acid composition of human brain). Sphingomyelin (*N*-acylsphingosine-1-phosphocholine) accounts for about 14.8% of the phospholipid content in the human brain (O'Brien & Sampson, 1965a, 1965b; Rouser, Feldman, et al., 1965; Rouser, Galli, et al., 1965). Higher concentrations of sphingomyelin are found in peripheral nerves (about 25%) and in white matter (20%) mainly because it is a major lipid of the myelin membrane. Sphingomyelin fatty acids comprise mainly stearic (18:0), lignoceric (24:0), and nervonic (24:1) acids. Cerebrosides are derivatives of ceramide in which a carbohydrate group is attached to the primary hydroxyl of sphingosine by a beta-glycosidic linkage. In human brain, cerebrosides amount to 15.8% of the total lipids (Rouser, Feldman, et al., 1965; Rouser, Galli, et al., 1965). Being a major component of myelin, cerebroside concentration in white matter is about 10-fold higher than in gray matter. Most of the cerebroside in brain is galactosylceramide. The fatty acid components of human brain cerebrosides characteristically contain hydroxyl fatty acids and these account for more than 50% of the total fatty acids. Among the nonhydroxyl fatty acids, lignoceric (24:0) and nervonic (24:1) are the major components, and cerebronic (24h:0) and hydroxynervonic (24h:1) are the most abundant hydroxyl fatty acids in human brain. Sulfatides are sulfate esters of galactocerebrosides in which the sulfate group is located at C-3 of the galactopyranoside moiety. Sulfatide is the only sulfosphingolipid present in brain. In human brain, the sulfatides are associated primarily with myelin and they account for about 6.2% of total lipids of brain (Rouser, Feldman, et al., 1965; Rouser, Galli, et al., 1965). The fatty acid composition of sulfatides is similar to that of cerebrosides. Gangliosides, sialic acid-containing glycosphingolipids, occur ubiquitously in cell plasma membranes and are particularly abundant in brain (Sastry, 1985; Sonnino & Chigorno, 2000). In human brain, they occur in substantially higher

**Table 1** Content and Fatty Acid Composition of Main Human Brain Glycerophospholipids

| Tissue | Content % Lipid-P | Fatty Acid Composition (mol%) | | | | | | | | | | |
|---|---|---|---|---|---|---|---|---|---|---|---|---|
| | | 14:0 | 16:0 | 16:1 | 18:0 | 18:1 | 18:2 | 20:1 | 20:4 +22:1 | 22:5 n-6 | 22:5 n-3 | 22:6 |
| PC human brain | 32.8 | – | 47.6 | – | 12.1 | 40.3 | – | – | – | – | – | – |
| PC human gray matter | 38.9 | 2.9 | 45.0 | 3.1 | 9.3 | 31.4 | 0.4 | 0.7 | 4.1 | – | – | 3.1 |
| PC human white matter | 30.2 | 1.3 | 34.3 | 1.0 | 13.4 | 45.2 | 0.4 | 1.1 | 1.3 | – | – | 0.1 |
| PE human brain | 35.6 | – | – | – | – | – | – | – | – | – | – | – |
| PE human gray matter | 42.2 | – | 6.7 | – | 26.0 | 11.9 | – | 1.5 | 13.8 | 14.3 | – | 24.3 |
| PE human white matter | 34.1 | – | 6.7 | – | 9.0 | 42.4 | - | 7.9 | 6.4 | 13.7 | 0.5 | 3.4 |
| PS human brain | 16.6 | – | – | – | – | – | – | – | – | – | – | – |
| PS human gray matter | 12.6 | – | 2.3 | – | 25.4 | 21.5 | – | 1.0 | 1.6 | 5.0 | 3.3 | 36.6 |
| PS human white matter | 15.7 | – | 1.7 | - | 35.8 | 39.7 | 0.3 | 5.3 | 2.0 | 4.8 | 0.9 | 5.6 |

Abbreviations: PC, phosphatidylcholine; PE, phosphatidylethanolamine; PS, phosphatidylserine.

Data from Rouser, Feldman, et al. (1965), Rouser, Galli, et al. (1965b), Rouser and Yamamoto (1968), O'Brien and Sampson (1965a, 1965b), and Panganamala et al. (1971).

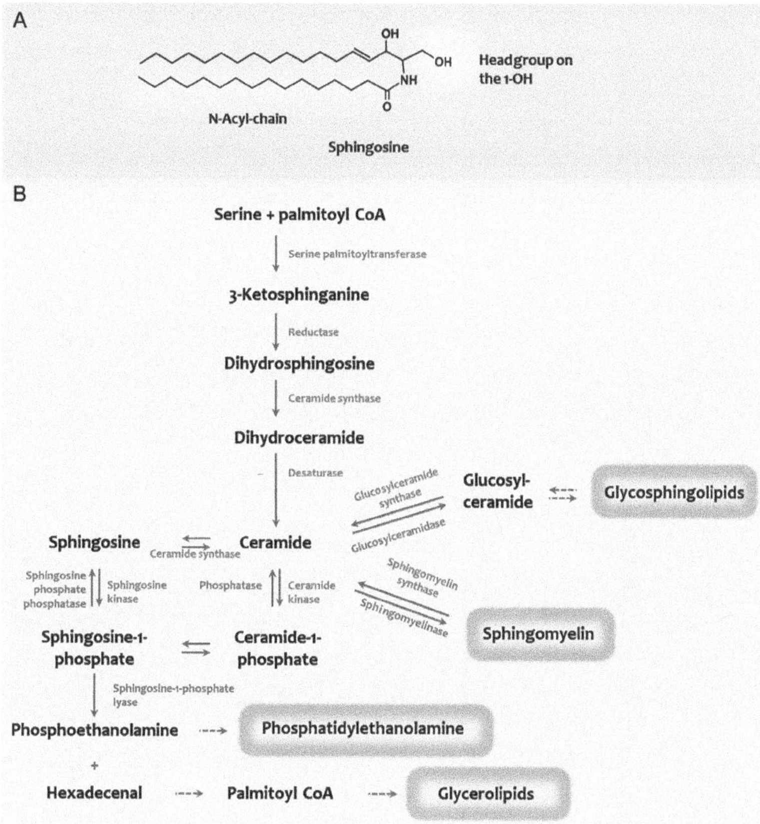


**Figure 3** Sphingolipid metabolism and interconnected bioactive sphingolipid metabolites. (A) Structure of ceramide, with a sphingosine backbone. (B) *De novo* sphingolipid biosynthesis pathway which starts with the condensation of palmitoyl coenzyme A (CoA) and serine. *Adapted with permission from Maceyka and Spiegel (2014).*

concentrations in gray matter as compared to white matter and spinal cord (Ando, Chang, & Yu, 1978; Ueno, Ando, & Yu, 1978). Gangliosides consist of a lipid moiety linked to a very large family of oligosaccharide structures differing in glycosidic linkage position, sugar configuration, neutral sugar, and sialic acid content. The main gangliosides of the brain belong to the ganglio series, a series characterized by the tetrasaccharide β-Gal-(1-3)-β-GalNAc-(1-4)-β-Gal-(1-4)-β-Glc to which residues of sialic acid are α-ketosidically linked. Sialic acid refers to all the derivatives of neuraminic acid, 5-amino-3,5-dideoxy-D-glycero-D-galactononulosonic acid. In human brain, the most represented structure is that of *N*-acetyl-neuraminic acid, followed by that of *N*-acetyl-9-*O*-acetylneuraminic acid (Ghidoni et al., 1980; Haverkamp et al., 1977; Sonnino & Chigorno, 2000). Ganglioside lactones, in which a sialic acid esterifies a primary hydroxyl group, have been found to occur in human brain. The lipid moiety of gangliosides, the ceramide, consists of a long-chain amino alcohol linked to a fatty acid by an amide linkage. The 18- and 20-carbon atom structures containing a *trans* double bond at position 4–5 are the most abundant long-chain amino alcohol components of brain gangliosides; they are generally called "sphingosine." The long-chain amino alcohols not containing a double bond at position 4–5 are generally called sphinganine. Stearic acid (18:0) is the main fatty acid of human brain gangliosides and forms over 80% of the total gangliosides fatty acid content (Sonnino & Chigorno, 2000).

### 2.3.1 Fatty Acids in Human Brain

In human brain, fatty acids are either saturated, monounsaturated, or polyunsaturated hydrocarbon chains that normally vary from 14 to 24 carbons in length, with an average chain length strictly maintained about 18 carbon atoms, and a relative distribution between saturated (SFA) and unsaturated (UFA, being UFA = PUFA series n-3 + PUFA series n-6) fatty acids of 40:60 (Naudí et al., 2013a, 2013b). Furthermore, the available data demonstrate the existence of cross-regional differences in human brain fatty acid composition. Thus, Table 2 reflects the fatty acid profile in five different regions of the adult human nervous system. The data are conclusive: despite maintaining an interregional stable average chain length (18 carbon atoms), a ratio of saturated:unsaturated practically identical (40:60), and a global content of DHA and AA of approximately 20% of fatty acid content, there are cross-regional differences with respect to the type of PUFA distribution affecting very specially to both monounsaturated (MUFA) and polyunsaturated (PUFA) fatty acids. So, it has been found that the higher the presence of MUFA for a given region, the lower the PUFA content. In any case, DHA (22:6n-3) is the most abundant PUFA in all regions with a mol% ranging from 8% to 13% (Naudi et al., 2012), in line with previous finding pointing out the very high level of DHA in the whole brain (O'Brien & Sampson, 1965a, 1965b; Salem, Kim, & Yergey, 1986; Svennerholm, 1968; Thudichum, 1962). This amount is not an exceptional concentration compared to other tissues, but has a relevant meaning for brain (see later). Figure 4 shows the long chain and very long-chain fatty acid (VLCFA) biosynthesis in humans.

**Table 2** Fatty Acid Composition (mol%) of Gray Matter from Human Central Nervous System: A Cross-Regional Comparative Approach

| | Frontal Cortex | Hippocampus | Substantia Nigra | Medulla Oblongata | Spinal Cord | *P*< |
|---|---|---|---|---|---|---|
| 14:0 | 0.51 ± 0.04 | 0.42 ± 0.05 | 0.54 ± 0.04 | 0.50 ± 0.04 | 0.48 ± 0.05 | ns |
| 16:0 | 21.13 ± 0.51 | 19.54 ± 0.27 | 12.68 ± 0.39 | 13.57 ± 0.38 | 14.75 ± 0.25 | 0.001 |
| 16:1n-7 | 0.98 ± 0.12 | 0.89 ± 0.10 | 1.68 ± 0.18 | 1.21 ± 0.03 | 0.94 ± 0.06 | 0.004 |
| 18:0 | 21.35 ± 1.23 | 21.89 ± 0.20 | 24.61 ± 0.27 | 25.64 ± 0.61 | 22.07 ± 1.72 | ns |
| 18:1n-9 | 23.78 ± 1.51 | 26.12 ± 0.50 | 33.57 ± 0.19 | 30.13 ± 0.87 | 33.51 ± 1.43 | 0.001 |
| 18:2n-6 | 0.77 ± 0.12 | 0.59 ± 0.04 | 0.33 ± 0.06 | 0.56 ± 0.01 | 0.96 ± 0.61 | ns |
| 18:3n-3 | 0.14 ± 0.01 | 0.23 ± 0.02 | 0.17 ± 0.003 | 0.23 ± 0.01 | 0.34 ± 0.05 | 0.002 |
| 20:0 | 1.25 ± 0.23 | 1.44 ± 0.09 | 4.95 ± 0.12 | 5.58 ± 0.23 | 7.62 ± 0.53 | 0.001 |
| 20:1 | 0.19 ± 0.04 | 0.37 ± 0.01 | 0.22 ± 0.02 | 0.45 ± 0.02 | 0.75 ± 0.09 | 0.001 |
| 20:2n-6 | 0.23 ± 0.01 | 0.23 ± 0.02 | 0.23 ± 0.03 | 0.31 ± 0.06 | 0.28 ± 0.01 | ns |
| 20:3n-6 | 0.63 ± 0.07 | 0.90 ± 0.10 | 0.61 ± 0.02 | 0.99 ± 0.03 | 0.87 ± 0.16 | ns |
| 20:4n-6 | 8.28 ± 0.19 | 8.05 ± 0.24 | 3.70 ± 0.29 | 3.95 ± 0.33 | 3.13 ± 0.09 | 0.001 |
| 22:4n-6 | 4.77 ± 0.14 | 6.24 ± 0.20 | 4.32 ± 0.15 | 4.07 ± 0.08 | 3.16 ± 0.17 | 0.001 |
| 22:5n-6 | 0.67 ± 0.09 | 0.92 ± 0.08 | 0.12 ± 0.007 | 0.40 ± 0.02 | 0.24 ± 0.04 | 0.001 |
| 22:5n-3 | 0.26 ± 0.03 | 0.33 ± 0.02 | 0.06 ± 0.006 | 0.09 ± 0.01 | 0.38 ± 0.14 | 0.055 |
| 22:6n-3 | 13.68 ± 0.17 | 10.97 ± 0.31 | 9.74 ± 0.28 | 9.28 ± 0.45 | 8.84 ± 0.71 | 0.001 |

*Continued*

**Table 2** Fatty Acid Composition (mol%) of Gray Matter from Human Central Nervous System: A Cross-Regional Comparative Approach—cont'd

| | Frontal Cortex | Hippocampus | Substantia Nigra | Medulla Oblongata | Spinal Cord | *P* < |
|---|---|---|---|---|---|---|
| 24:0 | 0.38 ± 0.06 | 0.45 ± 0.04 | 0.64 ± 0.06 | 1.19 ± 0.22 | 1.00 ± 0.08 | 0.001 |
| 24:1n-9 | 0.93 ± 0.23 | 0.33 ± 0.04 | 1.73 ± 0.18 | 1.75 ± 0.11 | 0.59 ± 0.10 | 0.001 |
| ACL | 18.60 ± 0.01 | 18.58 ± 0.008 | 18.59 ± 0.005 | 18.64 ± 0.03 | 18.52 ± 0.01 | ns |
| SFA | 44.64 ± 1.33 | 43.77 ± 0.37 | 43.43 ± 0.34 | 46.51 ± 0.47 | 45.95 ± 1.81 | ns |
| UFA | 55.35 ± 1.33 | 56.22 ± 0.37 | 56.56 ± 0.34 | 53.48 ± 0.47 | 54.04 ± 1.81 | ns |
| MUFA | 25.90 ± 1.70 | 27.74 ± 0.52 | 37.22 ± 0.24 | 33.56 ± 0.92 | 35.80 ± 1.53 | 0.001 |
| PUFA | 29.45 ± 0.46 | 28.48 ± 0.25 | 19.33 ± 0.42 | 19.92 ± 0.45 | 18.24 ± 0.43 | 0.001 |
| PUFAn-6 | 15.36 ± 0.36 | 16.95 ± 0.36 | 9.34 ± 0.26 | 10.30 ± 0.30 | 8.67 ± 0.81 | 0.001 |
| PUFAn-3 | 14.08 ± 0.18 | 11.53 ± 0.34 | 9.99 ± 0.28 | 9.61 ± 0.46 | 9.57 ± 0.57 | 0.001 |

Values: mean ± SEM; n × group: 3–9. ACL, average chain length; SFA, saturated fatty acids; UFA, unsaturated fatty acids; PUFA n-6/n-3, polyunsaturated fatty acids n-6 or n-3 series; MUFA, monounsaturated fatty acids; ns, not significant.

Adapted with permission from Naudí et al. (2013a, 2013b).

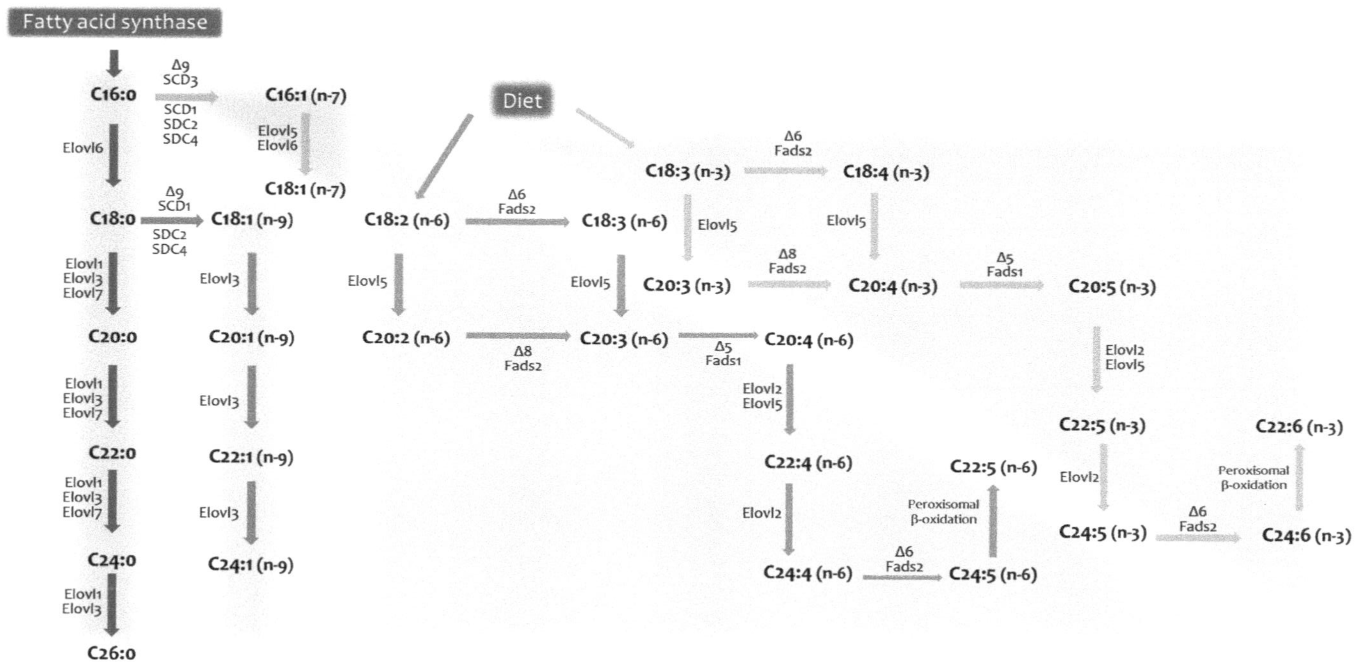


**Figure 4** See legend on next page.

Different fatty acid profiles necessarily imply different lipid molecular species, generating a region-specific lipidome. Reinforcing this possibility, it has been previously described how phospholipid composition is characteristic of the region in human brain (Söderberg et al., 1990). With regard to the specific differences in DHA content, it is relevant that these differences are due to variances in desaturase activities (Naudí et al., 2013a, 2013b). These differential desaturase activities seem to be key to support the interregional differences in fatty acid profiles and suggest the possibility that neurons can actively maintain their own compositional profile. This fact could be in conflict with the notion that neurons do not participate actively in DHA biosynthesis and that the 22:6 endowment is due to provisions proceeding from liver, endothelial cells, and astrocytes (Bazan, Molina, & Gordon, 2011; Chen, Allegood, et al., 2008; Chen, Green, et al., 2008; Kim, 2007; Spector, 2001). In this context, it is proposed that neurons can actively regulate DHA content through an active ability to synthesize DHA and to actively uptake DHA from different external sources. This

---

**Figure 4** Long-chain and very long-chain fatty acid biosynthesis in humans. The long-chain saturated fatty acids and unsaturated fatty acids of the n-10, n-7, and n-9 series can be synthesized from palmitic acid (C16:0) produced by the fatty acid synthase. Long-chain fatty acids of the n-6 and n-3 series can only be synthesized from precursors obtained from dietary precursors (DIET). It is well established that DHA can be biosynthesized from α-linolenic acid (18:3n-3), a shorter chain n-3 fatty acid precursor, through chain elongation and desaturation processes (Sprecher, 2000). Linolenic acid is desaturated to 18:4n-3 by Δ6-desaturase, chain-elongated to 20:4n-3, and subsequently converted to eicosapentaenoic acid (EPA, 20:5n-3) by Δ5-desaturase in the endoplasmic reticulum (ER). Human brain Δ5- and Δ6-desaturases have been identified and cloned (Cho, Nakamura, & Clarke, 1999a, 1999b). Then, EPA is elongated to 22:5n-3 which is further elongated to 24:5n-3 followed by desaturation by Δ6-desaturase to 24:6n-3. Subsequently, 24:6n-3 is transferred to peroxisomes and converted to 22:6n-3 by removing two carbon chains by β-oxidation (Ferdinandusse et al., 2001). DHA thus formed is transferred back to the ER and quickly incorporated into membrane lipids by esterification during *de novo* synthesis or by a deacylation–reacylation reaction. In neural membranes, DHA is found enriched in aminophospholipids, phosphatidylethanolamine (PE), and phosphatidylserine (PS), particularly as the 1-stearoyl-2-docosahexaenoyl (18:0/22:6) species (Murthy et al., 2002; Yabuuchi & O'Brien, 1968). Long-chain n-6 fatty acids are biosynthesized from linoleic acid (18:2n-6) using the analogous pathway and, apparently, the same enzyme system. In human brain, as in most tissues, the commonly observed long-chain n-6 fatty acid is arachidonic acid (AA, 20:4n-6). Docosapentaenoic acid (DPA, 22:5n-6) produced by further elongation and desaturation of AA and subsequent peroxisomal β-oxidation is a minor component. Elovl, elongation of very long-chain fatty acids (fatty acid elongase); Fads, fatty acid desaturases. *Adapted with permission from Naudí et al. (2013a, 2013b).*

would be a redundant adaptive mechanism to ensure an optimal DHA pool for neuronal needs, allowing independence from potential external fluctuations. Further studies are, however, needed to solidify these new concepts.

Using positron emission tomography (PET) and positron emitting tracers such as [1-$^{11}$C]AA and [1-$^{11}$C]DHA, PUFA incorporation or consumption rates in the human brain were measured as 17.8 mg/day/1500 g brain for AA and 4.6 mg/day/1500 g brain for DHA, respectively. The estimated whole-brain DHA concentration is 5.13 g with a half-life of 773 days (2.1 years), while the whole-brain AA concentration is 3.78 g with a half-life of 147 days (Rapoport, Rao, & Igarashi, 2007). These observations do not indicate that humans are poor DHA synthesizers on the very low turnover rate detected for DHA as suggested by some authors (Brenna, Salem, Sinclair, & Cunnane, 2009; Yamashima, 2012), but rather highlight the importance of the preservation and extreme conservation of DHA pool for the human brain. Indeed, the preservation of DHA in neural systems for 500–600 million years occurred despite enormous genomic changes since the beginning of animal evolution (Crawford et al., 2013). These authors have hypothesized that this extreme conservation implies that the DHA was actually dictating to DNA rather than the more conventional view of evolution occurring the other way round. That is, despite countless mutations that might have occurred, any mutation that sought to replace DHA with another molecule did not work. In that sense, DHA would be the master of DNA (Crawford et al., 2013). Irrespectively of these considerations, these data support an intimate relationship between DHA and brain function.

## 2.4 Functional Properties of Lipids in Human Brain

The functional properties of lipids in brain can be ascribed to their roles in the structural and functional integrity of neuronal and glial cell membranes, the generation of lipid mediators, and the chemical reactivity of the acyl chains.

### *2.4.1 Structural and Functional Integrity of Neuronal and Glial Cell Membranes*

The inherent propensity of the nonpolar acyl chains of lipids to self-assemble in water is the physical basis for spontaneous membrane formation and renders membranes virtually impermeable to polar solutes. While a single lipid species should be sufficient to generate a barrier, a cell membrane requires greater complexity and diversity in its lipid components to cover all the structural and functional needs demanded of a cell membrane. This structural diversity has profound implications by influencing generic chemical and physical membrane parameters such as geometry, curvature, fluidity, thickness, lipid-packing density, and surface charge. These properties of membrane lipids play crucial roles in neuronal and glial cell physiology, determining the regulation of ion channels and receptors, as well as the physiology of synaptic transmission, and even electrical properties (Piomelli et al., 2007).

Phospholipids constitute the bulk of the membrane's lipid matrix. A major factor determining the shape of phospholipids is the nature of their hydrophobic tail, the fatty acid residues linked to the *sn*-1 and *sn*-2 hydroxyl group on the glycerol backbone. At physiological temperatures, the length of a phospholipid molecule is directly proportional to the number of carbon atoms and inversely proportional to the number of double bonds present in its fatty acid chains. As described above, the adult human brain's average chain length is 18 carbon atoms and the average double bond index is 1.5. In addition, the molecular shape of a phospholipid within the bilayer, although influenced by the surrounding environment, is ultimately determined by the compatibility between the size of its polar head group and that of its hydrophobic tail: if the two are fully compatible, the lipid has a cylindrical form; if not, it is either conical (when the tail is larger) or inverted conical (when the head is larger). Conical lipids tend to form negatively curved monolayers, whereas inverted conical lipids tend to form positively curved monolayers (Mouritsen, 2005; McMahon & Gallop, 2005). Changes in the geometrical attributes of membrane lipids have major consequences in the functional properties of neurons.

The fatty acid chains in membrane lipids have the dominant influence on the physical properties of the membrane bilayer they constitute. Thus, for example, membrane bilayers consisting solely of PC(18:0/18:0) have a phase transition temperature of 55 °C (Silvius, 1982) which means that it is only at temperatures >55 °C that the membrane will be "fluid" (more precisely described as liquid-crystalline) and thus able to function normally. Changing the phospholipid head group, the phase transition temperature is little affected. For instance, PE(18:0/18:0) has a transition temperature of 74 °C, while for PS(18:0/18:0) it is 68 °C, and for PG(18:0/18:0) it is 55 °C (Silvius, 1982). However, replacing the fatty acids with either shorter chains or more unsaturated fatty acid chains would be a great help as it would significantly lower the transition temperature. For example, for PC(16:0/16:0) the transition temperature is 41 °C, while for

PC(18:0/18:1) it is 6 °C, and for PC(16:0/18:1) it is −2 °C, while for PC(16:1/16:1) it is −36 °C (Silvius, 1982). As indicated, adult human brain has an average chain length of 18 carbon atoms and an average double bond index of about 1.5 (Naudí et al., 2013a, 2013b). These are values that ensure an optimal fluidity and maintenance of the membrane functional properties in homeostatic conditions.

PC usually contains one *cis*-unsaturated acyl chain, such as oleic acid (18:1). The rigid kink of the *cis*-double bond lowers the packing density of the acyl chains, which increases membrane fluidity (Koynova & Caffrey, 1998). Facilitated by its cylindrical shape, PC self-assembles spontaneously into closed bilayers that adopt a liquid-crystalline state at physiological temperatures. Thus, PC is ideally suited to providing a stable and fluid matrix for cellular membranes. By contrast, PE is a conically shaped phospholipid that imposes negative curvature stress on the membrane owing to its relatively small polar head group. The nonbilayer propensity of PE increases with the degree of unsaturation of the acyl chain, creating lipid-packing defects that facilitate membrane fusion and influence the binding and activity of peripheral membrane proteins (Frolov, Shnyrova, & Zimmerberg, 2011; Marsh, 2007). Despite their relatively low abundance, PS and PI are key determinants of membrane surface charge and they mediate functional interactions with positively charged regions of peripheral and integral membrane proteins (Grinstein, 2010; Magalhaes & Glogauer, 2010).

Unlike phospholipids, sphingolipids contain primarily saturated or *trans*-monounsaturated acyl chains linked to a serine backbone. This hydrophobic structure, termed ceramide, is modified with a phosphocholine head group in the case of sphingomyelin or with saccharides in the case of glycosphingolipids. Owing to its acyl-chain composition, sphingomyelin forms a taller, narrower cylinder than PC, increasing its packing density in the membrane. Consequently, at physiological temperatures a sphingomyelin bilayer exists in a solid gel phase with tightly packed, immobile acyl chains (Koynova & Caffrey, 1998; Slotte, 2013; Van Meer, Voelker, & Feigenson, 2008). However, the addition of sterols renders these membranes fluid. Sterols (see Fig. 1B) are abundant apolar membrane lipids with an inflexible core formed by four fused rings, with cholesterol predominating in human brain. By interfering with acyl-chain packing, sterols inhibit the transition of the membrane to the solid gel state. At the same time, sterols rigidify fluid membranes by reducing the flexibility of neighboring unsaturated acyl chains, thereby increasing membrane thickness and impermeability to solutes (the so-called condensing effect of sterols)

(Yeagle, 1993). Thus, sterols allow cells to minimize unregulated solute movement across their membranes while keeping them fluid over a broad range of acyl-chain compositions and temperatures.

Together with cholesterol, sphingomyelin promotes the assembly of lateral membrane domains (lipid rafts) that may have important roles in cells (Piomelli et al., 2007). Lipid rafts are membrane microdomains intimately associated with cell signaling. These biochemical microstructures are characterized by their high contents of sphingolipids, cholesterol, and saturated fatty acids and a reduced content of PUFAs. The standard fluid-mosaic model of biological membranes does not predict this type of heterogeneity because it assigns complete freedom of lateral movement to lipids, and expects them to distribute randomly throughout the membrane. Nevertheless, lateral partitioning has been demonstrated in both artificial and natural lipid bilayers and may constitute an important organizing principle for cell membranes (Piomelli et al., 2007). Finally, in most cells, including neurons and glia, the two plasma membrane monolayers have different lipid compositions: the inner leaflet is enriched in phosphatidylserine, phosphatidylethanolamine, and phosphatidylinositol, whereas the outer leaflet is enriched in phosphatidylcholine and sphingomyelin.

Therefore, neuronal and glial cell membranes are dynamic, heterogeneous, and asymmetric entities that require continuous adjustments in the chemical structure and molecular shape of their lipid constituents, particularly phospholipids and sphingolipids. It is little appreciated that membrane lipids continually undergo very rapid cycles of deacylation and reacylation (i.e., phospholipid fatty acids are being continually removed and replaced at both the *sn*-1 and *sn*-2 carbons of the glycerol backbone of the lipid). This process is described as "membrane remodeling" and is the fundamental reason why membranes can respond very quickly to internal and external changes. It is also likely very important in the quality control of membrane lipid composition.

### 2.4.2 Lipid Signaling in the Human Brain

Lipids are information-carrying molecules in the human brain (for reviews, see Farooqui, 2009, 2012; Piomelli, 2005; Piomelli et al., 2007). Neural membrane lipids can be rapidly converted to lipid mediators or second messengers, which are lipophilic molecules that facilitate signal transduction processes, regulate cell–cell communication, and control molecular and cellular events in the brain. Lipid mediators are important endogenous regulators derived from enzymatic degradation of glycerophospholipids, sphingolipids, and cholesterol by phospholipases, sphingomyelinases, and cytochrome P450 hydroxylases, respectively. In neural cells, lipid mediators are associated with proliferation, differentiation, oxidative stress, inflammation, and apoptosis. A major group of lipid mediators, which originates in the enzymatic oxidation of arachidonic acid, is called the eicosanoids (i.e., prostaglandins, leukotrienes, thromboxanes, and lipoxins). The corresponding lipid mediators of DHA metabolism are named docosanoids. They include resolvins, protectins (neuroprotectins), and maresins. Docosanoids produce antioxidant, anti-inflammatory, and antiapoptotic effects in brain tissue. Other glycerophospholipid-derived lipid mediators are diacylglycerols (DAG), phosphatidylinositol 1,4,5-triphosphates, platelet-activating factor, lysophosphatidic acid, and endocannabinoids. Degradation of sphingolipids also results in the generation of sphingolipid-derived lipid mediators, such as ceramide, ceramide 1-phosphate, sphingosine, and sphingosine 1-phosphate. These mediators are involved in differentiation, growth, cell migration, and apoptosis. Similarly, cholesterol-derived lipid mediators including, 24- and 25-hydroxycholesterol, produce apoptosis. Abnormal metabolism of lipid mediators may be closely associated with pathogenesis of AD. Figure 5 shows representative glycerophospholipid-, sphingolipid-, and cholesterol-derived lipid mediators, and their roles in the human brain.

Lipid mediators have a peculiarity: whereas hydrophilic neurotransmitters and second messengers have limited access to the hydrophobic core of the membrane, lipids are amphipathic compounds that are generated within the bilayer and have the option to operate either inside or outside its boundaries. In other words, for this class of biomolecules the membrane is a conduit rather than a barrier (Piomelli et al., 2007). Furthermore, we can discern four additional key features of lipid-mediated signaling in the brain (Piomelli et al., 2007). First, the membrane lipid composition confers specific biophysical properties on its own membranes, but also becomes a reservoir than can be used to generate a host of intracellular and transcellular messengers on demand, in a similar way to the biosynthesis of steroid hormones. Second, such messengers are almost invariably produced through a "cascade" process in which a single biochemical route yields not one, but a sequence of functionally distinct signals. Third, lipid signals may achieve easily both nuclear and organelle receptors by virtue of its chemical properties. Finally, the system is designed to generate redundancy as different biochemical mechanisms can be used to generate the same lipid mediators. The coordination of this multiplicity of informational molecules and pathways likely stems from the

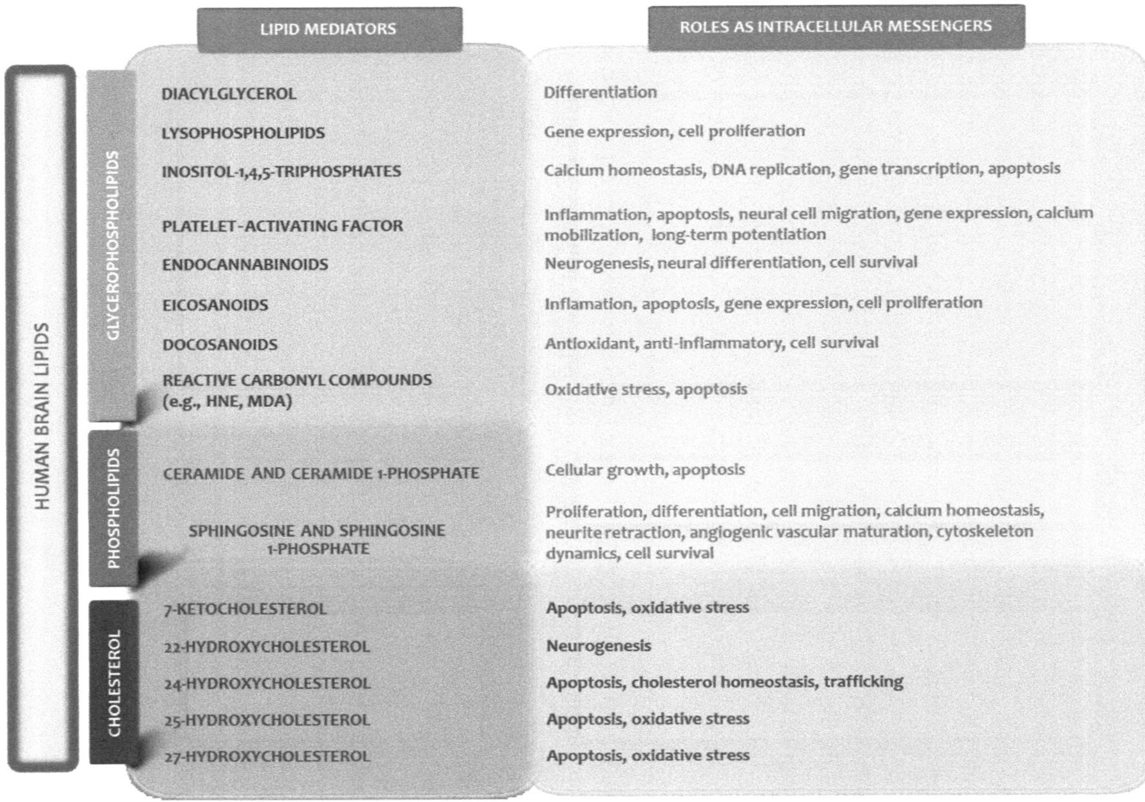


**Figure 5** Representative glycerophospholipid-, sphingolipid-, and cholesterol-derived lipid mediators, and their roles in the human brain.

temporal and spatial partitioning of lipid signaling within the heterogeneous layout of the membrane bilayer (Piomelli et al., 2007).

### 2.4.3 Chemical Reactivity of the Acyl Chains in the Human Brain

The physico-chemical properties of the membrane bilayer and the chemical reactivity of the fatty acids that compose the membrane are two inherent traits of the membrane lipids that determine their susceptibility to oxidative damage (Hulbert, Pamplona, Buffenstein, & Buttemer, 2007; Pamplona, 2008; Pamplona, Barja, & Portero-Otín, 2002). The first property is related to the fact that oxygen and reactive species physiologically generated by oxidative cell metabolism are more soluble in the fluid lipid bilayer than in the aqueous solution (Gamliel, Afri, & Frimer, 2008; Moller et al., 2005). The second and more significant property is related to the fact that PUFA residues of phospholipids are extremely sensitive to oxidation, their sensitivity increasing exponentially as a function of the number of double bonds per fatty acid molecule (Bielski, Arudi, & Sutherland, 1983; Holman, 1954). So, PUFA side chains (with two or more double bonds) are much more easily attacked by reactive species (e.g., free radicals) than are SFA (no double bonds) or MUFA (one double bond) side chains. Consequently, neural cell membrane lipids become primary targets of oxidative damage and the subsequent lipid peroxidation process.

Lipid peroxidation generates hydroperoxides as well as endoperoxides, which undergo fragmentation to produce a broad range of reactive intermediates called reactive carbonyl species (RCS) with three to nine carbons in length, the most reactive being α,β-unsaturated aldehydes [4-hydroxy-2-nonenal (HNE) and acrolein], dialdehydes [malondialdehyde (MDA) and glyoxal], and keto-aldehydes [4-oxo-2-nonenal (ONE) and isoketals] (Catalá, 2009; Esterbauer, Schaur, & Zollner, 1991; Fritz & Petersen, 2013; Zimniak, 2011) (Fig. 6A). 2-Hydroxyheptanal and 4-hydroxyhexenal are other significant aldehydic products of lipid peroxidation of PUFAs. These carbonyl compounds, ubiquitously generated in biological systems, have unique properties contrasted with other reactive species. For instance, compared with reactive oxygen species (ROS), reactive aldehydes have a much greater half-life (i.e., minutes to hours instead of nanoseconds to microseconds for most ROS). Further, the noncharged structure of RCS allows them to migrate easily through hydrophobic membranes and hydrophilic cytosolic media, thereby extending the migration distance far from the generation site (Pamplona, 2008). In addition to aldehyde formation, lipid hydroperoxyl radicals undergo endocyclization to produce fatty acid esters; two classes of these

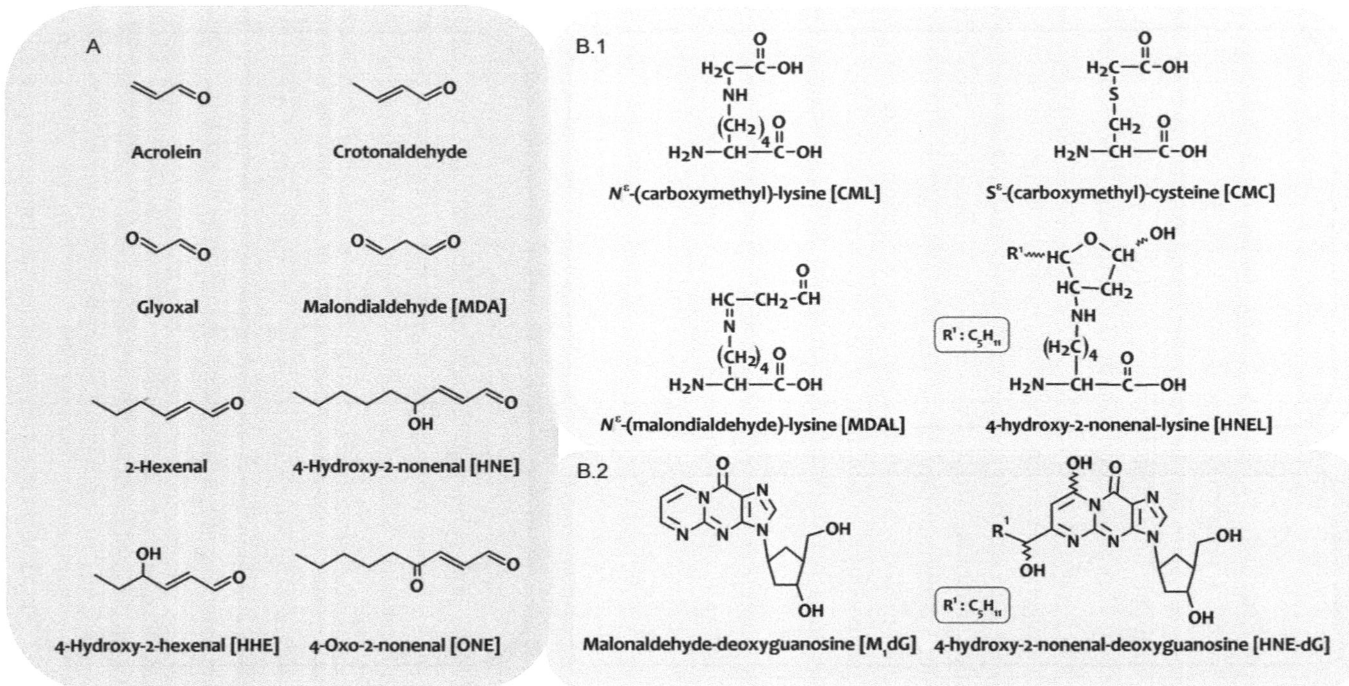


**Figure 6** (A) General structures of principal lipoxidation-derived reactive carbonyl species detected in human brain. (B) Reactive carbonyl species generated by lipid peroxidation react with nucleophilic groups in macromolecules (B.1, proteins; B.2, DNA) resulting in their chemical, nonenzymatic, irreversible modification, and formation of a variety of adducts and crosslinks collectively named advanced lipoxidation end-products (ALEs). ALE-proteins represented in the figure have been detected in adult human brain.

cyclized fatty acids are isoprostanes and neuroprostanes (Sultana, Perluigi, & Butterfield, 2013). All these compounds have been detected, characterized, and located (by MS and immunohistochemistry) in the human brain.

These compounds have specific physiological signaling roles inducing adaptive responses to decrease oxidative damage and improve antioxidant defenses (Higdon, Diers, Oh, Landar, & Darley-Usmar, 2012; Pamplona, 2008; Pamplona, 2011). Two of these mechanisms involved in the prevention of oxidative damage effects are (i) the regulation of uncoupling protein activity (Brand et al., 2004; Echtay et al., 2003) and (ii) the activation of the antioxidant response signaling pathway (Nrf2 pathway) that includes the expression of enzymes such as glutathione-*S*-transferase (GST) specifically designed to detoxify reactive carbonyl compounds (Copple, Goldring, Kitteringham, & Park, 2008; Giles, 2009; Maher & Yamamoto, 2010; Wakabayashi et al., 2004). As important as GST for these adaptive mechanisms is the role GPx4 (phospholipid hydroperoxide glutathione peroxidase) has in restoring reduced states of membrane fatty acids from phospholipids to ensure membrane lipid homeostasis (Brigelius-Flohé, 2006; Conrad, Schneider, Seiler, & Bornkamm, 2007; Imai & Nakagawa, 2003).

Based on the features mentioned above, these carbonyl compounds can be, however, more destructive than ROS and may have far-reaching damaging effects on target sites within or outside membranes. Carbonyl compounds react with nucleophilic groups in macromolecules (lipoxidation reactions) like proteins (Thorpe & Baynes, 2003), DNA (West & Marnett, 2006), and aminophospholipids (Naudí et al., 2013a, 2013b), among others, resulting in their chemical, nonenzymatic, and irreversible modification, and formation of a variety of adducts and crosslinks collectively named advanced lipoxidation endproducts (ALEs) (Pamplona, 2011; Thorpe & Baynes, 2003) (Fig. 6B.1 and 6B.2). The physico-chemical and biological effects derived from ALE formation include protein alterations in physico-chemical properties (conformation, charge, hydrophobicity, and solubility), formation of intra- and intermolecular protein crosslinks and aggregates, loss of enzymatic activity, and DNA damage and mutagenesis, among several others (Pamplona, 2008, 2011). Additionally, ALE formation is also involved in the generation of lipofuscin, a yellow-brown pigment already described in human neurons by Hannover in 1843 (Hannover, 1843; Ottis et al., 2012) (see later).

Consequently, the high concentration of PUFAs in neuronal and glial cell membrane phospholipids not only makes them prime targets for reaction with oxidizing agents but also enables them to participate in long free radical chain reactions. The regulatory function and cytotoxicity of the lipid peroxidation-derived aldehydes hinges on their abundance, reactivity, and half-life. In this scenario, from a given membrane fatty acid profile it is possible to calculate its peroxidizability index (PI) by combining this composition with the relative susceptibility of individual fatty acids to peroxidation. So, PI is an approach to the relative susceptibility of a given membrane fatty acid composition to peroxidative damage. The higher the number the more susceptible, the lower the value of PI, the more resistant to lipid peroxidation is the membrane bilayer (Hulbert et al., 2007; Pamplona et al., 2002). Figure 7 shows the presence of cross-regional differences in the PI in the human central nervous system and, consequently, establishes a cross-regional selective neuronal vulnerability (SNV).

The different cross-regionally PIs observed are due to changes in the type of unsaturated fatty acid that participates in membrane composition. So, there is a systematic redistribution between the types of PUFAs present from highly unsaturated fatty acids to the less unsaturated that is region-specific (see Table 2). Surprisingly, the change shows a gradient that follows the cranio-caudal axis considering the structural organization of the human central nervous system. The mechanism(s) responsible for the cross-regional-related differences in fatty acid profile could be related, in principle, to the fatty acid desaturation pathway, and the deacylation–reacylation cycle. The mechanism underlying the membrane unsaturation regulation could

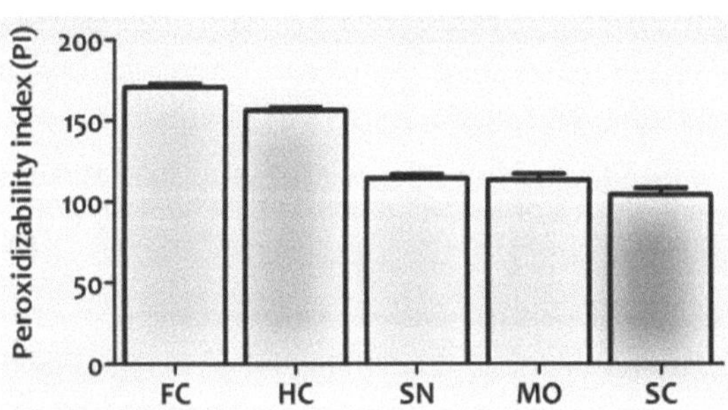


**Figure 7** Cross-regional differences in the peroxidizability index (PI) in the human central nervous system. FC, frontal cortex; HC, hippocampus; SN, substantia nigra; MO, medulla oblongata; SC, spinal cord. [PI = 0.025 × (% monoenoics) + 1 × (% dienoics) + 2 × (% trienoics) + 4 × (% tetraenoics) + 6 × (% pentaenoics) + 8 × (% hexaenoics)] (Hulbert et al., 2007). *Adapted with permission from Naudí et al. (2013a, 2013b).*

explain the differences in membrane fatty acid composition and, in turn, the PI, suggesting a region-specific regulatory mechanism that is expressed differentially in a cranio-caudal axis likely associated with the development process and even the evolution of the central nervous system.

## 3. LIPIDOMICS OF HUMAN BRAIN AGING

Human brain performs a wide range of motor, sensory, regulatory, behavioral, and cognitive functions which decline with advancing age and, especially in neurodegenerative conditions associated with aging, such as AD pathology. However, currently it became clear that neuronal cell number is largely preserved in the neocortex and hippocampus of the aging human brain, declining only in the setting of AD. Cells in the human brain are affected by, and respond to, aging much as cells in other organ systems do. Yet, deterioration in structure and function of the adult human brain during aging is not uniform throughout the brain. Consequently, human brain aging must be considered as a heterogeneous process probably subject to a region-specific (and even cell) SNV (Jové et al., 2014; Mattson & Magnus, 2006; Wang, Michaelis, & Michaelis, 2010). Yet, SNV is often ignored in the study of brain aging (and AD). By definition, SNV refers to the fact that select populations of neurons are more vulnerable to injury or death under adverse conditions, whereas other neurons are relatively resistant to such stresses in their environment. The selective vulnerability of some neurons is often manifested in structural and functional changes that may or may not lead to cell death. For example, vulnerable neurons often suffer loss of dendrites that leads to a significant impairment of synaptic transmission, but the cells may still survive for a time in this altered state. Therefore, understanding the mechanisms underlying SNV is an essential step in efforts to develop strategies to moderate the deleterious impact of aging (and AD) on the overall human quality of life. In this frame, it is plausible to hypothesize that cross-regional differences in human brain lipid composition could be responsible for this SNV which, in turn, leads to different rates of aging.

Human brain aging and AD pathology do not affect all neurons equally. Thus, for example, in the hippocampus, neurons in the CA1 region are vulnerable to brain aging and AD, but those in the nearby CA3 region are not nearly as heavily damaged as the CA1 neurons (Giannakopoulos, Gold,

Michel, & Bouras, 1998; Mueller et al., 2007; O'Banion, Coleman, & Callahan, 1994). In addition, a profile of selective loss of synapses and neurons in certain brain regions has been described for both the aging process (Morrison & Hof, 1997; Morrison, Hof, & Morrison, 1998; Terry, DeTeresa, & Hansen, 1987) and AD (Braak & Braak, 1991, 1992; Morrison & Hof, 2007; Price et al., 1987). These studies have been performed, for the most part, at the histological level and have identified relatively few neurochemical changes that correlate with either neuronal vulnerability or resistance to age- or AD-associated injury or death. This SNV of certain human brain neurons could be an intrinsic characteristic associated with the lipid pattern of these neurons.

Brain volumetric measurements (by noninvasive techniques such as structural brain imaging and functional magnetic resonance imaging) as well as the PET and measures of cerebral metabolic rate of glucose (CMRGl) reinforce the notion that aging affects some regions of the brain more than others. In addition to the volume changes in select regions of the brain during aging [the association cortex, the neostriatum, and the cerebellum are the most vulnerable regions to age-dependent loss of volume, whereas the primary sensory cortices (such as the visual cortex), the entorhinal cortex, the paleostriatum, and the pons show much less shrinkage (Raz & Rodrigue, 2006; Raz, Rodrigue, & Haacke, 2007)], it has been repeatedly shown that the frontal cortex shows the greatest and most consistent decrements in CMRGl as compared with all other regions in the cortex or subcortical components of the aging brain (Loessner et al., 1995; Reiman et al., 2010). These changes in metabolic activity in select cortical areas during aging are either related to altered neuronal expression of some key enzymes controlling the overall metabolic state of neurons and associated glial cells, or they are the result of altered activation of synapses or of the disruptive effects of abnormal neuronal excitability during aging (Wang et al., 2010). Gene expression analyses, in combination with neuroimaging studies, as well as detailed histological investigations, are providing new windows onto the molecular and cellular changes that might account for such differential patterns of neuronal susceptibility to the aging process and to AD (Wang et al., 2010). In these studies, however, the possible involvement of membrane lipids and lipid metabolism in the cellular alterations observed during aging is simply ignored. It should also be emphasized that neuronal losses during aging even in select, sensitive regions are relatively modest, whereas decreases in the number of synapses in the same regions appear to be a more prominent characteristic of brain aging. These observations have led to the assertion that most of the functional decline associated with normal aging is caused by relatively subtle changes, such as loss of dendrites, reductions in spine densities, altered spine morphologies, or changes in the molecular profile of synapses (Burke & Barnes, 2006; Mattson & Magnus, 2006; Morrison & Hof, 2002; West, Coleman, Flood, & Troncoso, 1994). All these changes have to be associated with or due to alterations in the neural membrane lipid profile.

In order to study how human brain regions differentially respond to the stresses associated with increasing age, some investigators have used functional genomics approaches (Berchtold et al., 2008; Evans et al., 2003; Fraser, Khaitovich, Plotkin, Pääbo, & Eisen, 2005; Khaitovich et al., 2004; Liang et al., 2007). Such studies have provided further support for the concept of regional heterogeneity with respect to the differential rates of aging-associated changes. Furthermore, these works demonstrate that the most prominent ontological categories among the differentially expressed genes were those of intracellular signaling, neurogenesis, synaptic transmission, transcription factor regulation, and calcium ion [$Ca^{2+}$] regulation. Other investigators have used lipidomics approaches, though the number of these studies is still rather limited.

The studies by Burger and Seidel (1958) and Rouser and Yamamoto (1968), both performed in whole-brain samples, were the first evidence that the membrane lipid composition of the human brain changes with aging. Burger and Seidel (1958) found that the amount of total lipids increased during the first two decades of life and then began to decrease. Rouser and Yamamoto (1968) also demonstrated a curvilinear regression of human brain lipid levels with age; however, as pointed out by Ledesma, Martin, and Dotti (2012), in both studies, the use of whole brains to analyze lipids resulted in variations in lipid content that also reflected changes in the proportions of gray and white matter.

More recent studies analyzing the lipid composition of different areas of human brain have confirmed the occurrence of age-related lipid alterations. Overall, all the described changes are perfectly aligned to the progressive and deleterious character of the aging process, and it seems that concentrations of most lipids in the human brain decrease after the age of 50. So, PI, PE, and PC brain levels decrease very slowly with age, with less than 10% loss in the period between age 40 and 100 (Farooqui, Liss, & Horrocks, 1988). In another study, 10–20% loss of phospholipids in different brain regions (gray matter, white matter, nucleus caudatus, hippocampus, pons, cerebellum, medulla oblongata) was observed only in individuals between age 89 and

92 compared to 33- to 36-year-old individuals, while phospholipid composition in various brain regions stayed unchanged during aging (Söderberg et al., 1990). Phospholipid decrease starts slowly after age 20 and, after age 80 becomes more pronounced, with no significant difference in lipid profile between male and female brains (Svennerholm, Boström, Helander, & Jungbjer, 1991; Svennerholm, Boström, Jungbjer, & Olsson, 1994). Additionally, no changes were observed in the mole percentage of lipid classes and fatty acids in lipid rafts from normal brains (human frontal brain cortex) throughout the lifespan (24–85 years) (Martín et al., 2010). In contrast, ethanolamine plasmalogen (PPE) brain levels decrease 18% (till the age of 70) and 29% (till the age of 100), and sphingomyelin brain levels decrease 12% and 20% in the same time period, respectively (Horrocks, VanRollins, & Yates, 1981). In line with these studies, a recent (and unique) study focused on the human brain fatty acid profile (McNamara, Liu, Jandacek, Rider, & Tso, 2008). The goal of this work was to examine whether orbitofrontal cortex (OFC, Brodmann area 10) gray matter fatty acid composition changed during normal aging in subjects aged 29–80 years ($n=30$). The results showed that increasing age was associated with a progressive decline in PUFA composition, including DHA and arachidonic acid (AA, 20:4n-6) (globally a decrease of 15% is documented), and transient, apparently compensatory, elevations in elongase and desaturase gene expression. The age-related reduction in PUFA composition was inversely correlated with stearoyl-CoA desaturase expression and activity resulting in elevations in MUFAs (an increase of 21% was observed). The authors proposed that these dynamic age-related changes in OFC gray matter fatty acid composition and biosynthetic gene expression may contribute to the progressive decline in OFC gray matter volume found with advancing age, though in transversal studies it is always difficult to establish cause–consequence relationships.

The described changes in the fatty acid pattern, despite being restricted to a unique human cerebral area (further studies are needed to learn the behavior of the fatty acid pattern across the aging process in different brain regions), seem to suggest that there is not an increase in the PI (because of the decrease in PUFA content). Consequently, no changes, or even a slight decrease in the steady-state levels of ALEs, would be detected. Unfortunately, no data are available on this issue, pointing to the need for further studies in this field. Yet, a recent work evaluating the human brain lipofuscin proteome was stimulating (Ottis et al., 2012). Lipofuscin, first described in neurons by Hannover (1843), is a yellow-brown pigment chemically and morphologically polymorphous and consists of electron-dense material and features autofluorescence with characteristic spectral properties (Seehafer & Pearce, 2006). These pigment granules consist of approximately two-thirds protein and one-third lipids (Jolly, Douglas, Davey, & Roiri, 1995; Porta, 1991). Lipofuscin, often referred to as "aging pigment," is located primarily in secondary lysosomes or residual bodies of neurons (Terman & Brunk, 1998) and accumulates in a linear relation to age but differing according to the neuronal subtypes (Mann, Yates, & Stamp, 1978). In this context, the work of Ottis et al. (2012) using a proteomics approach found in aged human brain major lipofuscin targets, proteins belonging to cytoskeleton, mitochondrial bioenergetics, synapse, and cell membrane receptors. This proteome is practically identical to the proteome derived from lipoxidation reactions described in the frontal cortex of aged humans (Pamplona et al., 2005), suggesting the existence of a pool of proteins (which play key roles in cell physiology) particularly vulnerable to lipoxidative damage.

Finally, the available evidence also suggests a region-specific effect of aging on brain cholesterol content. Thus, the studies of Svennerholm et al. (1994) and Söderberg et al. (1990)) report a reduction in cholesterol levels starting at 20 years of age in human frontal and temporal cortices, as well as hippocampus, nucleus caudatus, medulla oblongata, and cerebellum. Interestingly, the rate of reduction in cholesterol content is region-dependent, likely expressing differences in metabolic needs of each specific region, as well as different responses to aging. This decrease in cholesterol levels could be associated with a decreased synthesis (Thelen, Falkai, Bayer, & Lütjohann, 2006) and increased catabolism (Martin et al., 2008) of cholesterol during aging leading to an overall decrease in levels of this lipid.

Globally, the available evidence suggests that major adult human brain lipids undergo progressive and significant changes in their concentrations and distribution during the aging process. However, the individual contribution of these lipid patterns to the aging process is nowadays unknown. Therefore, a goal of future research is to define which types of lipids change with age in the different human brain areas and how they relate both to the function of the area and to the dysfunction leading to neuropathology. Indeed, it is not yet known whether the changes in the confirmed lipids represent neutral changes with age, changes causal to physiological aspects of aging, or beneficial responses to damaging agents. Furthermore, these studies make evident the power of lipidomics as a tool to better understand the phenotype of aging in the human population and to link this knowledge in functional studies to aging pathways. In summary, the described findings suggest that lipid species and their metabolism are closely linked to human brain aging.

## 4. LIPIDOMICS OF ALZHEIMER'S DISEASE PATHOLOGY

AD is a neurodegenerative disorder neuropathologically characterized by extracellular deposits of β-amyloid (Aβ40 and Aβ42 as the main species) in the brain parenchyma forming senile plaques and giving rise around cerebral blood vessels to β-amyloid angiopathy, and intraneuronal deposits of hyper-phosphorylated, abnormally conformed, and truncated tau structuring neurofibrillary tangles (NFTs), dystrophic neurites of senile plaques, and neuropil threads (Duyckaerts & Dickson, 2011). A minority of patients suffer from early-onset familial AD (EOFAD) linked to mutations of the genes encoding β-amyloid precursor protein (APP), presenilin 1 (PSN1), and presenilin 2 (PSN2) (Bertram & Tanzi, 2011). The majority of AD cases have a late onset (LOAD) which develops as sporadic AD (sAD or AD) in spite of the putative combination of low penetrating genetic factors and environmental factors that may be involved in their pathogenesis (Bertram & Tanzi, 2011).

In AD, early abnormal tau deposition appears in selected nuclei of the brainstem followed by the entorhinal cortex and olfactory bulb and tracts; later on, it extends to the hippocampal complex, basal forebrain, and limbic system, and eventually to the whole cerebral cortex and other regions such as the striatum and thalamus (Braak & Braak, 1991, 1999; Braak, Thal, Ghebremedhin, & del Tredici, 2011; Grinberg et al., 2009; Simic et al., 2009). Systematic anatomical studies have allowed the categorization of stages of disease progression based on the accumulation of lesions in the brain. Braak and Braak stages I–II are manifested by NFTs in the olfactory bulb and tracts, and entorhinal cortex, followed by the transentorhinal cortex and initial CA1; stages III–IV show increased number of NFTs in the preceding regions and extension of NFTs to the whole CA1 region of the hippocampus, subiculum, temporal cortex, magnocellular nuclei of the basal forebrain including Meynert nucleus, amygdala, anterodorsal thalamic nuclei, and tubero-mammillary nucleus; stages V–VI entail, in addition to the increased severity in the above-mentioned areas, the cortical association areas including the frontal and parietal cortices, the claustrum, reticular nuclei of the thalamus, and, finally, the primary sensory areas compromising the primary visual cortex (Braak & Braak, 1991, 1999; Braak et al., 2011). β-amyloid deposits first appear in the OFC and temporal cortex, and they then progress practically to the whole cerebral cortex, diencephalic nuclei, and lastly, the cerebellum Braak & Braak, 1991, 1999; Thal, Rüb, Orantes, & Braak, 2002). Regarding senile plaques, Braak and Braak stage A is characterized by plaques in the basal neocortex, particularly the orbitofrontal and temporal cortices; stage B involves, in addition, the association cortices; and stage C, the primary cortical areas (Braak & Braak, 1991, 1999).

Importantly, cognitive impairment clinically categorized as mild or moderate may occur at stages III–IV, whereas dementia can appear in individuals with AD pathology at stages V–VI (Markesbery, 2010; Nelson et al., 2012; Price et al., 2009). The time between the first appearance of AD-related pathology and the development of cognitive decline and dementia has been estimated to be several decades in those individuals in whom dementia eventually occurs (Ohm, Müller, Braak, & Bohl, 1995). It is worth stressing that AD-related pathology, including stages I–II, is present in about 85% of individuals aged 65 (Braak & Braak, 1997; Braak et al., 2011; Ferrer, 2012). Therefore, AD can be considered a very common and relatively well-tolerated degenerative process during a long period of time, but it may have devastating effects once thresholds are crossed (Ferrer, 2012). These facts highlight the need to gain information about the first silent stages of the neurodegenerative process with the aim of understanding early pathogenic mechanisms and identifying possible targets for therapeutic intervention geared to curbing or retarding progression to clinical stages (Ferrer, 2012; McGeer & McGeer, 2013; Selkoe, 2012).

In addition to these pathological hallmarks, multiple alterations converge in the pathogenesis of AD. Mitochondrial functional defects, increased production of oxidative and nitrosative reactive species (ROS and NOS), and damage to enzymes involved in energy metabolism are causative of nerve cell exhaustion (Ferrer, 2009; Jové et al., 2014; Pamplona et al., 2005; Sultana & Butterfield, 2010). Altered production of trophic factors, neurotransmitter, and neuromodulators, together with impaired function of degradation pathways such as those related to cytoplasmic proteolysis, autophagy, and the ubiquitin–proteasome system, play crucial roles as well (Cataldo, Paskevich, Kominami, & Nixon, 1991; Ferrer, 2012; Keller, Hanni, & Markesbery, 2000; Selkoe, 2012; Wang et al., 2010). Altered lipid composition of neural membranes also seems to play an important role.

## 4.1 Evidence for Disturbance of Human Brain Lipid Content in AD Pathology

Lipidomic analyses have uncovered multiple lipid alterations which are disease-specific in the brain of AD patients (Han, 2010; Haughey, Bandaru, Bae, & Mattson, 2010; Frisardi, Panza, Seripa, Farooqui, & Farooqui, 2011; Kosicek & Hecimovic, 2013; Sultana et al., 2013; Touboul & Gaudin, 2014; Wood, 2012). The disturbance of human brain lipid content in AD pathology can be grouped into four notions: (i) phospholipid classes, specifically plasmalogen PE (PPE) and plasmalogen PC (PPC) content, are significantly reduced at the earliest clinically recognizable stage of AD (i.e., mild cognitive impairment (MCI)), and impair as AD progresses; (ii) sulfatide content is specifically depleted in patients with MCI, and it is aggravated in the different AD stages; (iii) ceramide levels are significantly higher in subjects with MCI, increasing with advanced AD stages; and (iv) lipoxidative stress is significantly higher in AD patients, increasing with advanced AD stages. Altogether, the changes in brain lipidome induced by AD may play an important role in AD pathogenesis and may be linked to the pathological process of AD including oxidative molecular damage, synapse loss, synaptic dysfunction, alteration in lipid signaling that favors neuronal dysfunction and apoptosis, and neurodegeneration. Table 3 offers a comprehensive list of studies reporting lipid changes in the brain of individuals with AD pathology.

The origin and meaning of the specific PPE and PPC decrease with AD deserve special mention. At the present moment, these changes in phospholipid dynamics in AD [decreased PPE and PPC content (Ginsberg, Rafique, Xuereb, Rapoport, & Gershfeld, 1995; Goodenowe et al., 2007; Han, 2005; Han et al., 2001; Igarashi et al., 2011; Wood et al., 2010), decreased phospholipid precursors for their synthesis (Ellison, Beal, & Martin, 1987; Molina et al., 1998; Nitsch et al., 1992), as well as increased brain levels of their degradation product (Nitsch et al., 1992)] have been described as being the result of a peroxisomal dysfunction [the formation of PPE and PPC is conducted in peroxisomes (Wallner & Schmitz, 2011)] in both the liver and brain (Astarita et al., 2010; Grimm et al., 2011; Goodenowe et al., 2007; Kou et al., 2011), a conclusion further supported by the accumulation of VLCFAs in AD brain, also metabolized by peroxisomes (Kou et al., 2011). However, in addition to this explanation, additional mechanisms should be considered.

**Table 3** Studies Reporting Lipid Changes in the Brain of Individuals with AD Pathology

| Lipid Class | Analytical Method | Sample Size | Brain Regions | Change | References |
|---|---|---|---|---|---|
| PE | Spectrophotometry | 10AD vs. 10C | Frontal, primary auditory, and parietal cortices | Decreased | Nitsch et al. (1992) |
| PE | TLC | 9AD vs. 9Cs | Subiculum, superior-middle temporal gyrus, inferior parietal lobe, and cerebellum | Decreased | Prasad, Lovell, Yatin, Dhillon, and Markesbery (1998) |
| PPE | HPLC and TLC | 9AD vs. 9C | Middle temporal cortex | Decreased | Ginsberg et al. (1995) |
| PPE | HPLC and GC | 15AD vs. 13C | Frontal cortex, hippocampus, and white matter | Decreased | Guan et al. (1999) |
| PPE | $^{31}$P NMR | 45AD vs. 11C | Superior-middle frontal gyrus, superior temporal gyrus, inferior parietal lobe, occipital cortex, and cerebellum | Decreased | Pettegrew, Panchalingam, Hamilton, and McClure (2001) |
| PC | HPLC | 10AD vs. 10C | Frontal, primary auditory, and parietal cortices | Decreased | Nitsch et al. (1992) |
| PC | HPLC | 6AD vs. 4C | Frontal cortex, parietal, and temporal region | Unchanged | Wells, Farooqui, Liss, and Horrocks (1995) |
| PC | TLC | 9AD vs. 9C | Subiculum, superior-middle temporal gyrus, inferior parietal lobe, and cerebellum | Unchanged | Prasad et al. (1998) |

*Continued*

**Table 3** Studies Reporting Lipid Changes in the Brain of Individuals with AD Pathology—cont'd

| Lipid Class | Analytical Method | Sample Size | Brain Regions | Change | References |
|---|---|---|---|---|---|
| PC | HPLC and GC | 15AD vs. 13C | Frontal cortex, hippocampus, and white matter | Decreased | Guan et al. (1999) |
| PI | TLC | 9AD vs. 9C | Subiculum, superior-middle temporal gyrus, inferior parietal gyrus, and cerebellum | Decreased | Prasad et al. (1998) |
| PI | TLC | 17AD vs. 18C | Anterior temporal cortex | Decreased | Stokes and Hawthorne (1987) |
| PI | $^{31}P$ NMR | 45AD vs. 11C | Superior-middle frontal gyrus, superior temporal gyrus, inferior parietal lobe, occipital cortex, and cerebellum | Decreased | Pettegrew et al. (2001) |
| SM | $^{31}P$ NMR | 45AD vs. 11C | Superior-middle frontal gyrus, superior temporal gyrus, inferior parietal lobe, occipital cortex, and cerebellum | Increased | Pettegrew et al. (2001) |
| SM | ESI-MS | 7AD vs. 7C | Middle frontal gyrus, superior frontal gyrus, and cerebellum | Decreased | Cutler et al. (2004) |
| SM | ESI-MS | 30AD vs. 26C | Middle frontal gyrus, middle temporal gyrus, and cerebellum | Increased | Bandaru et al. (2009) |
| SM | HPLC | 9AD vs. 6C | Frontotemporal area | Decreased | He, Huang, Li, Gong, and Schuchman (2010) |

| | | | | | |
|---|---|---|---|---|---|
| Ceramide | HPLC | 9AD vs. 6C | Frontotemporal area | Increased | He et al. (2010) |
| Ceramide | ESI-MS | 7AD vs. 7C | Middle frontal gyrus, superior frontal gyrus, and cerebellum | Increased | Cutler et al. (2004) |
| Sulfatide | QqQ-MS | 6AD vs. 8C | Superior frontal gyrus | Decreased | Cheng, Wang, Li, Cairns, and Han (2013) |
| Gangliosides | TLC-Blot and MALDI-QIT-TOF MS | 4AD vs. 4C | Inferior frontal gyrus and hippocampus | Decreased/ increased | Valdes-Gonzalez et al. (2011) |

Abbreviations: AD, Alzheimer's disease; C, control healthy human subjects. Lipid classes: PE, phosphatidylethanolamine; PPE, plasmalogen phosphatidylethanolamine; PC, phosphatidylcholine; PI, phosphatidylinositol; SM, sphingomyelin. Analytical methods: HPLC, high-performance liquid chromatography; TLC, thin-layer chromatography; GC, gas chromatography; NMR, nuclear magnetic resonance.

Plasmalogens are a subclass of GPs that possess a vinyl ether fatty alcohol substituent at *sn*-1 position of the glycerol backbone. PE is quantitatively the major phospholipid in human brain (35.6%) and the predominant form is the PPE, accounting for 50–60% of the PE class of lipids in the whole human brain. PPC accounts for only about 2% of the total PC (32.8%) in human brain. Therefore, PPE represents the major structural phospholipid pool in human brain. It is well known that PPE plays an important role as an antioxidant in cellular membranes (Brosche & Platt, 1998) since the products of enol ether oxidation do not propagate the oxidation of PUFAs. Furthermore, in cellular membranes, the inner leaflet is enriched in the PE lipid class (and, consequently, PPE), whereas the outer leaflet is enriched in PC lipid class (where 2% should be PPC). Therefore, the inner leaflet, exposed to the intracellular milieu, is specifically enriched in a lipid with antioxidant properties. This characteristic should be considered as an adaptive evolutionary mechanism developed by neural cells in order to protect them in the face of oxidative stress, and evidence of the relevance of oxidative stress homeostasis in neural physiology (Jové et al., 2014; Pamplona & Costantini, 2011). In addition, in gray matter, the major PPE molecular species are enriched in DHA and AA at *sn*-2 position. DHA and AA are PUFAs with a high content in double bonds and, consequently, with a high PI. But, in addition, both unsaturated fatty acids are precursors of relevant lipid mediators. Therefore, DHA and AA are PUFAs that show a double face: a protective role (the adaptive responses derived from their lipid mediators) and a deleterious role (derived from their susceptibility to oxidation). In this frame, it is proposed that the disease-specific decrements in PPE (and PPC), as well as DHA and AA, reported in AD (particularly in very affected areas such as hippocampus, and apparently in contradiction to the levels reported in frontal cortex (see later)) are the result of two mechanisms: increased oxidative damage and an increased consumption of DHA and AA as precursors of eicosanoids and docosanoids—that is, lipid mediators that probably are trying to cope with the oxidative conditions in order to sustain neuronal survival.

In AD brain, and subjects with MCI, increased lipid peroxidation has been identified by measuring the levels of free and protein-bound 4-hydroxy-2-nonenal, F2-Isoprostanes, F4-neuroprostanes, isoprostane 8,12-iso-iPF2α-VI, MDA, and acrolein (reviewed in Martínez, Portero-Otin, Pamplona, & Ferrer, 2010; Sultana et al., 2013), suggesting that lipid peroxidation is an early event in the progression of AD. Furthermore, lipid peroxidation products, as mentioned above, react with cell components, resulting in the direct oxidation of amino acids, glycoxidation, and lipoxidation in AD brain as indexed by the presence and concentrations of glutamic and aminoadipic semialdehydes, carboxymethyl-lysine, carboxyethyllysine, and malondialdehyde-lysine (Martínez et al., 2010; Pamplona et al., 2005). Furthermore, this increased lipoxidative protein damage in AD patients preferentially affects a set of proteins related to cytoskeleton and metabolism/energy production (Pamplona et al., 2005) in a similar way to the lipofuscin proteome previously described (Ottis et al., 2012). And more interestingly, a recent study (Benseny-Cases, Klementieva, Cotte, Ferrer, & Cladera, 2014), using Fourier transform infrared microscopy, reported that in samples from patients diagnosed with AD, the plaques (amyloid peptides are the main component of one of the characteristic pathological hallmarks of AD: senile plaques) and their immediate surroundings are always characterized by the specific presence of oxidized lipids. In consequence, oxidative stress may be a major risk (or causal?) factor for AD origin and progression (Frisardi et al., 2011; Jové et al., 2014; Sultana et al., 2013) and the PPE deficiency in AD supports the oxidative stress hypothesis.

Lipid rafts are also affected by AD pathology. The presence of lipid alterations in lipid rafts from the frontal cortex in late stages of AD has been recently demonstrated. Thus, a recent study (Martín et al., 2010) revealed that lipid rafts from AD brains (frontal cortex) exhibit aberrant lipid profiles compared to healthy brains. In particular, lipid rafts from AD brains displayed abnormally low levels of PUFAn-3 (mainly DHA) and monoenes (mainly oleic acid), as well as reduced unsaturation and PIs. Also, multiple relationships between phospholipids and fatty acids were altered in AD lipid rafts. Significantly, the disruption of such mechanisms in AD brains leads to a considerable increase in lipid raft order and viscosity, which may explain the alterations in lipid raft signaling observed in AD. More importantly, these lipid alterations at the level of lipid rafts were observed in AD brains from the earliest stages of AD, namely, AD I/II (Fabelo et al., 2014). Thus, these changes in the lipid matrix of lipid rafts affected both lipid classes and fatty acids (reduced unsaturation index and increased saturate/polyunsaturated ratios in phospholipid acyl chains) and were also detected in the entorhinal cortex (in addition to frontal cortex), but not in the cerebellum from the same subjects. Paralleling these changes, lipid rafts from AD frontal and entorhinal cortices displayed higher anisotropy for environment-sensitive probes, indicating that lipid changes in AD lipid rafts increased membrane order and viscosity in these domains (Díaz et al., 2015; Fabelo et al., 2014). The pathophysiological consequences of these alterations in the development and progression of AD were strengthened by the significant, and specific, accumulation of β-secretase within the lipid rafts of AD subjects even at the earliest stages, providing a mechanistic connection between lipid alterations in these microdomains and amyloidogenic processing of amyloid precursor protein (Díaz et al., 2015; Fabelo et al., 2014).

## 4.2 Docosahexaenoic Acid and Alzheimer's Disease Pathology: An Allostatic Adaption

In the healthy state, the adult human brain lipidome is under strict homeostatic control. Lipidome is adapted to the structural and functional needs of the neural cells in a region-specific way. Some basic characteristics are shared between regions such as the average chain length (18 carbon atoms) and the ratio SFA:UFAs (40:60, respectively), but there are differences for other lipid traits such as the particular content of DHA which is strictly maintained in a range between 8% and 13% depending on the specific region. This DHA content ensures the specific and special structural and functional properties of the neural cells (and particularly neurons), covers the generation of lipid mediators that signal cells for specific functions and survival mechanisms and, additionally, functions as a target of oxidative damage based on the high susceptibility derived from the number of double bonds. Curiously, DHA synthesis requires oxidative conditions and, in its turn, DHA is a target of oxidative stress. To maintain this dynamic pool of DHA constant, cells offer several mechanisms including biosynthesis pathways (for DHA, lipid mediators, antioxidants), and lipid remodeling and repair mechanisms which are under homeostatic control.

During the aging process, this homeostatic system is under pressure. Thus, the persistence of oxidative stress in time induces a slow but progressive increase in the oxidative (and lipoxidative) molecular damage and the general oxidative conditions. This new and changing oxidative stress state demands an adaptive physiological response which will need to be maintained over time. Therefore, oxidative stress conditions force an allostatic response to maintain the homeostatic system. This allostatic adaption (to explore the concept of allostatic load, see Hyötyläinen & Orešič, 2014; Korte, Koolhaas, Wingfield, & McEwen, 2005) will imply a metabolic cost (an allostatic load) because the adaptive responses must be maintained throughout life. During normal aging, however, the success of this adaptive response is evidenced in the fact that neural cells survive and perform their functions. In this context, it is plausible to postulate that brain regions struggle to maintain their specific DHA content during aging.

In AD pathology, the pressure over the homeostatic system is exacerbated. Thus, it is evident that oxidative stress homeostasis is dysfunctional and the (lipo)oxidation-derived molecular damage is clearly and significantly higher. In this framework, in order to maintain homeostasis and cell survival neural cells activate adaptive responses to cope with oxidative stress. One of these mechanisms is to upregulate DHA synthesis, resulting in an increased DHA level in cell membrane, as well as in the content of DHA-derived lipid mediators. The aim is to protect the cell from oxidative stress and ensure cell survival. In AD, increased DHA levels have been described in target areas of AD in the earlier stages, as well as in apparently untargeted areas. However, the long-term persistence of the oxidative condition reaches a threshold where the allostatic adaption to maintain homeostasis fails and neural cells (particularly neurons) are heading for death. In this circumstance, a loss in DHA content and exacerbated lipoxidative damage is clearly manifested in affected areas, and especially in advanced stages of disease. Interestingly, AD progression and spreading throughout the brain is (like a shock wave) toward regions with higher DHA content, and in this expansion is progressively manifested the trilogy adaptation–overload–failure. The failure of the homeostatic system leads cells to neurodegeneration.

## 5. SUMMARY AND FUTURE PROSPECTS

Although generalizations should be treated with caution at this point, based on the need for replication of findings in larger populations, the current evidence regarding the neurons most affected in AD suggests that their specific-particular SNV expresses a lipidomic pattern prone to inducing neuronal dysfunction, which is aggravated by changes produced by the aging process, leading to the persistent activation of neuronal pathways that ultimately lead to neurodegeneration.

Elucidating how individual molecular species that participate in lipid metabolism homeostasis network are associated with AD will require further studies, but the current evidence is consistent with the existence of specific mechanistic associations among neuronal vulnerability, lipid profile, oxidative stress, aging, and neurodegeneration. Massive data obtained from systems biology, and particularly lipidomics, will allow, in coming years, for the emergence of an accurate definition of the role of lipids in defining the SNV of all cell types making up the human brain, as well as for identification of the key factors in the onset of brain aging and neurodegeneration. In addition, lipidomics may help to identify and evaluate biomarkers of AD that can be detected at the level of CSF, or even plasma, improving diagnosis and leading to the development of potential therapeutic interventions and treatments.

In spite of the potential of lipidomics in the study of the nervous system under physiological and pathological conditions, the present review has also revealed the tremendous lack of information regarding lipidomes in the different brain regions and in different physiological and pathological conditions. Focus on the study of lipidome at the cellular level in the future will lead to improved understanding of neuronal function in different settings. Obviously, these arguments are not limited to normal conditions; regional lipidomics and cellular lipidomics will also permit delineation of factors that sustain SNV.

## ACKNOWLEDGMENTS

The studies conducted at the Department of Experimental Medicine were supported in part by R&D grants from the Spanish Ministry of Economy and Competitiveness (BFU2009-11879/BFI, PI11/1532, PI13/00584, PI14/01115, and PI14/00328), and the Autonomous Government of Catalonia (2014SGR168). Studies at the Institute of Neuropathology were funded by the Spanish Ministry of Economy and Competitiveness (PI14/00757), and by the Seventh Framework Programme of the European Commission, grant agreement 278486: DEVELAGE. We thank T. Yohannan for editorial help.

*Competing Interests*: The authors declare that they have no competing interests.

## REFERENCES

Amoscato, A. A., Sparvero, L. J., He, R. R., Watkins, S., Bayir, H., & Kagan, V. E. (2014). Imaging mass spectrometry of diversified cardiolipin molecular species in the brain. *Analytical Chemistry, 86*, 6587–6595.

Ando, S., Chang, N. C., & Yu, R. K. (1978). High-performance thin-layer chromatography and densitometric determination of brain ganglioside compositions of several species. *Analytical Biochemistry, 89*, 437–450.

Astarita, G., Jung, K. M., Berchtold, N. C., Nguyen, V. Q., Gillen, D. L., Head, E., et al. (2010). Deficient liver biosynthesis of docosahexaenoic acid correlates with cognitive impairment in Alzheimer's disease. *PLoS One, 5*, e12538.

Bandaru, V. V., Troncoso, J., Wheeler, D., Pletnikova, O., Wang, J., Conant, K., et al. (2009). ApoE4 disrupts sterol and sphingolipid metabolism in Alzheimer's, but not normal brain. *Neurobiology of Aging, 30*, 591–599.

Bazan, N. G., Molina, M. F., & Gordon, W. C. (2011). Docosahexaenoic acid signalolipidomics in nutrition: Significance in aging, neuroinflammation, macular degeneration, Alzheimer's, and other neurodegenerative diseases. *Annual Review of Nutrition, 31*, 321–351.

Benseny-Cases, N., Klementieva, O., Cotte, M., Ferrer, I., & Cladera, J. (2014). Microspectroscopy (μFTIR) reveals co-localization of lipid oxidation and amyloid plaques in human Alzheimer disease brains. *Analytical Chemistry, 86*, 12047–12054.

Berchtold, N. C., Cribbs, D. H., Coleman, P. D., Rogers, J., Head, E., Kim, R., et al. (2008). Gene expression changes in the course of normal brain aging are sexually dimorphic.

*Proceedings of the National Academy of Sciences of the United States of America, 105*, 15605–15610.
Bertram, L., & Tanzi, R. E. (2011). Genetics of Alzheimer's disease. In D. Dickson, & R. Weller (Eds.), *Neurodegeneration: The molecular pathology of dementia and movement disorders* (pp. 51–61). West Sussex: Wiley-Blackwell.
Bielski, B. H., Arudi, R. L., & Sutherland, M. W. (1983). A study of the reactivity of HO2/O2- with unsaturated fatty acids. *The Journal of Biological Chemistry, 258*, 4759–4761.
Braak, H., & Braak, E. (1991). Neuropathological stageing of Alzheimer-related changes. *Acta Neuropathologica, 82*, 239–259.
Braak, H., & Braak, E. (1992). The human entorhinal cortex: Normal morphology and lamina-specific pathology in various diseases. *Neuroscience Research, 15*, 6–31.
Braak, H., & Braak, E. (1997). Frequency of stages of Alzheimer-related lesions in different age categories. *Neurobiology of Aging, 18*, 351–357.
Braak, H., & Braak, E. (1999). Temporal sequence of Alzheimer's disease-related pathology. In A. Peters, & J. H. Morrison (Eds.), *Cerebral cortex* (pp. 475–512). New York: Academic/Plenum Publishers.
Braak, H., Thal, D. R., Ghebremedhin, E., & del Tredici, K. (2011). Stages of the pathologic process in Alzheimer disease: Age categories from 1 to 100 years. *Journal of Neuropathology and Experimental Neurology, 70*, 960–969.
Brand, M. D., Affourtit, C., Esteves, T. C., Green, K., Lambert, A. J., Miwa, S., et al. (2004). Mitochondrial superoxide: Production, biological effects, and activation of uncoupling proteins. *Free Radical Biology and Medicine, 37*, 755–767.
Brenna, J. T., Salem, N., Jr., Sinclair, A. J., & Cunnane, S. C. (2009). International Society for the Study of Fatty Acids and Lipids, ISSFAL. alpha-Linolenic acid supplementation and conversion to n-3 long-chain polyunsaturated fatty acids in humans. *Prostaglandins, Leukotrienes and Essential Fatty Acids, 80*, 85–91.
Brigelius-Flohé, R. (2006). Glutathione peroxidases and redox-regulated transcription factors. *Biological Chemistry, 387*, 1329–1335.
Broadhurst, C. L., Wang, Y., Crawford, M. A., Cunnane, S. C., Parkington, J. E., & Schmidt, W. F. (2002). Brain-specific lipids from marine, lacustrine, or terrestrial food resources: Potential impact on early African Homo sapiens. *Comparative Biochemistry and Physiology, Part B: Biochemistry & Molecular Biology, 131*, 653–673.
Brosche, T., & Platt, D. (1998). The biological significance of plasmalogens in defense against oxidative damage. *Experimental Gerontology, 33*, 363–369.
Brown, H. A. (2007). Lipidomics and bioactive lipids: Specialized analytical methodsand lipids in disease. Preface. *Methods in Enzymology, 433*, XV–XVI.
Brown, H. A., Henage, L. G., Preininger, A. M., Xiang, Y., & Exton, J. H. (2007). Biochemical analysis of phospholipase D. *Methods in Enzymology, 434*, 49–87.
Buckingham, J. (2010). *Dictionary of natural products on CD-ROM, version 19.1*. London: Chapman and Hall.
Burger, M., & Seidel, K. (1958). Chemical biomorphosis of the human brain and sciatic nerve; a survey. *Zeitschrift für Alternsforschung, 12*, 52–79.
Burke, S. N., & Barnes, C. A. (2006). Neural plasticity in the ageing brain. *Nature Reviews Neuroscience, 7*, 30–40.
Catalá, A. (2009). Lipid peroxidation of membrane phospholipids generates hydroxyl-alkenals and oxidized phospholipids active in physiological and/or pathological conditions. *Chemistry and Physics of Lipids, 157*, 1–11.
Cataldo, A. M., Paskevich, P. A., Kominami, E., & Nixon, R. A. (1991). Lysosomal hydrolases of different classes are abnormally distributed in brains of patients with Alzheimer disease. *Proceedings of the National Academy of Sciences of the United States of America, 88*, 10998–111002.

Chen, Y., Allegood, J., Liu, Y., Wang, E., Cachón-Gonzalez, B., Cox, T. M., et al. (2008). Imaging MALDI mass spectrometry using an oscillating capillary nebulizer matrix coating system and its application to analysis of lipids in brain from a mouse model of Tay-Sachs/Sandhoff disease. *Analytical Chemistry*, *80*, 2780–2788.

Chen, C. T., Green, J. T., Orr, S. K., & Bazinet, R. P. (2008). Regulation of brain polyunsaturated fatty acid uptake and turnover. *Prostaglandins, Leukotrienes, and Essential Fatty Acids*, *79*, 85–91.

Cheng, H., Wang, M., Li, J. L., Cairns, N. J., & Han, X. (2013). Specific changes of sulfatide levels in individuals with pre-clinical Alzheimer's disease: An early event in disease pathogenesis. *Journal of Neurochemistry*, *127*, 733–738.

Cho, H. P., Nakamura, M., & Clarke, S. D. (1999a). Cloning, expression, and fatty acid regulation of the human delta-5 desaturase. *The Journal of Biological Chemistry*, *274*, 37335–37339.

Cho, H. P., Nakamura, M. T., & Clarke, S. D. (1999b). Cloning, expression, and nutritional regulation of the mammalian Delta-6 desaturase. *The Journal of Biological Chemistry*, *274*, 471–477.

Conrad, M., Schneider, M., Seiler, A., & Bornkamm, G. W. (2007). Physiological role of phospholipid hydroperoxide glutathione peroxidase in mammals. *Biological Chemistry*, *388*, 1019–1025.

Copple, I. M., Goldring, C. E., Kitteringham, N. R., & Park, B. K. (2008). The Nrf2-Keap1 defence pathway: Role in protection against drug-induced toxicity. *Toxicology*, *246*, 24–33.

Crawford, M. A., Broadhurst, C. L., Guest, M., Nagar, A., Wang, Y., Ghebremeskel, K., et al. (2013). A quantum theory for the irreplaceable role of docosahexaenoic acid in neural cell signalling throughout evolution. *Prostaglandins, Leukotrienes, and Essential Fatty Acids*, *88*, 5–13.

Cutler, R. G., Kelly, J., Storie, K., Pedersen, W. A., Tammara, A., Hatanpaa, K., et al. (2004). Involvement of oxidative stress-induced abnormalities in ceramide and cholesterol metabolism in brain aging and Alzheimer's disease. *Proceedings of the National Academy of Sciences of the United States of America*, *101*, 2070–2075.

Cyberlipid Center Website. http://www.cyberlipid.org.

Díaz, M., Fabelo, N., Martín, V., Ferrer, I., Gómez, T., & Marín, R. (2015). Biophysical alterations in lipid rafts from human cerebral cortex associate with increased BACE1/AβPP interaction in early stages of Alzheimer's disease. *Journal of Alzheimer's Disease*, *2015*(43), 1185–1198.

Dietschy, J. M., & Turley, S. D. (2001). Cholesterol metabolism in the brain. *Current Opinion in Lipidology*, *12*, 105–112.

Duyckaerts, C., & Dickson, D. (2011). Neuropathology of Alzheimer's disease and its variants. In D. Dickson, & R. Weller (Eds.), *Neurodegeneration: The molecular pathology of dementia and movement disorders* (pp. 62–91). West Sussex: Wiley-Blackwell.

Echtay, K. S., Esteves, T. C., Pakay, J. L., Jekabsons, M. B., Lambert, A. J., Portero-Otín, M., et al. (2003). A signalling role for 4-hydroxy-2-nonenal in regulation of mitochondrial uncoupling. *EMBO Journal*, *22*, 4103–4110.

Ellison, D. W., Beal, M. F., & Martin, J. B. (1987). Phosphoethanolamine and ethanolamine are decreased in Alzheimer's disease and Huntington's disease. *Brain Research*, *417*, 389–392.

Enriquez-Algeciras, M., & Bhattacharya, S. K. (2013). Lipidomic mass spectrometry and its application in neuroscience. *World Journal of Biological Chemistry*, *4*, 102–110.

Esterbauer, H., Schaur, R. J., & Zollner, H. (1991). Chemistry and biochemistry of 4-hydroxynonenal, malonaldehyde and related aldehydes. *Free Radical Biology and Medicine*, *11*, 81–128.

Evans, S. J., Choudary, P. V., Vawter, M. P., Li, J., Meador-Woodruff, J. H., Lopez, J. F., et al. (2003). DNA microarray analysis of functionally discrete human brain regions reveals divergent transcriptional profiles. *Neurobiology of Disease*, *14*, 240–250.

Fabelo, N., Martín, V., Marín, R., Moreno, D., Ferrer, I., & Díaz, M. (2014). Altered lipid composition in cortical lipid rafts occurs at early stages of sporadic Alzheimer's disease and facilitates APP/BACE1 interactions. *Neurobiology of Aging*, *35*, 1801–1812.

Fahy, E., Cotter, D., Sud, M., & Subramaniam, S. (2011). Lipid classification, structures and tools. *Biochimica et Biophysica Acta*, *1811*, 637–647.

Fahy, E., Subramaniam, S., Brown, H. A., Glass, C. K., Merrill, A. H., Murphy, R. C., et al. (2005). A comprehensive classification system for lipids. *Journal of Lipid Research*, *46*, 839–861.

Fahy, E., Subramaniam, S., Murphy, R. C., Nishijima, M., Raetz, C. R., Shimizu, T., et al. (2009). Update of the LIPID MAPS comprehensive classification system for lipids. *Journal of Lipid Research*, *50*(Suppl.), S9-14.

Farooqui, A. A. (2009). Lipid mediators in the neural cell nucleus: Their metabolism, signaling, and association with neurological disorders. *The Neuroscientist*, *15*, 392–407.

Farooqui, A. A. (2012). Lipid mediators and their metabolism in the nucleous: Implications for Alzheimer's disease. *Journal of Alzheimer's Disease*, *30*, S163–S178.

Farooqui, A. A., Liss, L., & Horrocks, L. A. (1988). Neurochemical aspects of Alzheimer's disease: Involvement of membrane phospholipids. *Metabolic Brain Disease*, *3*, 19–35.

Ferdinandusse, S., Denis, S., Mooijer, P. A., Zhang, Z., Reddy, J. K., Spector, A. A., et al. (2001). Identification of the peroxisomal beta-oxidation enzymes involved in the biosynthesis of docosahexaenoic acid. *Journal of Lipid Research*, *42*, 1987–1995.

Fernandez-Irigoyen, J., Labarga, A., Zabaleta, A., de Morentin, X. M., Perez-Valderrama, E., Zelaya, M. V., et al. (2014). Toward defining the anatomo-proteomic puzzle of the human brain: An integrative analysis. *Proteomics: Clinical Applications*. http://dx.doi.org/10.1002/prca.201400127.

Ferrer, I. (2009). Altered mitochondria, energy metabolism, voltage-dependent anion channel, and lipid rafts converge to exhaust neurons in *Alzheimer's disease*. *Journal of Bioenergetics and Biomembranes*, *41*, 425–431.

Ferrer, I. (2012). Defining Alzheimer as a common age-related neurodegenerative process not inevitably leading to dementia. *Progress in Neurobiology*, *97*, 38–51.

Fraser, H. B., Khaitovich, P., Plotkin, J. B., Pääbo, S., & Eisen, M. B. (2005). Aging and gene expression in the primate brain. *PLoS Biology*, *3*, e274.

Frisardi, V., Panza, F., Seripa, D., Farooqui, T., & Farooqui, A. A. (2011). Glycerophospholipids and glycerophospholipid-derived lipid mediators: A complex meshwork in Alzheimer's disease pathology. *Progress in Lipid Research*, *50*, 313–330.

Fritz, K. S., & Petersen, D. R. (2013). An overview of the chemistry and biology of reactive aldehydes. *Free Radical Biology and Medicine*, *59*, 85–91.

Frolov, V. A., Shnyrova, A. V., & Zimmerberg, J. (2011). Lipid polymorphisms and membrane shape. *Cold Spring Harbor Perspectives in Biology*, *3*, a004747.

Gamliel, A., Afri, M., & Frimer, A. A. (2008). Determining radical penetration of lipid bilayers with new lipophilic spin traps. *Free Radical Biology and Medicine*, *44*, 1394–1405.

Ghidoni, R., Sonnino, S., Tettamanti, G., Baumann, N., Reuter, G., & Schauer, R. (1980). Isolation and characterization of a trisialoganglioside from mouse brain, containing 9-O-acetyl-N-acetylneuraminic acid. *The Journal of Biological Chemistry*, *255*, 6990–6995.

Giannakopoulos, P., Gold, G., Michel, J. P., & Bouras, C. (1998). Cellular vulnerability in brain aging and Alzheimer's disease. Clinical correlates and molecular background. *Annales de Médecine Interne*, *149*, 187–191.

Giles, G. I. (2009). Redox-controlled transcription factors and gene expression. In C. Jacob, & P. G. Winyard (Eds.), *Redox signaling and regulation in biology and medicine* (pp. 245–270). Weinheim: Wiley-VCH Verlag GmbH&Co.

Ginsberg, L., Rafique, S., Xuereb, J. H., Rapoport, S. I., & Gershfeld, N. L. (1995). Disease and anatomic specificity of ethanolamine plasmalogen deficiency in Alzheimer's disease brain. *Brain Research*, *698*, 223–236.

Goodenowe, D. B., Cook, L. L., Liu, J., Lu, Y., Jayasinghe, D. A., Ahiahonu, P. W., et al. (2007). Peripheral ethanolamine plasmalogen deficiency: A logical causative factor in Alzheimer's disease and dementia. *Journal of Lipid Research*, *48*, 2485–2498.

Grimm, M. O., Kuchenbecker, J., Rothhaar, T. L., Grösgen, S., Hundsdörfer, B., Burg, V. K., et al. (2011). Plasmalogen synthesis is regulated via alkyl-dihydroxyacetonephosphate-synthase by amyloid precursor protein processing and is affected in Alzheimer's disease. *Journal of Neurochemistry*, *116*, 916–925.

Grinberg, L. T., Rüb, U., Ferretti, R. E., Nitrini, R., Farfel, J. M., Polichiso, L., et al. (2009). The dorsal raphe nucleus shows phospho-tau neurofibrillary changes before the transentorhinal region in Alzheimer's disease. A precocious onset? *Neuropathology and Applied Neurobiology*, *35*, 406–416.

Grinstein, S. (2010). Imaging signal transduction during phagocytosis: Phospholipids, surface charge, and electrostatic interactions. *American Journal of Physiology. Cell Physiology*, *299*, C876–C881.

Guan, Z. Z., Wang, Y. A., Cairns, N. J., Lantos, P. L., Dallner, G., & Sindelar, P. J. (1999). Decrease and structural modifications of phosphatidylethanolamine plasmalogen in the brain with Alzheimer disease. *Journal of Neuropathology and Experimental Neurology*, *58*, 740–747.

Han, X. (2002). Characterization and direct quantitation of ceramide molecular species from lipid extracts of biological samples by electrospray ionization tandem mass spectrometry. *Analytical Biochemistry*, *302*, 199–212.

Han, X. (2005). Lipid alterations in the earliest clinically recognizable stage of Alzheimer's disease: Implication of the role of lipids in the pathogenesis of Alzheimer's disease. *Current Alzheimer Research*, *2*, 65–77.

Han, X. (2007). Neurolipidomics: Challenges and developments. *Frontiers in Bioscience*, *12*, 2601–2615.

Han, X. (2010). Multi-dimensional mass spectrometry-based shotgun lipidomics and the altered lipids at the mild cognitive impairment stage of Alzheimer's disease. *Biochimica et Biophysica Acta*, *1801*, 774–783.

Han, X., & Gross, R. W. (2003). Global analyses of cellular lipidomes directly from crude extracts of biological samples by ESI mass spectrometry: A bridge to lipidomics. *Journal of Lipid Research*, *44*, 1071–1079.

Han, X., & Gross, R. W. (2005). Shotgun lipidomics: Electrospray ionization mass spectrometric analysis and quantitation of cellular lipidomes directly from crude extracts of biological samples. *Mass Spectrometry Reviews*, *24*, 367–412.

Han, X., Holtzman, D. M., & McKeel, D. W. (2001). Plasmalogen deficiency in early Alzheimer's disease subjects and in animal models: Molecular characterization using electrospray ionization mass spectrometry. *Journal of Neurochemistry*, *77*, 1168–1180.

Han, X., Yang, K., Cheng, H., Fikes, K. N., & Gross, R. W. (2005). Shotgun lipidomics of phosphoethanolamine-containing lipids in biological samples after one-step in situ derivatization. *Journal of Lipid Research*, *46*, 1548–1560.

Han, X., Yang, K., Yang, J., Cheng, H., & Gross, R. W. (2006). Shotgun lipidomics of cardiolipin molecular species in lipid extracts of biological samples. *Journal of Lipid Research*, *47*, 864–879.

Hannover, A. (1843). Mikroskopiske undersögelser af nervesysternet. *Det Kongelige Danske Videnskabernes Selskab Naturvidenskabelige og mathematiske Afkandlinger, 10*, 1–112.
Haughey, N. J., Bandaru, V. V., Bae, M., & Mattson, M. P. (2010). Roles for dysfunctional sphingolipid metabolism in Alzheimer's disease neuropathogenesis. *Biochimica et Biophysica Acta, 1801*, 878–886.
Haverkamp, J., Veh, R. W., Sander, M., Schauer, R., Kamerling, J. P., & Vliegenthart, J. G. (1977). Demonstration of 9-O-acetyl-N-acetylneuraminic acid in brain gangliosides from various vertebrates including man. *Hoppe-Seyler's Zeitschrift für Physiologische Chemie, 358*, 1609–1612.
Hawrylycz, M. J., Lein, E. S., Guillozet-Bongaarts, A. L., Shen, E. H., Ng, L., Miller, J. A., et al. (2012). An anatomically comprehensive atlas of the adult human brain transcriptome. *Nature, 489*, 391–399.
He, X., Huang, Y., Li, B., Gong, C. X., & Schuchman, E. H. (2010). Deregulation of sphingolipid metabolism in Alzheimer's disease. *Neurobiology of Aging, 31*, 398–408.
Higdon, A., Diers, A. R., Oh, J. Y., Landar, A., & Darley-Usmar, V. M. (2012). Cell signaling by reactive lipid species: New concepts and molecular mechanisms. *Biochemical Journal, 442*, 453–464.
Holman, R. T. (1954). Autoxidation of fats and related substances. In R. T. Holman, W. O. Lundberg, & T. Malkin (Eds.), *Progress in chemistry of fats and other lipids* (pp. 51–98). London: Pergamon Press.
Horrocks, L. A., VanRollins, M., & Yates, A. J. (1981). Lipid changes in the ageing brain. In A. N. Davinson, & R. H. S. Thompson (Eds.), *The molecular basis of neuropathology*. London: Edward Arnold.
Houjou, T., Yamatani, K., Imagawa, M., Shimizu, T., & Taguchi, R. (2005). A shotgun tandem mass spectrometric analysis of phospholipids with normal-phase and/or reverse-phase liquid chromatography/electrospray ionization mass spectrometry. *Rapid Communications in Mass Spectrometry, 19*, 654–666.
Hulbert, A. J., Kelly, M. A., & Abbott, S. K. (2014). Polyunsaturated fats, membrane lipids and animal longevity. *Journal of Comparative Physiology B, 184*, 149–166.
Hulbert, A. J., Pamplona, R., Buffenstein, R., & Buttemer, W. A. (2007). Life and death: Metabolic rate, membrane composition, and life span of animals. *Physiological Reviews, 87*, 1175–1213.
Hyötyläinen, T., & Orešič, M. (2014). Systems biology strategies to study lipidomes in health and disease. *Progress in Lipid Research, 55*, 43–60.
Igarashi, M., Ma, K., Gao, F., Kim, H. W., Rapoport, S. I., & Rao, J. S. (2011). Disturbed choline plasmalogen and phospholipid fatty acid concentrations in Alzheimer's disease prefrontal cortex. *Journal of Alzheimer's Disease, 24*, 507–517.
Imai, H., & Nakagawa, Y. (2003). Biological significance of phospholipid hydroperoxide glutathione peroxidase (PHGPx, GPx4) in mammalian cells. *Free Radical Biology and Medicine, 34*, 145–169.
Ivanova, P. T., Milne, S. B., Byrne, M. O., Xiang, Y., & Brown, H. A. (2007). Glycerophospholipid identification and quantitation by electrospray ionization mass spectrometry. *Methods in Enzymology, 432*, 21–57.
Jiye, A., Trygg, J., Gullberg, J., Johansson, A. I., Jonsson, P., Antti, H., et al. (2005). Extraction and GC/MS analysis of the human blood plasma metabolome. *Analytical Chemistry, 77*, 8086–8094.
Jolly, R. D., Douglas, B. V., Davey, P. M., & Roiri, J. E. (1995). Lipofuscin in bovine muscle and brain: A model for studying age pigment. *Gerontology, 41*, S283–S295.
Jové, M., Portero-Otín, M., Naudí, A., Ferrer, I., & Pamplona, R. (2014). Metabolomics of human brain aging and age-related neurodegenerative diseases. *Journal of Neuropathology and Experimental Neurology, 73*, 640–657.

Kahma, K., Brotherus, J., Haltia, M., & Renkonen, O. (1976). Low and moderate concentrations of lysobisphosphatidic acid in brain and liver of patients affected by some storage diseases. *Lipids, 11*, 539–544.
Keller, J. N., Hanni, K. B., & Markesbery, W. R. (2000). Impaired proteasome function in Alzheimer's disease. *Journal of Neurochemistry, 75*, 436–439.
Khaitovich, P., Muetzel, B., She, X., Lachmann, M., Hellmann, I., Dietzsch, J., et al. (2004). Regional patterns of gene expression in human and chimpanzee brains. *Genome Research, 14*, 1462–1473.
Kim, H. Y. (2007). Novel metabolism of docosahexaenoic acid in neural cells. *The Journal of Biological Chemistry, 282*, 18661–18665.
Korte, S. M., Koolhaas, J. M., Wingfield, J. C., & McEwen, B. S. (2005). The Darwinian concept of stress: Benefits of allostasis and costs of allostatic load and the trade-offs in health and disease. *Neuroscience & Biobehavioral Reviews, 29*, 3–38.
Kosicek, M., & Hecimovic, S. (2013). Phospholipids and Alzheimer's disease: Alterations, mechanisms and potential biomarkers. *International Journal of Molecular Sciences, 14*, 1310–1322.
Kou, J., Kovacs, G. G., Höftberger, R., Kulik, W., Brodde, A., Forss-Petter, S., et al. (2011). Peroxisomal alterations in Alzheimer's disease. *Acta Neuropathologica, 122*, 271–283.
Koynova, R., & Caffrey, M. (1998). Phases and phase transitions of the phosphatidylcholines. *Biochimica et Biophysica Acta, 1376*, 91–145.
Laaksonen, R., Katajamaa, M., Päivä, H., Sysi-Aho, M., Saarinen, L., Junni, P., et al. (2006). A systems biology strategy reveals biological pathways and plasma biomarker candidates for potentially toxic statin-induced changes in muscle. *PLoS One, 1*, e97.
Ledesma, M. D., Martin, M. G., & Dotti, C. G. (2012). Lipid changes in the aged brain: Effect on synaptic function and neuronal survival. *Progress in Lipid Research, 51*, 23–35.
Li, M., Yang, L., Bai, Y., & Liu, H. (2014). Analytical methods in lipidomics and their applications. *Analytical Chemistry, 86*, 161–175.
Liang, W. S., Dunckley, T., Beach, T. G., Grover, A., Mastroeni, D., Walker, D. G., et al. (2007). Gene expression profiles in anatomically and functionally distinct regions of the normal aged human brain. *Physiological Genomics, 28*, 311–322.
Lipid Bank Website. http://www.lipidbank.jp.
Lipid Library Website. http://lipidlibrary.aocs.org.
Loessner, A., Alavi, A., Lewandrowski, K. U., Mozley, D., Souder, E., & Gur, R. E. (1995). Regional cerebral function determined by FDG-PET in healthy volunteers: Normal patterns and changes with age. *Journal of Nuclear Medicine, 36*, 1141–1149.
Lombard, J., López-García, P., & Moreira, D. (2012). The early evolution of lipid membranes and the three domains of life. *Nature Reviews. Microbiology, 10*, 507–515.
Maceyka, M., & Spiegel, S. (2014). Sphingolipid metabolites in inflammatory disease. *Nature, 510*, 58–67.
Magalhaes, M. A., & Glogauer, M. (2010). Pivotal advance: Phospholipids determine net membrane surface charge resulting in differential localization of active Rac1 and Rac2. *Journal of Leukocyte Biology, 87*, 545–555.
Maher, J., & Yamamoto, M. (2010). The rise of antioxidant signaling-The evolution and hermetic actions of Nrf2. *Toxicology and Applied Pharmacology, 244*, 4–15.
Mann, D. M., Yates, P. O., & Stamp, J. E. (1978). The relationship between lipofuscin pigment and ageing in the human nervous system. *Journal of the Neurological Sciences, 37*, 83–93.
Markesbery, W. R. (2010). Neuropathologic alterations in mild cognitive impairment: A review. *Journal of Alzheimer's Disease, 19*, 221–228.
Marsh, D. (2007). Lateral pressure profile, spontaneous curvature frustration, and the incorporation and conformation of proteins in membranes. *Biophysical Journal, 93*, 3884–3899.

Martín, V., Fabelo, N., Santpere, G., Puig, B., Marín, R., Ferrer, I., et al. (2010). Lipid alterations in lipid rafts from Alzheimer's disease human brain cortex. *Journal of Alzheimer's Disease, 19*, 489–502.

Martin, M. G., Perga, S., Trovò, L., Rasola, A., Holm, P., Rantamäki, T., et al. (2008). Cholesterol loss enhances TrkB signaling in hippocampal neurons aging in vitro. *Molecular Biology of the Cell, 19*, 2101–2112.

Martínez, A., Portero-Otin, M., Pamplona, R., & Ferrer, I. (2010). Protein targets of oxidative damage in human neurodegenerative diseases with abnormal protein aggregates. *Brain Pathology, 20*, 281–297.

Mattson, M. P., & Magnus, T. (2006). Ageing and neuronal vulnerability. *Nature Reviews Neuroscience*, 7, 278–294.

McGeer, P. L., & McGeer, E. G. (2013). The amyloiod cascade-inflammatory hypothesis of Alzheimer disease: Implications for therapy. *Acta Neuropathologica, 126*, 479–497.

McMahon, H. T., & Gallop, J. L. (2005). Membrane curvature and mechanisms of dynamic cell membrane remodelling. *Nature, 438*, 590–596.

McNamara, R. K., Liu, Y., Jandacek, R., Rider, T., & Tso, P. (2008). The aging human orbitofrontal cortex: Decreasing polyunsaturated fatty acid composition and associated increases in lipogenic gene expression and stearoyl-CoA desaturase activity. *Prostaglandins, Leukotrienes, and Essential Fatty Acids, 78*, 293–304.

Merrill, A. H., Sullards, M. C., Allegood, J. C., Kelly, S., & Wang, E. (2005). Sphingolipidomics: High-throughput, structure-specific, and quantitative analysis of sphingolipids by liquid chromatography tandem mass spectrometry. *Methods, 36*, 207–224.

Molina, J. A., Jiménez-Jiménez, F. J., Vargas, C., Gómez, P., de Bustos, F., Ortí-Pareja, M., et al. (1998). Cerebrospinal fluid levels of non-neurotransmitter amino acids in patients with Alzheimer's disease. *Journal of Neural Transmission, 105*, 279–286.

Moller, M., Botti, H., Batthyany, C., Rubbo, H., Radi, R., & Denicola, A. (2005). Direct measurement of nitric oxide and oxygen partitioning into liposomes and low density lipoprotein. *The Journal of Biological Chemistry, 280*, 8850–8854.

Morrison, J. H., & Hof, P. R. (1997). Life and death of neurons in the aging brain. *Science, 278*, 412–419.

Morrison, J. H., & Hof, P. R. (2002). Selective vulnerability of corticocortical and hippocampal circuits in aging and Alzheimer's disease. *Progress in Brain Research, 136*, 467–486.

Morrison, J. H., & Hof, P. R. (2007). Life and death of neurons in the aging cerebral cortex. *International Review of Neurobiology, 81*, 41–57.

Morrison, B. M., Hof, P. R., & Morrison, J. H. (1998). Determinants of neuronal vulnerability in neurodegenerative diseases. *Annals of Neurology, 44*, S32–S44.

Mouritsen, O. G. (2005). *Life as a matter of fat: The emerging science of lipidomics*. Berlin, New York: Springer.

Mueller, S. G., Stables, L., Du, A. T., Schuff, N., Truran, D., Cashdollar, N., et al. (2007). Measurement of hippocampal subfields and age-related changes with high resolution MRI at 4T. *Neurobiology of Aging, 28*(5), 719–726.

Murthy, M., Hamilton, J., Greiner, R. S., Moriguchi, T., Salem, N., Jr., & Kim, H. Y. (2002). Differential effects of n-3 fatty acid deficiency on phospholipid molecular species composition in the rat hippocampus. *Journal of Lipid Research, 43*, 611–617.

Naudí, A., Jové, M., Ayala, V., Cabré, R., Portero-Otin, M., Ferrer, I., et al. (2013). A study of selective neuronal vulnerability in the human central nervous system. *Revista Española de Geriatría y Gerontología, 48*, 216–223.

Naudí, A., Jové, M., Ayala, V., Cabré, R., Portero-Otín, M., & Pamplona, R. (2013). Non-enzymatic modification of aminophospholipids by carbonyl-amine reactions. *International Journal of Molecular Sciences, 14*, 3285–3313.

Naudi, A., Jove, M., Ayala, V., Ramirez, O., Cabre, R., Prat, J., et al. (2012). Region specific vulnerability to lipid peroxidation in the human central nervous system. In A. Catala (Ed.), *Lipid peroxidation* (pp. 437–456). Rijeka: InTech-Open Access Publishers.

Nelson, P. T., Alafuzoff, I., Bigio, E. H., Bouras, C., Braak, H., Cairns, N. J., et al. (2012). Correlation of Alzheimer disease neuropathologic changes with cognitive status: A review of the literature. *Journal of Neuropathology and Experimental Neurology, 71*, 362–381.

Nitsch, R. M., Blusztajn, J. K., Pittas, A. G., Slack, B. E., Growdon, J. H., & Wurtman, R. J. (1992). Evidence for a membrane defect in Alzheimer disease brain. *Proceedings of the National Academy of Sciences of the United States of America, 89*, 1671–1675.

Norton, W. T., Poduslo, S. E., & Suzuki, K. (1996). Subacute sclerosing leukoencephalitis. II. Chemical studies including abnormal myelin and an abnormal ganglioside pattern. *Journal of Neuropathology and Experimental Neurology, 25*, 582–597.

O'Banion, M. K., Coleman, P. D., & Callahan, L. M. (1994). Regional neuronal loss in aging and Alzheimer's disease: A brief review. *Seminars in Neuroscience, 6*, 307–314.

O'Brien, J. S., & Sampson, E. L. (1965a). Fatty acid and fatty aldehyde composition of the major brain lipids in normal human gray matter, white matter, and myelin. *Journal of Lipid Research, 6*, 545–551.

O'Brien, J. S., & Sampson, E. L. (1965b). Lipid composition of the normal human brain: Gray matter, white matter, and myelin. *Journal of Lipid Research, 6*, 537–544.

Ohm, T. G., Müller, H., Braak, H., & Bohl, J. (1995). Close-meshed prevalence rates of different stages as a tool to uncover the rate of Alzheimer's disease-related neurofibrillary changes. *Neuroscience, 64*, 209–217.

Oresic, M., Hänninen, V. A., & Vidal-Puig, A. (2008). Lipidomics: A new window to biomedical frontiers. *Trends in Biotechnology, 26*, 647–652.

Ottis, P., Koppe, K., Onisko, B., Dynin, I., Arzberger, T., Kretzschmar, H., et al. (2012). Human and rat brain lipofuscin proteome. *Proteomics, 12*, 2445–2454.

Pamplona, R. (2008). Membrane phospholipids, lipoxidative damage and molecular integrity: A causal role in aging and longevity. *Biochimica et Biophysica Acta, 1777*, 1249–1262.

Pamplona, R. (2011). Advanced lipoxidation end-products. *Chemico-Biological Interactions, 192*, 14–20.

Pamplona, R., Barja, G., & Portero-Otín, M. (2002). Membrane fatty acid unsaturation, protection against oxidative stress, and maximum life span: A homeoviscous-longevity adaptation? *Annals of the New York Academy of Sciences, 959*, 475–490.

Pamplona, R., & Costantini, D. (2011). Molecular and structural antioxidant defenses against oxidative stress in animals. *American Journal of Physiology—Regulatory, Integrative and Comparative Physiology, 301*, R843–R863.

Pamplona, R., Dalfó, E., Ayala, V., Bellmunt, M. J., Prat, J., Ferrer, I., et al. (2005). Proteins in human brain cortex are modified by oxidation, glycoxidation, and lipoxidation: Effects of Alzheimer disease and identification of lipoxidation targets. *Journal of Biological Chemistry, 1280*, 21522–21530.

Panganamala, R. V., Horrocks, L. A., Geer, J. C., & Cornwell, D. G. (1971). Positions of double bonds in the monounsaturated alk-1-enyl groups from the plasmalogens of human heart and brain. *Chemistry and Physics of Lipids, 6*, 97–102.

Patti, G. J., Yanes, O., & Siuzdak, G. (2012). Innovation: Metabolomics: The apogee of the omics trilogy. *Nature Reviews Molecular Cell Biology, 13*, 263–269.

Pellegrino, R. M., Di Veroli, A., Valeri, A., Goracci, L., & Cruciani, G. (2014). LC/MS lipid profiling from human serum: A new method for global lipid extraction. *Analytical and Bioanalytical Chemistry, 406*, 7937–7948.

Pettegrew, J. W., Panchalingam, K., Hamilton, R. L., & McClure, R. J. (2001). Brain membrane phospholipid alterations in Alzheimer's disease. *Neurochemical Research, 26*, 771–782.

Piomelli, D. (2005). The challenge of brain lipidomics. *Prostaglandins & Other Lipid Mediators, 77*, 23–34.

Piomelli, D., Astarita, G., & Rapaka, R. (2007). A neuroscientist's guide to lipidomics. *Nature Reviews Neuroscience, 8*, 743–754.

Porta, E. A. (1991). Advances in age pigment research. *Archives of Gerontology and Geriatrics, 12*, 303–320.

Power, C., & Patel, K. D. (2004). Neurolipidomics: An inflammatory perspective on fat in the brain. *Neurology, 63*, 608–609.

Prasad, M. R., Lovell, M. A., Yatin, M., Dhillon, H., & Markesbery, W. R. (1998). Regional membrane phospholipid alterations in Alzheimer's disease. *Neurochemical Research, 23*, 81–88.

Price, D. L., Cork, L. C., Struble, R. G., Kitt, C. A., Walker, L. C., Powers, R. E., et al. (1987). Dysfunction and death of neurons in human degenerative neurological diseases and in animal models. *Ciba Foundation Symposium, 126*, 30–48.

Price, J. L., McKeel, D. W., Jr., Buckles, V. D., Roe, C. M., Xiong, C., Grundman, M., et al. (2009). Neuropathology of non-demented aging: Presumptive evidence for preclinical Alzheimer disease. *Neurobiology of Aging, 30*, 1026–1036.

Rapoport, S. I., Rao, J. S., & Igarashi, M. (2007). Brain metabolism of nutritionally essential polyunsaturated fatty acids depends on both the diet and the liver. *Prostaglandins, Leukotrienes, and Essential Fatty Acids*, 77, 251–261.

Raz, N., & Rodrigue, K. M. (2006). Differential aging of the brain: Patterns, cognitive correlates and modifiers. *Neuroscience & Biobehavioral Reviews, 30*, 730–748.

Raz, N., Rodrigue, K. M., & Haacke, E. M. (2007). Brain aging and its modifiers: Insights from in vivo neuromorphometry and susceptibility weighted imaging. *Annals of the New York Academy of Sciences, 1097*, 84–93.

Reiman, E. M., Chen, K., Langbaum, J. B., Lee, W., Reschke, C., Bandy, D., et al. (2010). Higher serum total cholesterol levels in late middle age are associated with glucose hypometabolism in brain regions affected by Alzheimer's disease and normal aging. *NeuroImage, 49*, 169–176.

Rouser, G., Feldman, G., & Galli, C. (1965). Fatty acid compositions of human brain lecithin and sphingomyelin in normal individuals, senile cerebral cortical atrophy, Alzheimer's disease, Metachromatic Leucodystrophy, Tay-Sachs and Niemann-Pick diseases. *Journal of the American Oil Chemists Society, 42*, 411–412.

Rouser, G., Galli, C., & Kritchevsky, G. (1965). Lipid class composition of normal human brain and variations in metachromatic leucodystrophy, Tay-Sachs, Niemann-Pick, Chronic Gaucher's and Alzheimer's diseases. *Journal of the American Oil Chemists Society, 42*, 404–410.

Rouser, G., & Yamamoto, A. (1968). Curvilinear regression course of human brain lipid composition changes with age. *Lipids, 3*, 284–287.

Rouser, G., & Yamamoto, A. (1969). *Handbook of neurochemistry*. New York: Plenum Press.

Salem, N., Jr., Kim, H. Y., & Yergey, J. A. (1986). Docosahexaenoic acid: Membrane function and metabolism. In A. P. Simopoulos, R. R. Kifer, & R. E. Martin (Eds.), *Health effects of polyunsaturated fatty acids in seafoods* (pp. 263–317). New York: Academic Press.

Sastry, P. S. (1985). Lipids of nervous tissue: Composition and metabolism. *Progress in Lipid Research, 24*, 69–176.

Schwudke, D., Oegema, J., Burton, L., Entchev, E., Hannich, J. T., Ejsing, C. S., et al. (2006). Lipid profiling by multiple precursor and neutral loss scanning driven by the data-dependent acquisition. *Analytical Chemistry, 78*, 585–595.

Seehafer, S. S., & Pearce, D. A. (2006). You say lipofuscin, we say ceroid: Defining autofluorescent storage material. *Neurobiology of Aging, 27*, 576–588.

Selkoe, D. J. (2012). Preventing Alzheimer's disease. *Science, 337*, 1488–1492.

Seppänen-Laakso, T., & Oresic, M. (2009). How to study lipidomes. *Journal of Molecular Endocrinology*, *42*, 185–190.

Silvius, J. R. (1982). Thermotropic phase transitions of pure lipids in model membranes and their modifications by membrane proteins. *Lipid-Protein Interaction*, *2*, 239–281.

Simic, G., Stanic, G., Mladinov, M., Jovanov-Milosevic, N., Kostovic, I., & Hof, P. R. (2009). Does Alzheimer's disease begin in the brainstem? *Neuropathology and Applied Neurobiology*, *35*, 532–554.

Slotte, J. P. (2013). Biological functions of sphingomyelins. *Progress in Lipid Research*, *52*, 424–437.

Smith, A. D. (2000). *Oxford dictionary of biochemistry and molecular biology*. Oxford: Oxford University Press.

Söderberg, M., Edlund, C., Kristensson, K., & Dallner, G. (1990). Lipid compositions of different regions of the human brain during aging. *Journal of Neurochemistry*, *54*, 415–423.

Sommer, U., Herscovitz, H., Welty, F. K., & Costello, C. E. (2006). LC-MS based method for the qualitative and quantitative analysis of complex lipid mixtures. *Journal of Lipid Research*, *47*, 804–814.

Sonnino, S., & Chigorno, V. (2000). Ganglioside molecular species containing C18- and C20-sphingosine in mammalian nervous tissues and neuronal cell cultures. *Biochimica et Biophysica Acta*, *1469*, 63–77.

Spector, A. A. (2001). Plasma free fatty acid and lipoproteins as sources of polyunsaturated fatty acid for the brain. *Journal of Molecular Neuroscience*, *16*, 159–165.

Sprecher, H. (2000). Metabolism of highly unsaturated n-3 and n-6 fatty acids. *Biochimica et Biophysica Acta*, *1486*, 219–231.

Stokes, C. E., & Hawthorne, J. N. (1987). Reduced phosphoinositide concentrations in anterior temporal cortex of Alzheimer-diseased brains. *Journal of Neurochemistry*, *48*, 1018–1021.

Subramaniam, S., Fahy, E., Gupta, S., Sud, M., Byrnes, R. W., Cotter, D., et al. (2011). Bioinformatics and systems biology of the lipidome. *Chemical Reviews*, *111*, 6452–6490.

Sultana, R., & Butterfield, D. A. (2010). Role of oxidative stress in the progression of Alzheimer's disease. *Journal of Alzheimer's Disease*, *19*, 341–353.

Sultana, R., Perluigi, M., & Butterfield, A. D. (2013). Lipid peroxidation triggers neurodegeneration: A redox proteomics view into the Alzheimer disease brain. *Free Radical Biology and Medicine*, *62*, 157–169.

Svennerholm, L. (1968). Distribution and fatty acid composition of phosphoglycerides in normal human brain. *Journal of Lipid Research*, *9*, 570–579.

Svennerholm, L., Boström, K., Helander, C. G., & Jungbjer, B. (1991). Membrane lipids in the aging human brain. *Journal of Neurochemistry*, *56*, 2051–2059.

Svennerholm, L., Boström, K., Jungbjer, B., & Olsson, L. (1994). Membrane lipids of adult human brain: Lipid composition of frontal and temporal lobe in subjects of age 20 to 100 years. *Journal of Neurochemistry*, *63*, 1802–1811.

Terman, A., & Brunk, U. T. (1998). Lipofuscin: Mechanisms of formation and increase with age. *APMIS (Acta Pathologica, Microbiologica et Immunologica Scandinavica)*, *106*, 265–276.

Terry, R. D., DeTeresa, R., & Hansen, L. A. (1987). Neocortical cell counts in normal human adult aging. *Annals of Neurology*, *21*, 530–539.

Thal, D. R., Rüb, U., Orantes, M., & Braak, H. (2002). Phases of Aβ-deposition in the human brain and its relevance for the development of AD. *Neurology*, *58*, 1791–1800.

Thelen, K. M., Falkai, P., Bayer, T. A., & Lütjohann, D. (2006). Cholesterol synthesis rate in human hippocampus declines with aging. *Neuroscience Letters*, *403*, 15–19.

Thorpe, S. R., & Baynes, J. W. (2003). Maillard reaction products in tissue proteins: New products and new perspectives. *Amino Acids, 25*, 275–281.

Thudichum, J. L. W. (1884). *A treatise on the chemical constitution of brain*. London: Bailliere and Cox.

Thudichum, J. L. W. (1962). *A treatise on the chemical constitution of the brain*. Hamden: Archon Books (pp. 7, 8, 87, 90).

Touboul, D., & Gaudin, M. (2014). Lipidomics of Alzheimer's disease. *Bioanalysis, 6*, 541–561.

Ueno, K., Ando, S., & Yu, R. K. (1978). Gangliosides of human, cat, and rabbit spinal cords and cord myelin. *Journal of Lipid Research, 19*, 863–871.

Valdes-Gonzalez, T., Goto-Inoue, N., Hirano, W., Ishiyama, H., Hayasaka, T., Setou, M., et al. (2011). New approach for glyco- and lipidomics-molecular scanning of human brain gangliosides by TLC-Blot and MALDI-QIT-TOF MS. *Journal of Neurochemistry, 116*, 678–683.

Van Meer, G., Voelker, D. R., & Feigenson, G. W. (2008). Membrane lipids: Where they are and how they behave. *Nature Reviews Molecular Cell Biology, 9*, 112–124.

Wakabayashi, N., Dinkova-Kostova, A. T., Holtzclaw, W. D., Kang, M. I., Kobayashi, A., Yamamoto, M., et al. (2004). Protection against electrophile and oxidant stress by induction of the phase 2 response: Fate of cysteines of the Keap1 sensor modified by inducers. *Proceedings of the National Academy of Sciences of the United States of America, 101*, 2040–2045.

Wallner, S., & Schmitz, G. (2011). Plasmalogens the neglected regulatory and scavenging lipid species. *Chemistry and Physics of Lipids, 164*, 573–589.

Wang, X., Michaelis, M. L., & Michaelis, E. K. (2010). Functional genomics of brain aging and Alzheimer's disease: Focus on selective neuronal vulnerability. *Current Genomics, 11*, 618–633.

Want, E. J., Cravatt, B. F., & Siuzdak, G. (2005). The expanding role of mass spectrometry in metabolite profiling and characterization. *ChemBioChem, 6*, 1941–1951.

Watson, A. D. (2006). A global approach to lipid analysis in biological systems. *Journal of Lipid Research, 47*, 2101–2111.

Wells, K., Farooqui, A. A., Liss, L., & Horrocks, L. A. (1995). Neural membrane phospholipids in Alzheimer disease. *Neurochemical Research, 20*, 1329–1333.

West, M. J., Coleman, P. D., Flood, D. G., & Troncoso, J. C. (1994). Differences in the pattern of hippocampal neuronal loss in normal ageing and Alzheimer's disease. *Lancet, 344*, 769–772.

West, J. D., & Marnett, L. J. (2006). Endogenous reactive intermediates as modulators of cell signaling and cell death. *Chemical Research in Toxicology, 19*, 173–194.

Wood, P. L. (2012). Lipidomics of Alzheimer's disease: Current status. *Alzheimer's Research & Therapy, 4*, 5.

Wood, P. L., Mankidy, R., Ritchie, S., Heath, D., Wood, J. A., Flax, J., et al. (2010). Circulating plasmalogen levels and Alzheimer disease assessment scale-cognitive scores in Alzheimer patients. *Journal of Psychiatry & Neuroscience, 35*, 59–62.

Yabuuchi, H., & O'Brien, J. S. (1968). Positional distribution of fatty acids in glycerophosphatides of bovine gray matter. *Journal of Lipid Research, 9*, 65–67.

Yamashima, T. (2012). 'PUFA-GPR40-CREB signaling' hypothesis for the adult primate neurogenesis. *Progress in Lipid Research, 51*, 221–231.

Yeagle, P. (1993). *The membranes of cells*. San Diego, CA: Academic Press.

Yetukuri, L., Ekroos, K., Vidal-Puig, A., & Oresic, M. (2008). Informatics and computational strategies for the study of lipids. *Molecular BioSystems, 4*, 121–127.

Zimniak, P. (2011). Relationship of electrophilic stress to aging. *Free Radical Biology and Medicine, 51*, 1087–1105.

# INDEX

Note: Page numbers followed by "*f*" indicate figures and "*t*" indicate tables.


## A

AD. *See* Alzheimer's disease (AD)
Advanced glycation end-products (AGEs), 161
Alzheimer's disease (AD)
  altered metabolic pathways, 111*f*
  autoantibodies, 18–19
  characterization, 168
  description, 61
  diagnostic test, 97–98
  glucose metabolism, 65
  metabolomics studies, 62*t*
  pathological processes, 98–99
Alzheimer's disease lipidomics
  docosahexaenoic acid, 176–177
  human brain lipid content, 170–176
  reporting studies, 171*t*
  systematic anatomical studies, 168–169
Alzheimer's disease metabolomics
  blood-based, 109–113
  CSF, 101–104
Amyotrophic lateral sclerosis (ALS)
  blood-based metabolomics, 115–116
  CSF metabolomics, 105–106
  diagnostic test, 97–98
  metabolomics biomarker, 71
  pathological processes, 98–99
  riluzole, 99
Anticitrullinated peptide antibodies (ACPAs), 4–5
Anti-GAGA4 antibodies, 15
Antigen microarray technologies, 27–28
Anti-NMDAR encephalitis, 16–18
Atmospheric pressure photo-ionization (APPI), 113
Autoantibodies
  AD, 18–19
  anti-NMDAR encephalitis, 16–18
  biological samples, 24–26
  biomarkers, 29–35
  cancer, 8–9
  fluid-phase immunoassays, 27
  history of, 3–4
  human protein microarrays, 28
  multiple sclerosis, 13–15
  myasthenia gravis, 11–13
  natural, 19–24
  neuromyelitis optica, 15–16
  nucleic acid programmable protein arrays, 28
  peptoid arrays, 28
  rheumatoid arthritis, 4–5
  SLE, 5–7
  systemic sclerosis, 7–8
  validation of biomarker candidates, 29
  whole human proteome, 26
Autoantibody biomarkers
  Alzheimer's disease, 30–31
  human protein microarrays, 33–35
  immunoglobulin-binding patterns, 32–33
  multiple sclerosis, 31–32
  Parkinson's disease, 31

## B

Blood-based metabolomics, 107*t*
  Alzheimer's disease, 109–113
  amyotrophic lateral sclerosis, 115–116
  Parkinson's disease, 113–115
Brain volumetric measurements, 164–165

## C

Cancer, autoantibodies, 8–9
Ceramide, 147*f*, 155–156
Cerebral metabolic rate of glucose (CMRGl), 164–165
Cerebrosides, 145–148
Condensing effect of sterols, 155–156

## D

Derived lipids, 136–138
Docosahexaenoic acid, 176–177

## E

Eicosanoids, 156–157
Electrospray ionization (ESI), 141–142
Ethanolamine phosphoglycerides, 143–145

## F

Fatty acids
  adult human nervous system, 148, 149*t*
  biosynthesis, 151*f*
  chemical reactivity, 159–163
  docosahexaenoic acid, 153
Fluid-phase immunoassays, 27

## G

Glutathione-S-transferase (GST), 161
Glycerophospholipids, 143–145

## H

1H MRS, 82–83
Human protein microarrays, 28
  description, 66–68
  metabolomics studies, 68*t*

## I

Inositol phosphoglycerides, 143–145

## L

Levodopa, 99
Lewy bodies, 97–98
Lipid mediators, 157–159, 158*f*
Lipid metabolites and pathways strategy (LIPID MAPS), 136–138
Lipidomics
  Alzheimer's disease pathology, 168–177
  analytical methods, brain lipidome, 139–143
  definition, 139
  electrospray ionization, 141–142
  extraction method, 141
  human brain, 143–153
    chemical reactivity, acyl chains, 159–163
    fatty acids, 148–153
    glycerophospholipids, 143–145, 146*t*
    lipid signaling, 156–159
    sphingolipids, 145–148, 147*f*
    structural and functional integrity, 153–156
  human brain aging, 163–168
  lipid and classification, 136–139
  mass spectrometry, 141
  platform stages, 140*f*
Lipofuscin, 166–167
Lipoxidation-derived reactive carbonyl species, 160*f*
Lou Gehrig's disease, 71
Luciferase immunoprecipitation system (LIPS), 27

## M

Magnetic resonance spectroscopy (MRS)
  1H, 82–83
  metabolite identification, 57–58
  phosphorus (*see* Phosphorus MRS)
  proton, 82
  metabolite identification, 58–59
Mass spectrometry (MS), 100–101
Metabolic fingerprinting approach, 101
Metabolomics
  advantages, 54–55
  biomarkers, 56–57
    Alzheimer's disease, 61–65
    amyotrophic lateral sclerosis, 71
    cerebrospinal fluid, 57–58
    Huntington's disease, 66–68
    multiple sclerosis, 68–71
    Parkinson's disease, 65–66
    platforms for discovery, 58–61
  blood-based (*see* Blood-based metabolomics)
  brain tissue, 117*t*, 121, 123
  CSF, 102*t*
    Alzheimer's disease, 101–104
    amyotrophic lateral sclerosis, 105–106
    Parkinson's disease, 104–105
  description, 54–55, 55*f*
  mass spectrometry, 100–101
  in medicine, 55–56
  nuclear magnetic resonance, 100–101
  urine, 116–121, 117*t*
Mitochondrial dysfunction, 89
MRS. *See* Magnetic resonance spectroscopy (MRS)
Multiple sclerosis (MS)
  autoantibodies, 13–15
  metabolomics biomarker, 68–71
Muscle-specific tyrosine kinase (MuSK) autoantibodies, 11–13
Myasthenia gravis (MG), 11–13
Myelin surface proteins, 14

## N

Natural autoantibodies
functions, 23–24
implications and opportunity, 24
isotype and reactivity of, 21–22
prevalence and stability of, 21
production, 22–23
rise of, 19–21
Neurodegenerative diseases, metabolomics biomarker
Alzheimer's disease, 61–65
amyotrophic lateral sclerosis, 71
Huntington's disease, 66–68
multiple sclerosis, 68–71
Parkinson's disease, 65–66
Neurolipidomics, 139
Neuromyelitis optica (NMO), 15–16
Neuronal and glial cell membranes, 153–156
Nuclear magnetic resonance (NMR), 59–60
Nucleic acid programmable protein arrays (NAPPAs), 28

## O

Oleic acid, 155
Oligoclonal IgG banding (OCB), 15
Orthogonal partial least squares discriminant analysis (OPLS-DA), 105–106, 112*f*

## P

Parkinson's disease (PD)
blood-based metabolomics, 113–115
CSF metabolomics, 104–105
diagnostic test, 97–98
experimental and postmortem studies, 84
high magnetic field, 90
idiopathic, 85
levodopa, 99
metabolomics biomarker, 65–66, 67*t*
mitochondrial dysfunction, 89
pathological processes, 98–99
PET studies, 85
progressive supranuclear paralysis, 89
Pathwaycentric approach, 60–61
Peptidylarginine deiminases (PADs Q6 ), 5
Peptoid arrays, 28
Peroxidizability index, 161–162, 162*f*
Phage immunoprecipitation sequencing (PhIP seq), 26
Phosphatidic acid, 143–145
Phosphorus MRS
high-energy phosphates, 84, 86
multicenter 1HMRS study, 88
Parkinson's disease pathogenesis, 84
phosphorylation/mitochondrial impairment, 86
PINK1, 84, 87–88
Plasmalogens, 174
Progressive supranuclear palsy (PSP), 33
Protein citrullination, 4–5
Proton MRS, 82

## R

Reactive carbonyl species (RCS), 159–161
Rheumatoid arthritis (RA), 4–5
Rheumatoid factor (RF), 4–5
Riluzole, 99

## S

Scleroderma. *See* Systemic sclerosis (SSc)
Selective neuronal vulnerability (SNV), 163
Shotgun lipidomics, 141
Sialic acid, 147*f*
Single-voxel proton MRS, 82
Sphingolipids, 145–148, 147*f*
Sulfatide, 145–148
Systemic lupus erythematosus (SLE), 5–7
Systemic sclerosis (SSc), 7–8

## W

Whole human proteome, 26

# CONTENTS OF RECENT VOLUMES


## Volume 37

Section I: Selectionist Ideas and Neurobiology

Selectionist and Instructionist Ideas in Neuroscience
*Olaf Sporns*

Population Thinking and Neuronal Selection: Metaphors or Concepts?
*Ernst Mayr*

Selection and the Origin of Information
*Manfred Eigen*

Section II: Development and Neuronal Populations

Morphoregulatory Molecules and Selectional Dynamics during Development
*Kathryn L. Crossin*

Exploration and Selection in the Early Acquisition of Skill
*Esther Thelen and Daniela Corbetta*

Population Activity in the Control of Movement
*Apostolos P. Georgopoulos*

Section III: Functional Segregation and Integration in the Brain

Reentry and the Problem of Cortical Integration
*Giulio Tononi*

Coherence as an Organizing Principle of Cortical Functions
*Wolf Singerl*

Temporal Mechanisms in Perception
*Ernst Pöppel*

Section IV: Memory and Models

Selection versus Instruction: Use of Computer Models to Compare Brain Theories
*George N. Reeke, Jr.*

Memory and Forgetting: Long-Term and Gradual Changes in Memory Storage
*Larry R. Squire*

Implicit Knowledge: New Perspectives on Unconscious Processes
*Daniel L. Schacter*

Section V: Psychophysics, Psychoanalysis, and Neuropsychology

Phantom Limbs, Neglect Syndromes, Repressed Memories, and Freudian Psychology
*V. S. Ramachandran*

Neural Darwinism and a Conceptual Crisis in Psychoanalysis
*Arnold H. Modell*

A New Vision of the Mind
*Oliver Sacks*

INDEX

## Volume 38

Regulation of $GABA_A$ Receptor Function and Gene Expression in the Central Nervous System
*A. Leslie Morrow*

Genetics and the Organization of the Basal Ganglia
*Robert Hitzemann, Yeang Olan, Stephen Kanes, Katherine Dains, and Barbara Hitzemann*

Structure and Pharmacology of Vertebrate $GABA_A$ Receptor Subtypes
*Paul J. Whiting, Ruth M. McKernan, and Keith A. Wafford*

Neurotransmitter Transporters: Molecular Biology, Function, and Regulation
*Beth Borowsky and Beth J. Hoffman*

Presynaptic Excitability
*Meyer B. Jackson*

Monoamine Neurotransmitters in Invertebrates and Vertebrates: An Examination of the Diverse Enzymatic Pathways Utilized to Synthesize and Inactivate Biogenic Amines
*B. D. Sloley and A. V. Juorio*

Neurotransmitter Systems in Schizophrenia
*Gavin P. Reynolds*

Physiology of Bergmann Glial Cells
*Thomas Müller and Helmut Kettenmann*

INDEX

## Volume 39

Modulation of Amino Acid-Gated Ion Channels by Protein Phosphorylation
*Stephen J. Moss and Trevor G. Smart*

Use-Dependent Regulation of $GABA_A$ Receptors
*Eugene M. Barnes, Jr.*

Synaptic Transmission and Modulation in the Neostriatum
*David M. Lovinger and Elizabeth Tyler*

The Cytoskeleton and Neurotransmitter Receptors
*Valerie J. Whatley and R. Adron Harris*

Endogenous Opioid Regulation of Hippocampal Function
*Michele L. Simmons and Charles Chavkin*

Molecular Neurobiology of the Cannabinoid Receptor
*Mary E. Abood and Billy R. Martin*

Genetic Models in the Study of Anesthetic Drug Action
*Victoria J. Simpson and Thomas E. Johnson*

Neurochemical Bases of Locomotion and Ethanol Stimulant Effects
*Tamara J. Phillips and Elaine H. Shen*

Effects of Ethanol on Ion Channels
*Fulton T. Crews, A. Leslie Morrow, Hugh Criswell, and George Breese*

Index

## Volume 40

Mechanisms of Nerve Cell Death: Apoptosis or Necrosis after Cerebral Ischemia
*R. M. E. Chalmers-Redman, A. D. Fraser, W. Y. H. Ju, J. Wadia, N. A. Tatton, and W. G. Tatton*

Changes in Ionic Fluxes during Cerebral Ischemia
*Tibor Kristian and Bo K. Siesjo*

Techniques for Examining Neuroprotective Drugs *in Vitro*
*A. Richard Green and Alan J. Cross*

Techniques for Examining Neuroprotective Drugs *in Vivo*
*Mark P. Goldberg, Uta Strasser, and Laura L. Dugan*

Calcium Antagonists: Their Role in Neuroprotection
*A. Jacqueline Hunter*

Sodium and Potassium Channel Modulators: Their Role in Neuroprotection
*Tihomir P. Obrenovich*

NMDA Antagonists: Their Role in Neuroprotection
*Danial L. Small*

Development of the NMDA Ion-Channel Blocker, Aptiganel Hydrochloride, as a Neuroprotective Agent for Acute CNS Injury
*Robert N. McBurney*

The Pharmacology of AMPA Antagonists and Their Role in Neuroprotection
*Rammy Gill and David Lodge*

GABA and Neuroprotection
*Patrick D. Lyden*

Adenosine and Neuroprotection
*Bertil B. Fredholm*

Interleukins and Cerebral Ischemia
*Nancy J. Rothwell, Sarah A. Loddick, and Paul Stroemer*

Nitrone-Based Free Radical Traps as Neuroprotective Agents in Cerebral Ischemia and Other Pathologies
*Kenneth Hensley, John M. Carney, Charles A. Stewart, Tahera Tabatabaie, Quentin Pye, and Robert A. Floyd*

Neurotoxic and Neuroprotective Roles of Nitric Oxide in Cerebral Ischemia
*Turgay Dalkara and Michael A. Moskowitz*

A Review of Earlier Clinical Studies on Neuroprotective Agents and Current Approaches
*Nils-Gunnar Wahlgren*

Index

## Volume 41

Section I: Historical Overview

Rediscovery of an Early Concept
*Jeremy D. Schmahmann*

Section II: Anatomic Substrates

The Cerebrocerebellar System
*Jeremy D. Schmahmann and Deepak N. Pandya*

Cerebellar Output Channels
*Frank A. Middleton and Peter L. Strick*

Cerebellar-Hypothalamic Axis: Basic Circuits and Clinical Observations
*Duane E. Haines, Espen Dietrichs, Gregory A. Mihailoff, and E. Frank McDonald*

Section III. Physiological Observations

Amelioration of Aggression: Response to Selective Cerebellar Lesions in the Rhesus Monkey
*Aaron J. Berman*

Autonomic and Vasomotor Regulation
*Donald J. Reis and Eugene V. Golanov*

Associative Learning
*Richard F. Thompson, Shaowen Bao, Lu Chen, Benjamin D. Cipriano, Jeffrey S. Grethe, Jeansok J. Kim, Judith K. Thompson, Jo Anne Tracy, Martha S. Weninger, and David J. Krupa*

Visuospatial Abilities
*Robert Lalonde*

Spatial Event Processing
*Marco Molinari, Laura Petrosini, and Liliana G. Grammaldo*

Section IV: Functional Neuroimaging Studies

Linguistic Processing
*Julie A. Fiez and Marcus E. Raichle*

Sensory and Cognitive Functions
*Lawrence M. Parsons and Peter T. Fox*

Skill Learning
*Julien Doyon*

Section V: Clinical and Neuropsychological Observations

Executive Function and Motor Skill Learning
*Mark Hallett and Jordon Grafman*

Verbal Fluency and Agrammatism
*Marco Molinari, Maria G. Leggio, and Maria C. Silveri*

Classical Conditioning
*Diana S. Woodruff-Pak*

Early Infantile Autism
*Margaret L. Bauman, Pauline A. Filipek, and Thomas L. Kemper*

Olivopontocerebellar Atrophy and Friedreich's Ataxia: Neuropsychological Consequences of Bilateral versus Unilateral Cerebellar Lesions
*Thérèse Botez-Marquard and Mihai I. Botez*

Posterior Fossa Syndrome
*Ian F. Pollack*

Cerebellar Cognitive Affective Syndrome
*Jeremy D. Schmahmann and Janet C. Sherman*

Inherited Cerebellar Diseases
*Claus W. Wallesch and Claudius Bartels*

Neuropsychological Abnormalities in Cerebellar Syndromes—Fact or Fiction?
*Irene Daum and Hermann Ackermann*

Section VI: Theoretical Considerations

Cerebellar Microcomplexes
*Masao Ito*

Control of Sensory Data Acquisition
*James M. Bower*

Neural Representations of Moving Systems
*Michael Paulin*

How Fibers Subserve Computing Capabilities: Similarities between Brains and Machines
*Henrietta C. Leiner and Alan L. Leiner*

Cerebellar Timing Systems
*Richard Ivry*

Attention Coordination and Anticipatory Control
*Natacha A. Akshoomoff, Eric Courchesne, and Jeanne Townsend*

Context-Response Linkage
*W. Thomas Thach*

Duality of Cerebellar Motor and Cognitive Functions
*James R. Bloedel and Vlastislav Bracha*

Section VII: Future Directions

Therapeutic and Research Implications
*Jeremy D. Schmahmann*

## Volume 42

Alzheimer Disease
*Mark A. Smith*

Neurobiology of Stroke
*W. Dalton Dietrich*

Free Radicals, Calcium, and the Synaptic Plasticity-Cell Death Continuum: Emerging Roles of the Trascription Factor NF$\kappa$B
*Mark P. Mattson*

AP-I Transcription Factors: Short- and Long-Term Modulators of Gene Expression in the Brain
*Keith Pennypacker*

Ion Channels in Epilepsy
*Istvan Mody*

Posttranslational Regulation of Ionotropic Glutamate Receptors and Synaptic Plasticity
*Xiaoning Bi, Steve Standley, and Michel Baudry*

Heritable Mutations in the Glycine, $GABA_A$, and Nicotinic Acetylcholine Receptors Provide New Insights into the Ligand-Gated Ion Channel Receptor Superfamily
*Behnaz Vafa and Peter R. Schofield*

INDEX

## Volume 43

Early Development of the *Drosophila* Neuromuscular Junction: A Model for Studying Neuronal Networks in Development
*Akira Chiba*

Development of Larval Body Wall Muscles
*Michael Bate, Matthias Landgraf, and Mar Ruiz Gómez Bate*

Development of Electrical Properties and Synaptic Transmission at the Embryonic Neuromuscular Junction
*Kendal S. Broadie*

Ultrastructural Correlates of Neuromuscular Junction Development
*Mary B. Rheuben, Motojiro Yoshihara, and Yoshiaki Kidokoro*

Assembly and Maturation of the *Drosophila* Larval Neuromuscular Junction
*L. Sian Gramates and Vivian Budnik*

Second Messenger Systems Underlying Plasticity at the Neuromuscular Junction
*Frances Hannan and Yi Zhong*

Mechanisms of Neurotransmitter Release
*J. Troy Littleton, Leo Pallanck, and Barry Ganetzky*

Vesicle Recycling at the *Drosophila* Neuromuscular Junction
*Daniel T. Stimson and Mani Ramaswami*

Ionic Currents in Larval Muscles of *Drosophila*
*Satpal Singh and Chun-Fang Wu*

Development of the Adult Neuromuscular System
*Joyce J. Fernandes and Haig Keshishian*

Controlling the Motor Neuron
*James R. Trimarchi, Ping Jin, and Rodney K. Murphey*

## Volume 44

Human Ego-Motion Perception
*A. V. van den Berg*

Optic Flow and Eye Movements
*M. Lappe and K.-P. Hoffman*

The Role of MST Neurons during Ocular Tracking in 3D Space
*K. Kawano, U. Inoue, A. Takemura, Y. Kodaka, and F. A. Miles*

Visual Navigation in Flying Insects
*M. V. Srinivasan and S.-W. Zhang*

Neuronal Matched Filters for Optic Flow Processing in Flying Insects
*H. G. Krapp*

A Common Frame of Reference for the Analysis of Optic Flow and Vestibular Information
*B. J. Frost and D. R. W. Wylie*

Optic Flow and the Visual Guidance of Locomotion in the Cat
*H. Sherk and G. A. Fowler*

Stages of Self-Motion Processing in Primate Posterior Parietal Cortex
*F. Bremmer, J.-R. Duhamel, S. B. Hamed, and W. Graf*

Optic Flow Analysis for Self-Movement Perception
*C. J. Duffy*

Neural Mechanisms for Self-Motion Perception in Area MST
*R. A. Andersen, K. V. Shenoy, J. A. Crowell, and D. C. Bradley*

Computational Mechanisms for Optic Flow Analysis in Primate Cortex
*M. Lappe*

Human Cortical Areas Underlying the Perception of Optic Flow: Brain Imaging Studies
*M. W. Greenlee*

What Neurological Patients Tell Us about the Use of Optic Flow
*L. M. Vaina and S. K. Rushton*

INDEX

## Volume 45

Mechanisms of Brain Plasticity: From Normal Brain Function to Pathology
*Philip. A. Schwartzkroin*

Brain Development and Generation of Brain Pathologies
*Gregory L. Holmes and Bridget McCabe*

Maturation of Channels and Receptors: Consequences for Excitability
*David F. Owens and Arnold R. Kriegstein*

Neuronal Activity and the Establishment of Normal and Epileptic Circuits during Brain Development
*John W. Swann, Karen L. Smith, and Chong L. Lee*

The Effects of Seizures of the Hippocampus of the Immature Brain
*Ellen F. Sperber and Solomon L. Moshe*

Abnormal Development and Catastrophic Epilepsies: The Clinical Picture and Relation to Neuroimaging
*Harry T. Chugani and Diane C. Chugani*

Cortical Reorganization and Seizure Generation in Dysplastic Cortex
*G. Avanzini, R. Preafico, S. Franceschetti, G. Sancini, G. Battaglia, and V. Scaioli*

Rasmussen's Syndrome with Particular Reference to Cerebral Plasticity: A Tribute to Frank Morrell
*Fredrick Andermann and Yuonne Hart*

Structural Reorganization of Hippocampal Networks Caused by Seizure Activity
*Daniel H. Lowenstein*

Epilepsy-Associated Plasticity in gamma-Amniobutyric Acid Receptor Expression, Function and Inhibitory Synaptic Properties
*Douglas A. Coulter*

Synaptic Plasticity and Secondary Epileptogenesis
*Timothy J. Teyler, Steven L. Morgan, Rebecca N. Russell, and Brian L. Woodside*

Synaptic Plasticity in Epileptogenesis: Cellular Mechanisms Underlying Long-Lasting Synaptic Modifications that Require New Gene Expression
*Oswald Steward, Christopher S. Wallace, and Paul F. Worley*

Cellular Correlates of Behavior
*Emma R. Wood, Paul A. Dudchenko, and Howard Eichenbaum*

Mechanisms of Neuronal Conditioning
*David A. T. King, David J. Krupa, Michael R. Foy, and Richard F. Thompson*

Plasticity in the Aging Central Nervous System
*C. A. Barnes*

Secondary Epileptogenesis, Kindling, and Intractable Epilepsy: A Reappraisal from the Perspective of Neuronal Plasticity
*Thomas P. Sutula*

Kindling and the Mirror Focus
*Dan C. McIntyre and Michael O. Poulter*

Partial Kindling and Behavioral Pathologies
*Robert E. Adamec*

The Mirror Focus and Secondary Epileptogenesis
*B. J. Wilder*

Hippocampal Lesions in Epilepsy: A Historical Review
*Robert Naquet*

Clinical Evidence for Secondary Epileptogensis
*Hans O. Luders*

Epilepsy as a Progressive (or Nonprogressive "Benign") Disorder
*John A. Wada*

Pathophysiological Aspects of Landau-Kleffner Syndrome: From the Active Epileptic Phase to Recovery
*Marie-Noelle Metz-Lutz, Pierre Maquet, Annd De Saint Martin, Gabrielle Rudolf, Norma Wioland, Edouard Hirsch, and Chriatian Marescaux*

Local Pathways of Seizure Propagation in Neocortex
*Barry W. Connors, David J. Pinto, and Albert E. Telefeian*

Multiple Subpial Transection: A Clinical Assessment
*C. E. Polkey*

The Legacy of Frank Morrell
*Jerome Engel, Jr.*

## Volume 46

Neurosteroids: Beginning of the Story
*Etienne E. Baulieu, P. Robel, and M. Schumacher*

Biosynthesis of Neurosteroids and Regulation of Their Synthesis
*Synthia H. Mellon and Hubert Vaudry*

Neurosteroid 7-Hydroxylation Products in the Brain
*Robert Morfin and Luboslav Stárka*

Neurosteroid Analysis
*Ahmed A. Alomary, Robert L. Fitzgerald, and Robert H. Purdy*

Role of the Peripheral-Type Benzodiazepine Receptor in Adrenal and Brain Steroidogenesis
*Rachel C. Brown and Vassilios Papadopoulos*

Formation and Effects of Neuroactive Steroids in the Central and Peripheral Nervous System
*Roberto Cosimo Melcangi, Valerio Magnaghi, Mariarita Galbiati, and Luciano Martini*

Neurosteroid Modulation of Recombinant and Synaptic $GABA_A$ Receptors
*Jeremy J. Lambert, Sarah C. Harney, Delia Belelli, and John A. Peters*

$GABA_A$-Receptor Plasticity during Long-Term Exposure to and Withdrawal from Progesterone
*Giovanni Biggio, Paolo Follesa, Enrico Sanna, Robert H. Purdy, and Alessandra Concas*

Stress and Neuroactive Steroids
*Maria Luisa Barbaccia, Mariangela Serra, Robert H. Purdy, and Giovanni Biggio*

Neurosteroids in Learning and Memory Processes
*Monique Vallée, Willy Mayo, George F. Koob, and Michel Le Moal*

Neurosteroids and Behavior
*Sharon R. Engel and Kathleen A. Grant*

Ethanol and Neurosteroid Interactions in the Brain
*A. Leslie Morrow, Margaret J. VanDoren, Rebekah Fleming, and Shannon Penland*

Preclinical Development of Neurosteroids as Neuroprotective Agents for the Treatment of Neurodegenerative Diseases
*Paul A. Lapchak and Dalia M. Araujo*

Clinical Implications of Circulating Neurosteroids
*Andrea R. Genazzani, Patrizia Monteleone, Massimo Stomati, Francesca Bernardi, Luigi Cobellis, Elena Casarosa, Michele Luisi, Stefano Luisi, and Felice Petraglia*

Neuroactive Steroids and Central Nervous System Disorders
*Mingde Wang, Torbjörn Bäckström, Inger Sundström, Göran Wahlström, Tommy Olsson, Di Zhu, Inga-Maj Johansson, Inger Björn, and Marie Bixo*

Neuroactive Steroids in Neuropsychopharmacology
*Rainer Rupprecht and Florian Holsboer*

Current Perspectives on the Role of Neurosteroids in PMS and Depression
*Lisa D. Griffin, Susan C. Conrad, and Synthia H. Mellon*

Index

## Volume 47

Introduction: Studying Gene Expression in Neural Tissues by *in Situ* Hybridization
*W. Wisden and B. J. Morris*

Part I: *In Situ* Hybridization with Radiolabelled Oligonucleotides
*In Situ* Hybridization with Oligonucleotide Probes
*Wl. Wisden and B. J. Morris*

Cryostat Sectioning of Brains
*Victoria Revilla and Alison Jones*

Processing Rodent Embryonic and Early Postnatal Tissue for *in Situ* Hybridization with Radiolabelled Oligonucleotides
*David J. Laurie, Petra C. U. Schrotz, Hannah Monyer, and Ulla Amtmann*

Processing of Retinal Tissue for *in Situ* Hybridization
*Frank Müller*

Processing the Spinal Cord for *in Situ* Hybridization with Radiolabelled Oligonucleotides
*A. Berthele and T. R. Tölle*

Processing Human Brain Tissue for *in Situ* Hybridization with Radiolabelled Oligonucleotides
*Louise F. B. Nicholson*

*In Situ* Hybridization of Astrocytes and Neurons Cultured *in Vitro*
*L. A. Arizza-McNaughton, C. De Felipe, and S. P. Hunt*

*In Situ* Hybridization on Organotypic Slice Cultures
*A. Gerfin-Moser and H. Monyer*

Quantitative Analysis of *in Situ* Hybridization Histochemistry
*Andrew L. Gundlach and Ross D. O'Shea*

Part II: Nonradioactive *in Situ* hybridization

Nonradioactive *in Situ* Hybridization Using Alkaline Phosphatase-Labelled Oligonucleotides
*S. J. Augood, E. M. McGowan, B. R. Finsen, B. Heppelmann, and P. C. Emson*

Combining Nonradioactive *in Situ* Hybridization with Immunohistological and Anatomical Techniques
*Petra Wahle*

Nonradioactive *in Situ* Hybridization: Simplified Procedures for Use in Whole Mounts of Mouse and Chick Embryos
*Linda Ariza-McNaughton and Robb Krumlauf*

INDEX

## Volume 48

Assembly and Intracellular Trafficking of $GABA_A$ Receptors Eugene
*Barnes*

Subcellular Localization and Regulation of $GABA_A$ Receptors and Associated Proteins Bernhard Lüscher and Jean-Marc Fritschy $D_1$ Dopamine Receptors
*Richard Mailman*

Molecular Modeling of Ligand-Gated Ion Channels: Progress and Challenges
*Ed Bertaccini and James R. Trudel*

Alzheimer's Disease: Its Diagnosis and Pathogenesis
*Jillian J. Kril and Glenda M. Halliday*

DNA Arrays and Functional Genomics in Neurobiology
*Christelle Thibault, Long Wang, Li Zhang, and Michael F. Miles*

INDEX

## Volume 49

What Is West Syndrome?
*Olivier Dulac, Christine Soufflet, Catherine Chiron, and Anna Kaminski*

The Relationship between encephalopathy and Abnormal Neuronal Activity in the Developing Brain
*Frances E. Jensen*

Hypotheses from Functional Neuroimaging Studies
*Csaba Juhász, Harry T. Chugani, Ouo Muzik, and Diane C. Chugani*

Infantile Spasms: Unique Sydrome or General Age-Dependent Manifestation of a Diffuse Encephalopathy?
*M. A. Koehn and M. Duchowny*

Histopathology of Brain Tissue from Patients with Infantile Spasms
*Harry V. Vinters*

Generators of Ictal and Interictal Electroencephalograms Associated with Infantile Spasms: Intracellular Studies of Cortical and Thalamic Neurons
*M. Steriade and I. Timofeev*

Cortical and Subcortical Generators of Normal and Abnormal Rhythmicity
*David A. McCormick*

Role of Subcortical Structures in the Pathogenesis of Infantile Spasms: What Are Possible Subcortical Mediators?
*F. A. Lado and S. L. Moshé*

What Must We Know to Develop Better Therapies?
*Jean Aicardi*

The Treatment of Infantile Spasms: An Evidence-Based Approach
*Mark Mackay, Shelly Weiss, and O. Carter Snead III*

ACTH Treatment of Infantile Spasms: Mechanisms of Its Effects in Modulation of Neuronal Excitability
*K. L. Brunson, S. Avishai-Eliner, and T. Z. Baram*

Neurosteroids and Infantile Spasms: The Deoxycorticosterone Hypothesis
*Michael A. Rogawski and Doodipala S. Reddy*

Are there Specific Anatomical and/or Transmitter Systems (Cortical or Subcortical) That Should Be Targeted?
*Phillip C. Jobe*

Medical versus Surgical Treatment: Which Treatment When
*W. Donald Shields*

Developmental Outcome with and without Successful Intervention
*Rochelle Caplan, Prabha Siddarth, Gary Mathern, Harry Vinters, Susan Curtiss, Jennifer Levitt, Robert Asarnow, and W. Donald Shields*

Infantile Spasms versus Myoclonus: Is There a Connection?
*Michael R. Pranzatelli*

Tuberous Sclerosis as an Underlying Basis for Infantile Spasm
*Raymond S. Yeung*

Brain Malformation, Epilepsy, and Infantile Spasms
*M. Elizabeth Ross*

Brain Maturational Aspects Relevant to Pathophysiology of Infantile Spasms
*G. Auanzini, F. Panzica, and S. Franceschetti*

Gene Expression Analysis as a Strategy to Understand the Molecular Pathogenesis of Infantile Spasms
*Peter B. Crino*

Infantile Spasms: Criteria for an Animal Model
*Carl E. Stafstrom and Gregory L. Holmes*

INDEX

## Volume 50

Part I: Primary Mechanisms

How Does Glucose Generate Oxidative Stress In Peripheral Nerve?
*Irina G. Obrosova*

Glycation in Diabetic Neuropathy: Characteristics, Consequences, Causes, and Therapeutic Options
*Paul J. Thornalley*

Part II: Secondary Changes

Protein Kinase C Changes in Diabetes: Is the Concept Relevant to Neuropathy?
*Joseph Eichberg*

Are Mitogen-Activated Protein Kinases Glucose Transducers for Diabetic Neuropathies?
*Tertia D. Purves and David R. Tomlinson*

Neurofilaments in Diabetic Neuropathy
*Paul Fernyhough and Robert E. Schmidt*

Apoptosis in Diabetic Neuropathy
*Aviva Tolkovsky*

Nerve and Ganglion Blood Flow in Diabetes: An Appraisal
*Douglas W. Zochodne*

Part III: Manifestations

Potential Mechanisms of Neuropathic Pain in Diabetes
*Nigel A. Calcutt*

Electrophysiologic Measures of Diabetic Neuropathy: Mechanism and Meaning
*Joseph C. Arezzo and Elena Zotova*

Neuropathology and Pathogenesis of Diabetic Autonomic Neuropathy
*Robert E. Schmidt*

Role of the Schwann Cell in Diabetic Neuropathy
*Luke Eckersley*

Part IV: Potential Treatment

Polyol Pathway and Diabetic Peripheral Neuropathy
*Peter J. Oates*

Nerve Growth Factor for the Treatment of Diabetic Neuropathy: What Went Wrong, What Went Right, and What Does the Future Hold?
*Stuart C. Apfel*

Angiotensin-Converting Enzyme Inhibitors: Are there Credible Mechanisms for Beneficial Effects in Diabetic Neuropathy?
*Rayaz A. Malik and David R. Tomlinson*

Clinical Trials for Drugs Against Diabetic Neuropathy: Can We Combine Scientific Needs With Clinical Practicalities?
*Dan Ziegler and Dieter Luft*

INDEX

## Volume 51

Energy Metabolism in the Brain
*Leif Hertz and Gerald A. Dienel*

The Cerebral Glucose-Fatty Acid Cycle: Evolutionary Roots, Regulation, and (Patho) physiological Importance
*Kurt Heininger*

Expression, Regulation, and Functional Role of Glucose Transporters (GLUTs) in Brain
*Donard S. Dwyer, Susan J. Vannucci, and Ian A. Simpson*

Insulin-Like Growth Factor-1 Promotes Neuronal Glucose Utilization During Brain Development and Repair Processes
*Carolyn A. Bondy and Clara M. Cheng*

CNS Sensing and Regulation of Peripheral Glucose Levels
*Barry E. Levin, Ambrose A. Dunn-Meynell, and Vanessa H. Routh*

Glucose Transporter Protein Syndromes
*Darryl C. De Vivo, Dong Wang, Juan M. Pascual, and Yuan Yuan Ho*

Glucose, Stress, and Hippocampal Neuronal Vulnerability
*Lawrence P. Reagan*

Glucose/Mitochondria in Neurological Conditions
*John P. Blass*

Energy Utilization in the Ischemic/Reperfused Brain
*John W. Phillis and Michael H. O'Regan*

Diabetes Mellitus and the Central Nervous System
*Anthony L. McCall*

Diabetes, the Brain, and Behavior: Is There a Biological Mechanism Underlying the Association between Diabetes and Depression?
*A. M. Jacobson, J. A. Samson, K. Weinger, and C. M. Ryan*

Schizophrenia and Diabetes
*David C. Henderson and Elissa R. Ettinger*

Psychoactive Drugs Affect Glucose Transport and the Regulation of Glucose Metabolism
*Donard S. Dwyer, Timothy D. Ardizzone, and Ronald J. Bradley*

INDEX

## Volume 52

Neuroimmune Relationships in Perspective
*Frank Hucklebridge and Angela Clow*

Sympathetic Nervous System Interaction with the Immune System
*Virginia M. Sanders and Adam P. Kohm*

Mechanisms by Which Cytokines Signal the Brain
*Adrian J. Dunn*

Neuropeptides: Modulators of Immune Responses in Health and Disease
*David S. Jessop*

Brain–Immune Interactions in Sleep
*Lisa Marshall and Jan Born*

Neuroendocrinology of Autoimmunity
*Michael Harbuz*

Systemic Stress-Induced Th2 Shift and Its Clinical Implications
*Ibia J. Elenkov*

Neural Control of Salivary S-IgA Secretion
*Gordon B. Proctor and Guy H. Carpenter*

Stress and Secretory Immunity
*Jos A. Bosch, Christopher Ring, Eco J. C. de Geus, Enno C. I. Veerman, and Arie V. Nieuw Amerongen*

Cytokines and Depression
*Angela Clow*

Immunity and Schizophrenia: Autoimmunity, Cytokines, and Immune Responses
*Fiona Gaughran*

Cerebral Lateralization and the Immune System
*Pierre J. Neveu*

Behavioral Conditioning of the Immune System
*Frank Hucklebridge*

Psychological and Neuroendocrine Correlates of Disease Progression
*Julie M. Turner-Cobb*

The Role of Psychological Intervention in Modulating Aspects of Immune Function in Relation to Health and Well-Being
*J. H. Gruzelier*

INDEX

## Volume 53

Section I: Mitochondrial Structure and Function

Mitochondrial DNA Structure and Function
*Carlos T. Moraes, Sarika Srivastava, Ilias Kirkinezos, Jose Oca-Cossio, Corina van Waveren, Markus Woischnick, and Francisca Diaz*

Oxidative Phosphorylation: Structure, Function, and Intermediary Metabolism
*Simon J. R. Heales, Matthew E. Gegg, and John B. Clark*

Import of Mitochondrial Proteins
*Matthias F. Bauer, Sabine Hofmann, and Walter Neupert*

Section II: Primary Respiratory Chain Disorders

Mitochondrial Disorders of the Nervous System: Clinical, Biochemical, and Molecular Genetic Features
*Dominic Thyagarajan and Edward Byrne*

Section III: Secondary Respiratory Chain Disorders

Friedreich's Ataxia
*J. M. Cooper and J. L. Bradley*

Wilson Disease
*C. A. Davie and A. H. V. Schapira*

Hereditary Spastic Paraplegia
*Christopher J. McDermott and Pamela J. Shaw*

Cytochrome c Oxidase Deficiency
*Giacomo P. Comi, Sandra Strazzer, Sara Galbiati, and Nereo Bresolin*

Section IV: Toxin Induced Mitochondrial Dysfunction

Toxin-Induced Mitochondrial Dysfunction
*Susan E. Browne and M. Flint Beal*

Section V: Neurodegenerative Disorders

Parkinson's Disease
*L. V. P. Korlipara and A. H. V. Schapira*

Huntington's Disease: The Mystery Unfolds?
*Åsa Petersén and Patrik Brundin*

Mitochondria in Alzheimer's Disease
*Russell H. Swerdlow and Stephen J. Kish*

Contributions of Mitochondrial Alterations, Resulting from Bad Genes and a Hostile Environment, to the Pathogenesis of Alzheimer's Disease
*Mark P. Mattson*

Mitochondria and Amyotrophic Lateral Sclerosis
*Richard W. Orrell and Anthony H. V. Schapira*

Section VI: Models of Mitochondrial Disease

Models of Mitochondrial Disease
*Danae Liolitsa and Michael G. Hanna*

Section VII: Defects of $\beta$ Oxidation Including Carnitine Deficiency

Defects of $\beta$ Oxidation Including Carnitine Deficiency
*K. Bartlett and M. Pourfarzam*

Section VIII: Mitochondrial Involvement in Aging

The Mitochondrial Theory of Aging: Involvement of Mitochondrial DNA Damage and Repair
*Nadja C. de Souza-Pinto and Vilhelm A. Bohr*

INDEX

## Volume 54

Unique General Anesthetic Binding Sites Within Distinct Conformational States of the Nicotinic Acetylcholine Receptor
*Hugo R. Ariaas, William, R. Kem, James R. Truddell, and Michael P. Blanton*

Signaling Molecules and Receptor Transduction Cascades That Regulate NMDA Receptor-Mediated Synaptic Transmission
*Suhas. A. Kotecha and John F. MacDonald*

Behavioral Measures of Alcohol Self-Administration and Intake Control: Rodent Models
*Herman H. Samson and Cristine L. Czachowski*

Dopaminergic Mouse Mutants: Investigating the Roles of the Different Dopamine Receptor Subtypes and the Dopamine Transporter
*Shirlee Tan, Bettina Hermann, and Emiliana Borrelli*

*Drosophila melanogaster*, A Genetic Model System for Alcohol Research
*Douglas J. Guarnieri and Ulrike Heberlein*

INDEX

## Volume 55

Section I: Virsu Vectors For Use in the Nervous System

Non-Neurotropic Adenovirus: a Vector for Gene Transfer to the Brain and Gene Therapy of Neurological Disorders
*P. R. Lowenstein, D. Suwelack, J. Hu, X. Yuan, M. Jimenez-Dalmaroni, S. Goverdhama, and M.G. Castro*

Adeno-Associated Virus Vectors
*E. Lehtonen and L. Tenenbaum*

Problems in the Use of Herpes Simplex Virus as a Vector
*L. T. Feldman*

Lentiviral Vectors
*J. Jakobsson, C. Ericson, N. Rosenquist, and C. Lundberg*

Retroviral Vectors for Gene Delivery to Neural Precursor Cells
*K. Kageyama, H. Hirata, and J. Hatakeyama*

Section II: Gene Therapy with Virus Vectors for Specific Disease of the Nervous System

The Principles of Molecular Therapies for Glioblastoma
*G. Karpati and J. Nalbatonglu*

Oncolytic Herpes Simplex Virus
*J. C. C. Hu and R. S. Coffin*

Recombinant Retrovirus Vectors for Treatment of Brain Tumors
*N. G. Rainov and C. M. Kramm*

Adeno-Associated Viral Vectors for Parkinson's Disease
*I. Muramatsu, L. Wang, K. Ikeguchi, K-i Fujimoto, T. Okada, H. Mizukami, Y. Hanazono, A. Kume, I. Nakano, and K. Ozawa*

HSV Vectors for Parkinson's Disease
*D. S. Latchman*

Gene Therapy for Stroke
*K. Abe and W. R. Zhang*

Gene Therapy for Mucopolysaccharidosis
*A. Bosch and J. M. Heard*

INDEX

## Volume 56

Behavioral Mechanisms and the Neurobiology of Conditioned Sexual Responding
*Mark Krause*

NMDA Receptors in Alcoholism
*Paula L. Hoffman*

Processing and Representation of Species-Specific Communication Calls in the Auditory System of Bats
*George D. Pollak, Achim Klug, and Eric E. Bauer*

Central Nervous System Control of Micturition
*Gert Holstege and Leonora J. Mouton*

The Structure and Physiology of the Rat Auditory System: An Overview
*Manuel Malmierca*

Neurobiology of Cat and Human Sexual Behavior
*Gert Holstege and J. R. Georgiadis*

INDEX

## Volume 57

Cumulative Subject Index of Volumes 1–25

## Volume 58

Cumulative Subject Index of Volumes 26–50

## Volume 59

Loss of Spines and Neuropil
*Liesl B. Jones*

Schizophrenia as a Disorder of Neuroplasticity
*Robert E. McCullumsmith, Sarah M. Clinton, and James H. Meador-Woodruff*

The Synaptic Pathology of Schizophrenia: Is Aberrant Neurodevelopment and Plasticity to Blame?
*Sharon L. Eastwood*

Neurochemical Basis for an Epigenetic Vision of Synaptic Organization
*E. Costa, D. R. Grayson, M. Veldic, and A. Guidotti*

Muscarinic Receptors in Schizophrenia: Is There a Role for Synaptic Plasticity?
*Thomas J. Raedler*

Serotonin and Brain Development
*Monsheel S. K. Sodhi and Elaine Sanders-Bush*

Presynaptic Proteins and Schizophrenia
*William G. Honer and Clint E. Young*

Mitogen-Activated Protein Kinase Signaling
*Svetlana V. Kyosseva*

Postsynaptic Density Scaffolding Proteins at Excitatory Synapse and Disorders of Synaptic Plasticity: Implications for Human Behavior Pathologies
*Andrea de Bartolomeis and Germano Fiore*

Prostaglandin-Mediated Signaling in Schizophrenia
*S. Smesny*

Mitochondria, Synaptic Plasticity, and Schizophrenia
*Dorit Ben-Shachar and Daphna Laifenfeld*

Membrane Phospholipids and Cytokine Interaction in Schizophrenia
*Jeffrey K. Yao and Daniel P. van Kammen*

Neurotensin, Schizophrenia, and Antipsychotic Drug Action
*Becky Kinkead and Charles B. Nemeroff*

Schizophrenia, Vitamin D, and Brain Development
*Alan Mackay-Sim, François FÉron, Darryl Eyles, Thomas Burne, and John McGrath*

Possible Contributions of Myelin and Oligodendrocyte Dysfunction to Schizophrenia
*Daniel G. Stewart and Kenneth L. Davis*

Brain-Derived Neurotrophic Factor and the Plasticity of the Mesolimbic Dopamine Pathway
*Oliver Guillin, Nathalie Griffon, Jorge Diaz, Bernard Le Foll, Erwan Bezard, Christian Gross, Chris Lammers, Holger Stark, Patrick Carroll, Jean-Charles Schwartz, and Pierre Sokoloff*

S100B in Schizophrenic Psychosis
*Matthias Rothermundt, Gerald Ponath, and Volker Arolt*

*Oct-6* Transcription Factor
*Maria Ilia*

NMDA Receptor Function, Neuroplasticity, and the Pathophysiology of Schizophrenia
*Joseph T. Coyle and Guochuan Tsai*

INDEX

## Volume 60

Microarray Platforms: Introduction and Application to Neurobiology
*Stanislav L. Karsten, Lili C. Kudo, and Daniel H. Geschwind*

Experimental Design and Low-Level Analysis of Microarray Data
*B. M. Bolstad, F. Collin, K. M. Simpson, R. A. Irizarry, and T. P. Speed*

Brain Gene Expression: Genomics and Genetics
*Elissa J. Chesler and Robert W. Williams*

DNA Microarrays and Animal Models of Learning and Memory
*Sebastiano Cavallaro*

Microarray Analysis of Human Nervous System Gene Expression in Neurological Disease
*Steven A. Greenberg*

DNA Microarray Analysis of Postmortem Brain Tissue
*Károly Mirnics, Pat Levitt, and David A. Lewis*

INDEX

## Volume 61

Section I: High-Throughput Technologies

Biomarker Discovery Using Molecular Profiling Approaches
*Stephen J. Walker and Arron Xu*

Proteomic Analysis of Mitochondrial Proteins
*Mary F. Lopez, Simon Melov, Felicity Johnson, Nicole Nagulko, Eva Golenko, Scott Kuzdzal, Suzanne Ackloo, and Alvydas Mikulskis*

Section II: Proteomic Applications

NMDA Receptors, Neural Pathways, and Protein Interaction Databases
*Holger Husi*

Dopamine Transporter Network and Pathways
*Rajani Maiya and R. Dayne Mayfield*

Proteomic Approaches in Drug Discovery and Development
*Holly D. Soares, Stephen A. Williams, Peter J. Snyder, Feng Gao, Tom Stiger, Christian Rohlff, Athula Herath, Trey Sunderland, Karen Putnam, and W. Frost White*

Section III: Informatics

Proteomic Informatics
*Steven Russell, William Old, Katheryn Resing, and Lawrence Hunter*

Section IV: Changes in the Proteome by Disease

Proteomics Analysis in Alzheimer's Disease: New Insights into Mechanisms of Neurodegeneration
*D. Allan Butterfield and Debra Boyd-Kimball*

Proteomics and Alcoholism
*Frank A. Witzmann and Wendy N. Strother*

Proteomics Studies of Traumatic Brain Injury
*Kevin K. W. Wang, Andrew Ottens, William Haskins, Ming Cheng Liu, Firas Kobeissy, Nancy Denslow, SuShing Chen, and Ronald L. Hayes*

Influence of Huntington's Disease on the Human and Mouse Proteome
*Claus Zabel and Joachim Klose*

Section V: Overview of the Neuroproteome

Proteomics—Application to the Brain
*Katrin Marcus, Oliver Schmidt, Heike Schaefer, Michael Hamacher, AndrÅ van Hall, and Helmut E. Meyer*

INDEX

## Volume 62

$GABA_A$ Receptor Structure–Function Studies: A Reexamination in Light of New Acetylcholine Receptor Structures
*Myles H. Akabas*

Dopamine Mechanisms and Cocaine Reward
*Aiko Ikegami and Christine L. Duvauchelle*

Proteolytic Dysfunction in Neurodegenerative Disorders
*Kevin St. P. McNaught*

Neuroimaging Studies in Bipolar Children and Adolescents
*Rene L. Olvera, David C. Glahn, Sheila C. Caetano, Steven R. Pliszka, and Jair C. Soares*

Chemosensory G-Protein-Coupled Receptor Signaling in the Brain
*Geoffrey E. Woodard*

Disturbances of Emotion Regulation after Focal Brain Lesions
*Antoine Bechara*

The Use of *Caenorhabditis elegans* in Molecular Neuropharmacology
*Jill C. Bettinger, Lucinda Carnell, Andrew G. Davies, and Steven L. McIntire*

INDEX

## Volume 63

Mapping Neuroreceptors at work: On the Definition and Interpretation of Binding Potentials after 20 years of Progress
*Albert Gjedde, Dean F. Wong, Pedro Rosa-Neto, and Paul Cumming*

Mitochondrial Dysfunction in Bipolar Disorder: From $^{31}$P-Magnetic Resonance Spectroscopic Findings to Their Molecular Mechanisms
*Tadafumi Kato*

Large-Scale Microarray Studies of Gene Expression in Multiple Regions of the Brain in Schizophrenia and Alzeimer's Disease
*Pavel L. Katsel, Kenneth L. Davis, and Vahram Haroutunian*

Regulation of Serotonin 2C Receptor PRE-mRNA Editing By Serotonin
*Claudia Schmauss*

The Dopamine Hypothesis of Drug Addiction: Hypodopaminergic State
*Miriam Melis, Saturnino Spiga, and Marco Diana*

Human and Animal Spongiform Encephalopathies are Autoimmune Diseases: A Novel Theory and Its supporting Evidence
*Bao Ting Zhu*

Adenosine and Brain Function
*Bertil B. Fredholm, Jiang-Fan Chen, Rodrigo A. Cunha, Per Svenningsson, and Jean-Marie Vaugeois*

INDEX

## Volume 64

Section I. The Cholinergic System
*John Smythies*

Section II. The Dopamine System
*John Symythies*

Section III. The Norepinephrine System
*John Smythies*

Section IV. The Adrenaline System
*John Smythies*

Section V. Serotonin System
*John Smythies*

INDEX

## Volume 65

Insulin Resistance: Causes and Consequences
*Zachary T. Bloomgarden*

Antidepressant-Induced Manic Conversion: A Developmentally Informed Synthesis of the Literature
*Christine J. Lim, James F. Leckman, Christopher Young, and AndrÉs Martin*

Sites of Alcohol and Volatile Anesthetic Action on Glycine Receptors
*Ingrid A. Lobo and R. Adron Harris*

Role of the Orbitofrontal Cortex in Reinforcement Processing and Inhibitory Control: Evidence from Functional Magnetic Resonance Imaging Studies in Healthy Human Subjects
*Rebecca Elliott and Bill Deakin*

Common Substrates of Dysphoria in Stimulant Drug Abuse and Primary Depression: Therapeutic Targets
*Kate Baicy, Carrie E. Bearden, John Monterosso, Arthur L. Brody, Andrew J. Isaacson, and Edythe D. London*

The Role of cAMP Response Element–Binding Proteins in Mediating Stress-Induced Vulnerability to Drug Abuse
*Arati Sadalge Kreibich and Julie A. Blendy*

G-Protein–Coupled Receptor Deorphanizations
*Yumiko Saito and Olivier Civelli*

Mechanistic Connections Between Glucose/Lipid Disturbances and Weight Gain Induced by Antipsychotic Drugs
*Donard S. Dwyer, Dallas Donohoe, Xiao-Hong Lu, and Eric J. Aamodt*

Serotonin Firing Activity as a Marker for Mood Disorders: Lessons from Knockout Mice
*Gabriella Gobbi*

INDEX

## Volume 66

Brain Atlases of Normal and Diseased Populations
*Arthur W. Toga and Paul M. Thompson*

Neuroimaging Databases as a Resource for Scientific Discovery
*John Darrell Van Horn, John Wolfe, Autumn Agnoli, Jeffrey Woodward, Michael Schmitt, James Dobson, Sarene Schumacher, and Bennet Vance*

Modeling Brain Responses
*Karl J. Friston, William Penny, and Olivier David*

Voxel-Based Morphometric Analysis Using Shape Transformations
*Christos Davatzikos*

The Cutting Edge of fMRI and High-Field fMRI
*Dae-Shik Kim*

Quantification of White Matter Using Diffusion-Tensor Imaging
*Hae-Jeong Park*

Perfusion fMRI for Functional Neuroimaging
*Geoffrey K. Aguirre, John A. Detre, and Jiongjiong Wang*

Functional Near-Infrared Spectroscopy: Potential and Limitations in Neuroimaging Studies
*Yoko Hoshi*

Neural Modeling and Functional Brain Imaging: The Interplay Between the Data-Fitting and Simulation Approaches
*Barry Horwitz and Michael F. Glabus*

Combined EEG and fMRI Studies of Human Brain Function
*V. Menon and S. Crottaz-Herbette*

INDEX

## Volume 67

Distinguishing Neural Substrates of Heterogeneity Among Anxiety Disorders
*Jack B. Nitschke and Wendy Heller*

Neuroimaging in Dementia
*K. P. Ebmeier, C. Donaghey, and N. J. Dougall*

Prefrontal and Anterior Cingulate Contributions to Volition in Depression
*Jack B. Nitschke and Kristen L. Mackiewicz*

Functional Imaging Research in Schizophrenia
*H. Tost, G. Ende, M. Ruf, F. A. Henn, and A. Meyer-Lindenberg*

Neuroimaging in Functional Somatic Syndromes
*Patrick B. Wood*

Neuroimaging in Multiple Sclerosis
*Alireza Minagar, Eduardo Gonzalez-Toledo, James Pinkston, and Stephen L. Jaffe*

Stroke
*Roger E. Kelley and Eduardo Gonzalez-Toledo*

Functional MRI in Pediatric Neurobehavioral Disorders
*Michael Seyffert and F. Xavier Castellanos*

Structural MRI and Brain Development
*Paul M. Thompson, Elizabeth R. Sowell, Nitin Gogtay, Jay N. Giedd, Christine N. Vidal, Kiralee M. Hayashi, Alex Leow, Rob Nicolson, Judith L. Rapoport, and Arthur W. Toga*

Neuroimaging and Human Genetics
*Georg Winterer, Ahmad R. Hariri, David Goldman, and Daniel R. Weinberger*

Neuroreceptor Imaging in Psychiatry: Theory and Applications
*W. Gordon Frankle, Mark Slifstein, Peter S. Talbot, and Marc Laruelle*

INDEX

## Volume 68

Fetal Magnetoencephalography: Viewing the Developing Brain *In Utero*
*Hubert Preissl, Curtis L. Lowery, and Hari Eswaran*

Magnetoencephalography in Studies of Infants and Children
*Minna Huotilainen*

Let's Talk Together: Memory Traces Revealed by Cooperative Activation in the Cerebral Cortex
*Jochen Kaiser, Susanne Leiberg, and Werner Lutzenberger*

Human Communication Investigated With Magnetoencephalography: Speech, Music, and Gestures
*Thomas R. Knösche, Burkhard Maess, Akinori Nakamura, and Angela D. Friederici*

Combining Magnetoencephalography and Functional Magnetic Resonance Imaging
*Klaus Mathiak and Andreas J. Fallgatter*

Beamformer Analysis of MEG Data
*Arjan Hillebrand and Gareth R. Barnes*

Functional Connectivity Analysis in Magnetoencephalography
*Alfons Schnitzler and Joachim Gross*

Human Visual Processing as Revealed by Magnetoencephalographys
*Yoshiki Kaneoke, Shoko Watanabe, and Ryusuke Kakigi*

A Review of Clinical Applications of Magnetoencephalography
*Andrew C. Papanicolaou, Eduardo M. Castillo, Rebecca Billingsley-Marshall, Ekaterina Pataraia, and Panagiotis G. Simos*

INDEX

## Volume 69

Nematode Neurons: Anatomy and Anatomical Methods in Caenorhabditis elegans
*David H. Hall, Robyn Lints, and Zeynep Altun*

Investigations of Learning and Memory in Caenorhabditis elegans
*Andrew C. Giles, Jacqueline K. Rose, and Catharine H. Rankin*

Neural Specification and Differentiation
*Eric Aamodt and Stephanie Aamodt*

Sexual Behavior of the Caenorhabditis elegans Male
*Scott W. Emmons*

The Motor Circuit
*Stephen E. Von Stetina, Millet Treinin, and David M. Miller III*

Mechanosensation in Caenorhabditis elegans
*Robert O'Hagan and Martin Chalfie*

## Volume 70

Spectral Processing by the Peripheral Auditory System Facts and Models
*Enrique A. Lopez-Poveda*

Basic Psychophysics of Human Spectral Processing
*Brian C. J. Moore*

Across-Channel Spectral Processing
*John H. Grose, Joseph W. Hall III, and Emily Buss*

Speech and Music Have Different Requirements for Spectral Resolution
*Robert V. Shannon*

Non-Linearities and the Representation of Auditory Spectra
*Eric D. Young, Jane J. Yu, and Lina A. J. Reiss*

Spectral Processing in the Inferior Colliculus
*Kevin A. Davis*

Neural Mechanisms for Spectral Analysis in the Auditory Midbrain, Thalamus, and Cortex
*Monty A. Escabí and Heather L. Read*

Spectral Processing in the Auditory Cortex
*Mitchell L. Sutter*

Processing of Dynamic Spectral Properties of Sounds
*Adrian Rees and Manuel S. Malmierca*

Representations of Spectral Coding in the Human Brain
*Deborah A. Hall, PhD*

Spectral Processing and Sound Source Determination
*Donal G. Sinex*

Spectral Information in Sound Localization
*Simon Carlile, Russell Martin, and Ken McAnally*

Plasticity of Spectral Processing
*Dexter R. F. Irvine and Beverly A. Wright*

Spectral Processing In Cochlear Implants
*Colette M. McKay*

INDEX

## Volume 71

Autism: Neuropathology, Alterations of the GABAergic System, and Animal Models
*Christoph Schmitz, Imke A. J. van Kooten, Patrick R. Hof, Herman van Engeland, Paul H. Patterson, and Harry W. M. Steinbusch*

The Role of GABA in the Early Neuronal Development
*Marta Jelitai and Emı́'lia Madarasz*

GABAergic Signaling in the Developing Cerebellum
*Chitoshi Takayama*

Insights into GABA Functions in the Developing Cerebellum
*Mo'nica L. Fiszman*

Role of GABA in the Mechanism of the Onset of Puberty in Non-Human Primates
*Ei Terasawa*

Rett Syndrome: A Rosetta Stone for Understanding the Molecular Pathogenesis of Autism
*Janine M. LaSalle, Amber Hogart, and Karen N. Thatcher*

GABAergic Cerebellar System in Autism: A Neuropathological and Developmental Perspective
*Gene J. Blatt*

Reelin Glycoprotein in Autism and Schizophrenia
*S. Hossein Fatemi*

Is There A Connection Between Autism, Prader-Willi Syndrome, Catatonia, and GABA?
*Dirk M. Dhossche, Yaru Song, and Yiming Liu*

Alcohol, GABA Receptors, and Neurodevelopmental Disorders
*Ujjwal K. Rout*

Effects of Secretin on Extracellular GABA and Other Amino Acid Concentrations in the Rat Hippocampus
*Hans-Willi Clement, Alexander Pschibul, and Eberhard Schulz*

Predicted Role of Secretin and Oxytocin in the Treatment of Behavioral and Developmental Disorders: Implications for Autism
*Martha G. Welch and David A. Ruggiero*

Immunological Findings in Autism
*Hari Har Parshad Cohly and Asit Panja*

Correlates of Psychomotor Symptoms in Autism
*Laura Stoppelbein, Sara Sytsma-Jordan, and Leilani Greening*

GABRB3 Gene Deficient Mice: A Potential Model of Autism Spectrum Disorder
*Timothy M. DeLorey*

The Reeler Mouse: Anatomy of a Mutant
*Gabriella D'Arcangelo*

Shared Chromosomal Susceptibility Regions Between Autism and Other Mental Disorders
*Yvon C. Chagnon index*

Index

## Volume 72

Classification Matters for Catatonia and Autism in Children
*Klaus-Jürgen Neumärker*

A Systematic Examination of Catatonia-Like Clinical Pictures in Autism Spectrum Disorders
*Lorna Wing and Amitta Shah*

Catatonia in Individuals with Autism Spectrum Disorders in Adolescence and Early Adulthood: A Long-Term Prospective Study
*Masataka Ohta, Yukiko Kano, and Yoko Nagai*

Are Autistic and Catatonic Regression Related? A Few Working Hypotheses Involving GABA, Purkinje Cell Survival, Neurogenesis, and ECT
*Dirk Marcel Dhossche and Ujjwal Rout*

Psychomotor Development and Psychopathology in Childhood
*Dirk M. J. De Raeymaecker*

The Importance of Catatonia and Stereotypies in Autistic Spectrum Disorders
*Laura Stoppelbein, Leilani Greening, and Angelina Kakooza*

Prader–Willi Syndrome: Atypical Psychoses and Motor Dysfunctions
*Willem M. A. Verhoeven and Siegfried Tuinier*

Towards a Valid Nosography and Psychopathology of Catatonia in Children and Adolescents
*David Cohen*

Is There a Common Neuronal Basis for Autism and Catatonia?
*Dirk Marcel Dhossche, Brendan T. Carroll, and Tressa D. Carroll*

Shared Susceptibility Region on Chromosome 15 Between Autism and Catatonia
*Yvon C. Chagnon*

Current Trends in Behavioral Interventions for Children with Autism
*Dorothy Scattone and Kimberly R. Knight*

Case Reports with a Child Psychiatric Exploration of Catatonia, Autism, and Delirium
*Jan N. M. Schieveld*

ECT and the Youth: Catatonia in Context
*Frank K. M. Zaw*

Catatonia in Autistic Spectrum Disorders: A Medical Treatment Algorithm
*Max Fink, Michael A. Taylor, and Neera Ghaziuddin*

Psychological Approaches to Chronic Catatonia-Like Deterioration in Autism Spectrum Disorders
*Amitta Shah and Lorna Wing*

Section V: Blueprints

Blueprints for the Assessment, Treatment, and Future Study of Catatonia in Autism Spectrum Disorders
*Dirk Marcel, Dhossche, Amitta Shah, and Lorna Wing*

Index

## Volume 73

Chromosome 22 Deletion Syndrome and Schizophrenia
*Nigel M. Williams, Michael C. O'Donovan, and Michael J. Owen*

Characterization of Proteome of Human Cerebrospinal Fluid
*Jing Xu, Jinzhi Chen, Elaine R. Peskind, Jinghua Jin, Jimmy Eng, Catherine Pan, Thomas J. Montine, David R. Goodlett, and Jing Zhang*

Hormonal Pathways Regulating Intermale and Interfemale Aggression
*Neal G. Simon, Qianxing Mo, Shan Hu, Carrie Garippa, and Shi-Fang Lu*

Neuronal GAP Junctions: Expression, Function, and Implications for Behavior
*Clinton B. McCracken and David C. S. Roberts*

Effects of Genes and Stress on the Neurobiology of Depression
*J. John Mann and Dianne Currier*

Quantitative Imaging with the Micropet Small-Animal Pet Tomograph
*Paul Vaska, Daniel J. Rubins, David L. Alexoff, and Wynne K. Schiffer*

Understanding Myelination through Studying its Evolution
*Rüdiger Schweigreiter, Betty I. Roots, Christine Bandtlow, and Robert M. Gould*

INDEX

## Volume 74

Evolutionary Neurobiology and Art
*C. U. M. Smith*

Section I: Visual Aspects

Perceptual Portraits
*Nicholas Wade*

The Neuropsychology of Visual Art: Conferring Capacity
*Anjan Chatterjee*

Vision, Illusions, and Reality
*Christopher Kennard*

Localization in the Visual Brain
*George K. York*

Section II: Episodic Disorders

Neurology, Synaesthesia, and Painting
*Amy Ione*

Fainting in Classical Art
*Philip Smith*

Migraine Art in the Internet: A Study of 450 Contemporary Artists
*Klaus Podoll*

Sarah Raphael's Migraine with Aura as Inspiration for the Foray of Her Work into Abstraction
*Klaus Podoll and Debbie Ayles*

The Visual Art of Contemporary Artists with Epilepsy
*Steven C. Schachter*

Section III: Brain Damage

Creativity in Painting and Style in Brain-Damaged Artists
*Julien Bogousslavsky*

Artistic Changes in Alzheimer's Disease
*Sebastian J. Crutch and Martin N. Rossor*

Section IV: Cerebrovascular Disease

Stroke in Painters
*H. Bäzner and M. Hennerici*

Visuospatial Neglect in Lovis Corinth's Self-Portraits
*Olaf Blanke*

Art, Constructional Apraxia, and the Brain
*Louis Caplan*

Section V: Genetic Diseases

Neurogenetics in Art
*Alan E. H. Emery*

A Naïve Artist of St Ives
*F. Clifford Rose*

Van Gogh's Madness
*F. Clifford Rose*

Absinthe, The Nervous System and Painting
*Tiina Rekand*

Section VI: Neurologists as Artists

Sir Charles Bell, KGH, FRS, FRSE (1774–1842)
*Christopher Gardner-Thorpe*

Section VII: Miscellaneous

Peg Leg Frieda
*Espen Dietrichs*

The Deafness of Goya (1746–1828)
*F. Clifford Rose*

INDEX

## Volume 75

Introduction on the Use of the *Drosophila* Embryonic/Larval Neuromuscular Junction as a Model System to Study Synapse Development and Function, and a Brief Summary of Pathfinding and Target Recognition
*Catalina Ruiz-Cañada and Vivian Budnik*

Development and Structure of Motoneurons
*Matthias Landgraf and Stefan Thor*

The Development of the *Drosophila* Larval Body Wall Muscles
*Karen Beckett and Mary K. Baylies*

Organization of the Efferent System and Structure of Neuromuscular Junctions in *Drosophila*
*Andreas Prokop*

Development of Motoneuron Electrical Properties and Motor Output
*Richard A. Baines*

Transmitter Release at the Neuromuscular Junction
*Thomas L. Schwarz*

Vesicle Trafficking and Recycling at the Neuromuscular Junction: Two Pathways for Endocytosis
*Yoshiaki Kidokoro*

Glutamate Receptors at the *Drosophila* Neuromuscular Junction
*Aaron DiAntonio*

Scaffolding Proteins at the *Drosophila* Neuromuscular Junction
*Bulent Ataman, Vivian Budnik, and Ulrich Thomas*

Synaptic Cytoskeleton at the Neuromuscular Junction
*Catalina Ruiz-Cañada and Vivian Budnik*

Plasticity and Second Messengers During Synapse Development
*Leslie C. Griffith and Vivian Budnik*

Retrograde Signaling that Regulates Synaptic Development and Function at the *Drosophila* Neuromuscular Junction
*Guillermo Marqués and Bing Zhang*

Activity-Dependent Regulation of Transcription During Development of Synapses
*Subhabrata Sanyal and Mani Ramaswami*

Experience-Dependent Potentiation of Larval Neuromuscular Synapses
*Christoph M. Schuster*

Selected Methods for the Anatomical Study of *Drosophila* Embryonic and Larval Neuromuscular Junctions
*Vivian Budnik, Michael Gorczyca, and Andreas Prokop*

Index

## Volume 76

Section I: Physiological Correlates of Freud's Theories

The ID, the Ego, and the Temporal Lobe
*Shirley M. Ferguson and Mark Rayport*

ID, Ego, and Temporal Lobe Revisited
*Shirley M. Ferguson and Mark Rayport*

Section II: Stereotaxic Studies

Olfactory Gustatory Responses Evoked by Electrical Stimulation of Amygdalar Region in Man Are Qualitatively Modifiable by Interview Content: Case Report and Review
*Mark Rayport, Sepehr Sani, and Shirley M. Ferguson*

Section III: Controversy in Definition of Behavioral Disturbance

Pathogenesis of Psychosis in Epilepsy. The "Seesaw" Theory: Myth or Reality?
*Shirley M. Ferguson and Mark Rayport*

Section IV: Outcome of Temporal Lobectomy

Memory Function After Temporal Lobectomy for Seizure Control: A Comparative Neuropsy chiatric and Neuropsychological Study
*Shirley M. Ferguson, A. John McSweeny, and Mark Rayport*

Life After Surgery for Temporolimbic Seizures
*Shirley M. Ferguson, Mark Rayport, and Carolyn A. Schell*

Appendix I
*Mark Rayport*

Appendix II: Conceptual Foundations of Studies of Patients Undergoing Temporal Lobe Surgery for Seizure Control
*Mark Rayport*

Index

## Volume 77

Regenerating the Brain
*David A. Greenberg and Kunlin Jin*

Serotonin and Brain: Evolution, Neuroplasticity, and Homeostasis
*Efrain C. Azmitia*

Therapeutic Approaches to Promoting Axonal Regeneration in the Adult Mammalian Spinal Cord
*Sari S. Hannila, Mustafa M. Siddiq, and Marie T. Filbin*

Evidence for Neuroprotective Effects of Antipsychotic Drugs: Implications for the Pathophysiology and Treatment of Schizophrenia
*Xin-Min Li and Haiyun Xu*

Neurogenesis and Neuroenhancement in the Pathophysiology and Treatment of Bipolar Disorder
*Robert J. Schloesser, Guang Chen, and Husseini K. Manji*

Neuroreplacement, Growth Factor, and Small Molecule Neurotrophic Approaches for Treating Parkinson's Disease
*Michael J. O'Neill, Marcus J. Messenger, Viktor Lakics, Tracey K. Murray, Eric H. Karran, Philip G. Szekeres, Eric S. Nisenbaum, and Kalpana M. Merchant*

Using *Caenorhabditis elegans* Models of Neurodegenerative Disease to Identify Neuroprotective Strategies
*Brian Kraemer and Gerard D. Schellenberg*

Neuroprotection and Enhancement of Neurite Outgrowth With Small Molecular Weight Compounds From Screens of Chemical Libraries
*Donard S. Dwyer and Addie Dickson*

INDEX

## Volume 78

Neurobiology of Dopamine in Schizophrenia
*Olivier Guillin, Anissa Abi-Dargham, and Marc Laruelle*

The Dopamine System and the Pathophysiology of Schizophrenia: A Basic Science Perspective
*Yukiori Goto and Anthony A. Grace*

Glutamate and Schizophrenia: Phencyclidine, *N*-methyl-D-aspartate Receptors, and Dopamine–Glutamate Interactions
*Daniel C. Javitt*

Deciphering the Disease Process of Schizophrenia: The Contribution of Cortical GABA Neurons
*David A. Lewis and Takanori Hashimoto*

Alterations of Serotonin Transmission in Schizophrenia
*Anissa Abi-Dargham*

Serotonin and Dopamine Interactions in Rodents and Primates: Implications for Psychosis and Antipsychotic Drug Development
*Gerard J. Marek*

Cholinergic Circuits and Signaling in the Pathophysiology of Schizophrenia
*Joshua A. Berman, David A. Talmage, and Lorna W. Role*

Schizophrenia and the α7 Nicotinic Acetylcholine Receptor
*Laura F. Martin and Robert Freedman*

Histamine and Schizophrenia
*Jean-Michel Arrang*

Cannabinoids and Psychosis
*Deepak Cyril D'Souza*

Involvement of Neuropeptide Systems in Schizophrenia: Human Studies
*Ricardo Cáceda, Becky Kinkead, and Charles B. Nemeroff*

Brain-Derived Neurotrophic Factor in Schizophrenia and Its Relation with Dopamine
*Olivier Guillin, Caroline Demily, and Florence Thibaut*

Schizophrenia Susceptibility Genes: In Search of a Molecular Logic and Novel Drug Targets for a Devastating Disorder
*Joseph A. Gogos*

INDEX

## Volume 79

The Destructive Alliance: Interactions of Leukocytes, Cerebral Endothelial Cells, and the Immune Cascade in Pathogenesis of Multiple Sclerosis
*Alireza Minagar, April Carpenter, and J. Steven Alexander*

Role of B Cells in Pathogenesis of Multiple Sclerosis
*Behrouz Nikbin, Mandana Mohyeddin Bonab, Farideh Khosravi, and Fatemeh Talebian*

The Role of CD4 T Cells in the Pathogenesis of Multiple Sclerosis
*Tanuja Chitnis*

The CD8 T Cell in Multiple Sclerosis: Suppressor Cell or Mediator of Neuropathology?
*Aaron J. Johnson, Georgette L. Suidan, Jeremiah McDole, and Istvan Pirko*

Immunopathogenesis of Multiple Sclerosis
*Smriti M. Agrawal and V. Wee Yong*

Molecular Mimicry in Multiple Sclerosis
*Jane E. Libbey, Lori L. McCoy, and Robert S. Fujinami*

Molecular "Negativity" May Underlie Multiple Sclerosis: Role of the Myelin Basic Protein Family in the Pathogenesis of MS
*Abdiwahab A. Musse and George Harauz*

Microchimerism and Stem Cell Transplantation in Multiple Sclerosis
*Behrouz Nikbin, Mandana Mohyeddin Bonab, and Fatemeh Talebian*

The Insulin-Like Growth Factor System in Multiple Sclerosis
*Daniel Chesik, Nadine Wilczak, and Jacques De Keyser*

Cell-Derived Microparticles and Exosomes in Neuroinflammatory Disorders
*Lawrence L. Horstman, Wenche Jy, Alireza Minagar, Carlos J. Bidot, Joaquin J. Jimenez, J. Steven Alexander, and Yeon S. Ahn*

Multiple Sclerosis in Children: Clinical, Diagnostic, and Therapeutic Aspects
*Kevin Rostásy*

Migraine in Multiple Sclerosis
*Debra G. Elliott*

Multiple Sclerosis as a Painful Disease
*Meghan Kenner, Uma Menon, and Debra Elliott*

Multiple Sclerosis and Behavior
*James B. Pinkston, Anita Kablinger, and Nadejda Alekseeva*

Cerebrospinal Fluid Analysis in Multiple Sclerosis
*Francisco A. Luque and Stephen L. Jaffe*

Multiple Sclerosis in Isfahan, Iran
*Mohammad Saadatnia, Masoud Etemadifar, and Amir Hadi Maghzi*

Gender Issues in Multiple Sclerosis
*Robert N. Schwendimann and Nadejda Alekseeva*

Differential Diagnosis of Multiple Sclerosis
*Halim Fadil, Roger E. Kelley, and Eduardo Gonzalez-Toledo*

Prognostic Factors in Multiple Sclerosis
*Roberto Bergamaschi*

Neuroimaging in Multiple Sclerosis
*Robert Zivadinov and Jennifer L. Cox*

Detection of Cortical Lesions Is Dependent on Choice of Slice Thickness in Patients with Multiple Sclerosis
*Ondrej Dolezal, Michael G. Dwyer, Dana Horakova, Eva Havrdova, Alireza Minagar, Srivats Balachandran, Niels Bergsland, Zdenek Seidl, Manuela Vaneckova, David Fritz, Jan Krasensky, and Robert Zivadinov*

The Role of Quantitative Neuroimaging Indices in the Differentiation of Ischemia from Demyelination: An Analytical Study with Case Presentation
*Romy Hoque, Christina Ledbetter, Eduardo Gonzalez-Toledo, Vivek Misra, Uma Menon, Meghan Kenner, Alejandro A. Rabinstein, Roger E. Kelley, Robert Zivadinov, and Alireza Minagar*

HLA-DRB1*1501, -DQB1*0301, -DQB1*0302, -DQB1*0602, and -DQB1*0603 Alleles Are Associated with More Severe Disease Outcome on MRI in Patients with Multiple Sclerosis
*Robert Zivadinov, Laura Uxa, Alessio Bratina, Antonio Bosco, Bhooma Srinivasaraghavan, Alireza Minagar, Maja Ukmar, Su yen Benedetto, and Marino Zorzon*

Glatiramer Acetate: Mechanisms of Action in Multiple Sclerosis
*Tjalf Ziemssen and Wiebke Schrempf*

Evolving Therapies for Multiple Sclerosis
*Elena Korniychuk, John M. Dempster, Eileen O'Connor, J. Steven Alexander, Roger E. Kelley, Meghan Kenner, Uma Menon, Vivek Misra, Romy Hoque, Eduardo C. Gonzalez-Toledo, Robert N. Schwendimann, Stacy Smith, and Alireza Minagar*

Remyelination in Multiple Sclerosis
*Divya M. Chari*

Trigeminal Neuralgia: A Modern-Day Review
*Kelly Hunt and Ravish Patwardhan*

Optic Neuritis and the Neuro-Ophthalmology of Multiple Sclerosis
*Paramjit Kaur and Jeffrey L. Bennett*

Neuromyelitis Optica: New Findings on Pathogenesis
*Dean M. Wingerchuk*

INDEX

## Volume 80

Epilepsy in the Elderly: Scope of the Problem
*Ilo E. Leppik*

Animal Models in Gerontology Research
*Nancy L. Nadon*

Animal Models of Geriatric Epilepsy
*Lauren J. Murphree, Lynn M. Rundhaugen, and Kevin M. Kelly*

Life and Death of Neurons in the Aging Cerebral Cortex
*John H. Morrison and Patrick R. Hof*

An In Vitro Model of Stroke-Induced Epilepsy: Elucidation of the Roles of Glutamate and Calcium in the Induction and Maintenance of Stroke-Induced Epileptogenesis
*Robert J. DeLorenzo, David A. Sun, Robert E. Blair, and Sompong Sambati*

Mechanisms of Action of Antiepileptic Drugs
*H. Steve White, Misty D. Smith, and Karen S. Wilcox*

Epidemiology and Outcomes of Status Epilepticus in the Elderly
*Alan R. Towne*

Diagnosing Epilepsy in the Elderly
*R. Eugene Ramsay, Flavia M. Macias, and A. James Rowan*

Pharmacoepidemiology in Community-Dwelling Elderly Taking Antiepileptic Drugs
*Dan R. Berlowitz and Mary Jo V. Pugh*

Use of Antiepileptic Medications in Nursing Homes
*Judith Garrard, Susan L. Harms, Lynn E. Eberly, and Ilo E. Leppik*

Differential Diagnosis of Multiple Sclerosis
*Halim Fadil, Roger E. Kelley, and Eduardo Gonzalez-Toledo*

Prognostic Factors in Multiple Sclerosis
*Roberto Bergamaschi*

Neuroimaging in Multiple Sclerosis
*Robert Zivadinov and Jennifer L. Cox*

Detection of Cortical Lesions Is Dependent on Choice of Slice Thickness in Patients with Multiple Sclerosis
*Ondrej Dolezal, Michael G. Dwyer, Dana Horakova, Eva Havrdova, Alireza Minagar, Srivats Balachandran, Niels Bergsland, Zdenek Seidl, Manuela Vaneckova, David Fritz, Jan Krasensky, and Robert Zivadinov*

The Role of Quantitative Neuroimaging Indices in the Differentiation of Ischemia from Demyelination: An Analytical Study with Case Presentation
*Romy Hoque, Christina Ledbetter, Eduardo Gonzalez-Toledo, Vivek Misra, Uma Menon, Meghan Kenner, Alejandro A. Rabinstein, Roger E. Kelley, Robert Zivadinov, and Alireza Minagar*

HLA-DRB1*1501, -DQB1*0301,-DQB1 *0302,-DQB1*0602, and -DQB1*0603 Alleles Are Associated with More Severe Disease Outcome on MRI in Patients with Multiple Sclerosis
*Robert Zivadinov, Laura Uxa, Alessio Bratina, Antonio Bosco, Bhooma Srinivasaraghavan, Alireza Minagar, Maja Ukmar, Su yen Benedetto, and Marino Zorzon*

Glatiramer Acetate: Mechanisms of Action in Multiple Sclerosis
*Tjalf Ziemssen and Wiebke Schrempf*

Evolving Therapies for Multiple Sclerosis
*Elena Korniychuk, John M. Dempster, Eileen O'Connor, J. Steven Alexander, Roger E. Kelley, Meghan Kenner, Uma Menon, Vivek Misra, Romy Hoque, Eduardo C. Gonzalez-Toledo, Robert N. Schwendimann, Stacy Smith, and Alireza Minagar*

Remyelination in Multiple Sclerosis
*Divya M. Chari*

Trigeminal Neuralgia: A Modern-Day Review
*Kelly Hunt and Ravish Patwardhan*

Optic Neuritis and the Neuro-Ophthalmology of Multiple Sclerosis
*Paramjit Kaur and Jeffrey L. Bennett*

Neuromyelitis Optica: New Findings on Pathogenesis
*Dean M. Wingerchuk*

INDEX

## Volume 81

Epilepsy in the Elderly: Scope of the Problem
*Ilo E. Leppik*

Animal Models in Gerontology Research
*Nancy L. Nadon*

Animal Models of Geriatric Epilepsy
*Lauren J. Murphree, Lynn M. Rundhaugen, and Kevin M. Kelly*

Life and Death of Neurons in the Aging Cerebral Cortex
*John H. Morrison and Patrick R. Hof*

An In Vitro Model of Stroke-Induced Epilepsy: Elucidation of the Roles of Glutamate and Calcium in the Induction and Maintenance of Stroke-Induced Epileptogenesis
*Robert J. DeLorenzo, David A. Sun, Robert E. Blair, and Sompong Sambati*

Mechanisms of Action of Antiepileptic Drugs
*H. Steve White, Misty D. Smith, and Karen S. Wilcox*

Epidemiology and Outcomes of Status Epilepticus in the Elderly
*Alan R. Towne*

Diagnosing Epilepsy in the Elderly
*R. Eugene Ramsay, Flavia M. Macias, and A. James Rowan*

Pharmacoepidemiology in Community-Dwelling Elderly Taking Antiepileptic Drugs
*Dan R. Berlowitz and Mary Jo V. Pugh*

Use of Antiepileptic Medications in Nursing Homes
*Judith Garrard, Susan L. Harms, Lynn E. Eberly, and Ilo E. Leppik*

Age-Related Changes in Pharmacokinetics: Predictability and Assessment Methods
*Emilio Perucca*

Factors Affecting Antiepileptic Drug Pharmacokinetics in Community-Dwelling Elderly
*James C. Cloyd, Susan Marino, and Angela K. Birnbaum*

Pharmacokinetics of Antiepileptic Drugs in Elderly Nursing Home Residents
*Angela K. Birnbaum*

The Impact of Epilepsy on Older Veterans
*Mary Jo V. Pugh, Dan R. Berlowitz, and Lewis Kazis*

Risk and Predictability of Drug Interactions in the Elderly
*René H. Levy and Carol Collins*

Outcomes in Elderly Patients With Newly Diagnosed and Treated Epilepsy
*Martin J. Brodie and Linda J. Stephen*

Recruitment and Retention in Clinical Trials of the Elderly
*Flavia M. Macias, R. Eugene Ramsay, and A. James Rowan*

Treatment of Convulsive Status Epilepticus
*David M. Treiman*

Treatment of Nonconvulsive Status Epilepticus
*Matthew C. Walker*

Antiepileptic Drug Formulation and Treatment in the Elderly: Biopharmaceutical Considerations
*Barry E. Gidal*

INDEX

## Volume 82

Inflammatory Mediators Leading to Protein Misfolding and Uncompetitive/Fast Off-Rate Drug Therapy for Neurodegenerative Disorders
*Stuart A. Lipton, Zezong Gu, and Tomohiro Nakamura*

Innate Immunity and Protective Neuroinflammation: New Emphasis on the Role of Neuroimmune Regulatory Proteins
*M. Griffiths, J. W. Neal, and P. Gasque*

Glutamate Release from Astrocytes in Physiological Conditions and in Neurodegenerative Disorders Characterized by Neuroinflammation
*Sabino Vesce, Daniela Rossi, Liliana Brambilla, and Andrea Volterra*

The High-Mobility Group Box 1 Cytokine Induces Transporter-Mediated Release of Glutamate from Glial Subcellular Particles (Gliosomes) Prepared from *In Situ*-Matured Astrocytes
*Giambattista Bonanno, Luca Raiteri, Marco Milanese, Simona Zappettini, Edon Melloni, Marco Pedrazzi, Mario Passalacqua, Carlo Tacchetti, Cesare Usai, and Bianca Sparatore*

The Role of Astrocytes and Complement System in Neural Plasticity
*Milos Pekny, Ulrika Wilhelmsson, Yalda Rahpeymai Bogestål, and Marcela Pekna*

New Insights into the Roles of Metalloproteinases in Neurodegeneration and Neuroprotection
*A. J. Turner and N. N. Nalivaeva*

Relevance of High-Mobility Group Protein Box 1 to Neurodegeneration
*Silvia Fossati and Alberto Chiarugi*

Early Upregulation of Matrix Metalloproteinases Following Reperfusion Triggers Neuroinflammatory Mediators in Brain Ischemia in Rat
*Diana Amantea, Rossella Russo, Micaela Gliozzi, Vincenza Fratto, Laura Berliocchi, G. Bagetta, G. Bernardi, and M. Tiziana Corasaniti*

The (Endo)Cannabinoid System in Multiple Sclerosis and Amyotrophic Lateral Sclerosis
*Diego Centonze, Silvia Rossi, Alessandro Finazzi-Agrò, Giorgio Bernardi, and Mauro Maccarrone*

Chemokines and Chemokine Receptors: Multipurpose Players in Neuroinflammation
*Richard M. Ransohoff, LiPing Liu, and Astrid E. Cardona*

Systemic and Acquired Immune Responses in Alzheimer's Disease
*Markus Britschgi and Tony Wyss-Coray*

Neuroinflammation in Alzheimer's Disease and Parkinson's Disease: Are Microglia Pathogenic in Either Disorder?
*Joseph Rogers, Diego Mastroeni, Brian Leonard, Jeffrey Joyce, and Andrew Grover*

Cytokines and Neuronal Ion Channels in Health and Disease
*Barbara Viviani, Fabrizio Gardoni, and Marina Marinovich*

Cyclooxygenase-2, Prostaglandin $E_2$, and Microglial Activation in Prion Diseases
*Luisa Minghetti and Maurizio Pocchiari*

Glia Proinflammatory Cytokine Upregulation as a Therapeutic Target for Neurodegenerative Diseases: Function-Based and Target-Based Discovery Approaches
*Linda J. Van Eldik, Wendy L. Thompson, Hantamalala Ralay Ranaivo, Heather A. Behanna, and D. Martin Watterson*

Oxidative Stress and the Pathogenesis of Neurodegenerative Disorders
*Ashley Reynolds, Chad Laurie, R. Lee Mosley, and Howard E. Gendelman*

Differential Modulation of Type 1 and Type 2 Cannabinoid Receptors Along the Neuroimmune Axis
*Sergio Oddi, Paola Spagnuolo, Monica Bari, Antonella D'Agostino, and Mauro Maccarrone*

Effects of the HIV-1 Viral Protein Tat on Central Neurotransmission: Role of Group I Metabotropic Glutamate Receptors
*Elisa Neri, Veronica Musante, and Anna Pittaluga*

Evidence to Implicate Early Modulation of Interleukin-1β Expression in the Neuroprotection Afforded by 17β-Estradiol in Male Rats Undergone Transient Middle Cerebral Artery Occlusion
*Olga Chiappetta, Micaela Gliozzi, Elisa Siviglia, Diana Amantea, Luigi A. Morrone, Laura Berliocchi, G. Bagetta, and M. Tiziana Corasaniti*

A Role for Brain Cyclooxygenase-2 and Prostaglandin-$E_2$ in Migraine: Effects of Nitroglycerin
*Cristina Tassorelli, Rosaria Greco, Marie Therèse Armentero, Fabio Blandini, Giorgio Sandrini, and Giuseppe Nappi*

The Blockade of K+-ATP Channels has Neuroprotective Effects in an *In Vitro* Model of Brain Ischemia
*Robert Nisticò, Silvia Piccirilli, L. Sebastianelli, Giuseppe Nisticò, G. Bernardi, and N. B. Mercuri*

Retinal Damage Caused by High Intraocular Pressure-Induced Transient Ischemia is Prevented by Coenzyme Q10 in Rat
*Carlo Nucci, Rosanna Tartaglione, Angelica Cerulli, R. Mancino, A. Spanò, Federica Cavaliere, Laura Rombolà, G. Bagetta, M. Tiziana Corasaniti, and Luigi A. Morrone*

Evidence Implicating Matrix Metalloproteinases in the Mechanism Underlying Accumulation of IL-1β and Neuronal Apoptosis in the Neocortex of HIV/gp120-Exposed Rats
*Rossella Russo, Elisa Siviglia, Micaela Gliozzi, Diana Amantea, Annamaria Paoletti, Laura Berliocchi, G. Bagetta, and M. Tiziana Corasaniti*

Neuroprotective Effect of Nitroglycerin in a Rodent Model of Ischemic Stroke: Evaluation of Bcl-2 Expression
*Rosaria Greco, Diana Amantea, Fabio Blandini, Giuseppe Nappi, Giacinto Bagetta, M. Tiziana Corasaniti, and Cristina Tassorelli*

INDEX

## Volume 83

Gender Differences in Pharmacological Response
*Gail D. Anderson*

Epidemiology and Classification of Epilepsy: Gender Comparisons
*John C. McHugh and Norman Delanty*

Hormonal Influences on Seizures: Basic Neurobiology
*Cheryl A. Frye*

Catamenial Epilepsy
*Patricia E. Penovich and Sandra Helmers*

Epilepsy in Women: Special Considerations for Adolescents
*Mary L. Zupanc and Sheryl Haut*

Contraception in Women with Epilepsy: Pharmacokinetic Interactions, Contraceptive Options, and Management
*Caryn Dutton and Nancy Foldvary-Schaefer*

Reproductive Dysfunction in Women with Epilepsy: Menstrual Cycle Abnormalities, Fertility, and Polycystic Ovary Syndrome
*Jürgen Bauer and Déirdre Cooper-Mahkorn*

Sexual Dysfunction in Women with Epilepsy: Role of Antiepileptic Drugs and Psychotropic Medications
*Mary A. Gutierrez, Romila Mushtaq, and Glen Stimmel*

Pregnancy in Epilepsy: Issues of Concern
*John DeToledo*

Teratogenicity and Antiepileptic Drugs: Potential Mechanisms
*Mark S. Yerby*

Antiepileptic Drug Teratogenesis: What are the Risks for Congenital Malformations and Adverse Cognitive Outcomes?
*Cynthia L. Harden*

Teratogenicity of Antiepileptic Drugs: Role of Pharmacogenomics
*Raman Sankar and Jason T. Lerner*

Antiepileptic Drug Therapy in Pregnancy I: Gestation-Induced Effects on AED Pharmacokinetics
*Page B. Pennell and Collin A. Hovinga*

Antiepileptic Drug Therapy in Pregnancy II: Fetal and Neonatal Exposure
*Collin A. Hovinga and Page B. Pennell*

Seizures in Pregnancy: Diagnosis and Management
*Robert L. Beach and Peter W. Kaplan*

Management of Epilepsy and Pregnancy: An Obstetrical Perspective
*Julian N. Robinson and Jane Cleary-Goldman*

Pregnancy Registries: Strengths, Weaknesses, and Bias Interpretation of Pregnancy Registry Data
*Marianne Cunnington and John Messenheimer*

Bone Health in Women With Epilepsy: Clinical Features and Potential Mechanisms
*Alison M. Pack and Thaddeus S. Walczak*

Metabolic Effects of AEDs: Impact on Body Weight, Lipids and Glucose Metabolism
*Raj D. Sheth and Georgia Montouris*

Psychiatric Comorbidities in Epilepsy
*W. Curt Lafrance, Jr., Andres M. Kanner, and Bruce Hermann*

Issues for Mature Women with Epilepsy
*Cynthia L. Harden*

Pharmacodynamic and Pharmacokinetic Interactions of Psychotropic Drugs with Antiepileptic Drugs
*Andres M. Kanner and Barry E. Gidal*

Health Disparities in Epilepsy: How Patient-Oriented Outcomes in Women Differ from Men
*Frank Gilliam*

INDEX

## Volume 84

Normal Brain Aging: Clinical, Immunological, Neuropsychological, and Neuroimaging Features
*Maria T. Caserta, Yvonne Bannon, Francisco Fernandez, Brian Giunta, Mike R. Schoenberg, and Jun Tan*

Subcortical Ischemic Cerebrovascular Dementia
*Uma Menon and Roger E. Kelley*

Cerebrovascular and Cardiovascular Pathology in Alzheimer's Disease
*Jack C. de la Torre*

Neuroimaging of Cognitive Impairments in Vascular Disease
*Carol Di Perri, Turi O. Dalaker, Mona K. Beyer, and Robert Zivadinov*

Contributions of Neuropsychology and Neuroimaging to Understanding Clinical Subtypes of Mild Cognitive Impairment
*Amy J. Jak, Katherine J. Bangen, Christina E. Wierenga, Lisa Delano-Wood, Jody Corey-Bloom, and Mark W. Bondi*

Proton Magnetic Resonance Spectroscopy in Dementias and Mild Cognitive Impairment
*H. Randall Griffith, Christopher C. Stewart, and Jan A. den Hollander*

Application of PET Imaging to Diagnosis of Alzheimer's Disease and Mild Cognitive Impairment
*James M. Noble and Nikolaos Scarmeas*

The Molecular and Cellular Pathogenesis of Dementia of the Alzheimer's Type: An Overview
*Francisco A. Luque and Stephen L. Jaffe*

Alzheimer's Disease Genetics: Current Status and Future Perspectives
*Lars Bertram*

Frontotemporal Lobar Degeneration: Insights from Neuropsychology and Neuroimaging
*Andrea C. Bozoki and Muhammad U. Farooq*

Lewy Body Dementia
*Jennifer C. Hanson and Carol F. Lippa*

Dementia in Parkinson's Disease
*Bradley J. Robottom and William J. Weiner*

Early Onset Dementia
*Halim Fadil, Aimee Borazanci, Elhachmia Ait Ben Haddou, Mohamed Yahyaoui, Elena Korniychuk, Stephen L. Jaffe, and Alireza Minagar*

Normal Pressure Hydrocephalus
*Glen R. Finney*

Reversible Dementias
*Anahid Kabasakalian and Glen R. Finney*

INDEX

## Volume 85

Involvement of the Prefrontal Cortex in Problem Solving
*Hajime Mushiake, Kazuhiro Sakamoto, Naohiro Saito, Toshiro Inui, Kazuyuki Aihara, and Jun Tanji*

GluK1 Receptor Antagonists and Hippocampal Mossy Fiber Function
*Robert Nisticò, Sheila Dargan, Stephen M. Fitzjohn, David Lodge, David E. Jane, Graham L. Collingridge, and Zuner A. Bortolotto*

Monoamine Transporter as a Target Molecule for Psychostimulants
*Ichiro Sora, BingJin Li, Setsu Fumushima, Asami Fukui, Yosefu Arime, Yoshiyuki Kasahara, Hiroaki Tomita, and Kazutaka Ikeda*

Targeted Lipidomics as a Tool to Investigate Endocannabinoid Function
*Giuseppe Astarita, Jennifer Geaga, Faizy Ahmed, and Daniele Piomelli*

The Endocannabinoid System as a Target for Novel Anxiolytic and Antidepressant Drugs
*Silvana Gaetani, Pasqua Dipasquale, Adele Romano, Laura Righetti, Tommaso Cassano, Daniele Piomelli, and Vincenzo Cuomo*

$GABA_A$ Receptor Function and Gene Expression During Pregnancy and Postpartum
*Giovanni Biggio, Maria Cristina Mostallino, Paolo Follesa, Alessandra Concas, and Enrico Sanna*

Early Postnatal Stress and Neural Circuit Underlying Emotional Regulation
*Machiko Matsumoto, Mitsuhiro Yoshioka, and Hiroko Togashi*

Roles of the Histaminergic Neurotransmission on Methamphetamine-Induced Locomotor Sensitization and Reward: A Study of Receptors Gene Knockout Mice
*Naoko Takino, Eiko Sakurai, Atsuo Kuramasu, Nobuyuki Okamura, and Kazuhiko Yanai*

Developmental Exposure to Cannabinoids Causes Subtle and Enduring Neurofunctional Alterations
*Patrizia Campolongo, Viviana Trezza, Maura Palmery, Luigia Trabace, and Vincenzo Cuomo*

Neuronal Mechanisms for Pain-Induced Aversion: Behavioral Studies Using a Conditioned Place Aversion Test
*Masabumi Minami*

Bv8/Prokineticins and their Receptors: A New Pronociceptive System
*Lucia Negri, Roberta Lattanzi, Elisa Giannini, Michela Canestrelli, Annalisa Nicotra, and Pietro Melchiorri*

$P2Y_6$-Evoked Microglial Phagocytosis
*Kazuhide Inoue, Schuichi Koizumi, Ayako Kataoka, Hidetoshi Tozaki-Saitoh, and Makoto Tsuda*

PPAR and Pain
*Takehiko Maeda and Shiroh Kishioka*

Involvement of Inflammatory Mediators in Neuropathic Pain Caused by Vincristine
*Norikazu Kiguchi, Takehiko Maeda, Yuka Kobayashi, Fumihiro Saika, and Shiroh Kishioka*

Nociceptive Behavior Induced by the Endogenous Opioid Peptides Dynorphins in Uninjured Mice: Evidence with Intrathecal *N*-ethylmaleimide Inhibiting Dynorphin Degradation
*Koichi Tan-No, Hiroaki Takahashi, Osamu Nakagawasai, Fukie Niijima, Shinobu Sakurada, Georgy Bakalkin, Lars Terenius, and Takeshi Tadano*

Mechanism of Allodynia Evoked by Intrathecal Morphine-3-Glucuronide in Mice
*Takaaki Komatsu, Shinobu Sakurada, Sou Katsuyama, Kengo Sanai, and Tsukasa Sakurada*

(–)-Linalool Attenuates Allodynia in Neuropathic Pain Induced by Spinal Nerve Ligation in C57/Bl6 Mice
*Laura Berliocchi, Rossella Russo, Alessandra Levato, Vincenza Fratto, Giacinto Bagetta, Shinobu Sakurada, Tsukasa Sakurada, Nicola Biagio Mercuri, and Maria Tiziana Corasaniti*

Intraplantar Injection of Bergamot Essential Oil into the Mouse Hindpaw: Effects on Capsaicin-Induced Nociceptive Behaviors
*Tsukasa Sakurada, Hikari Kuwahata, Soh Katsuyama, Takaaki Komatsu, Luigi A. Morrone, M. Tiziana Corasaniti, Giacinto Bagetta, and Shinobu Sakurada*

New Therapy for Neuropathic Pain
*Hirokazu Mizoguchi, Chizuko Watanabe, Akihiko Yonezawa, and Shinobu Sakurada*

Regulated Exocytosis from Astrocytes: Physiological and Pathological Related Aspects
*Corrado Calì, Julie Marchaland, Paola Spagnuolo, Julien Gremion, and Paola Bezzi*

Glutamate Release from Astrocytic Gliosomes Under Physiological and Pathological Conditions
*Marco Milanese, Tiziana Bonifacino, Simona Zappettini, Cesare Usai, Carlo Tacchetti, Mario Nobile, and Giambattista Bonanno*

Neurotrophic and Neuroprotective Actions of an Enhancer of Ganglioside Biosynthesis
*Jin-ichi Inokuchi*

Involvement of Endocannabinoid Signaling in the Neuroprotective Effects of Subtype 1 Metabotropic Glutamate Receptor Antagonists in Models of Cerebral Ischemia
*Elisa Landucci, Francesca Boscia, Elisabetta Gerace, Tania Scartabelli, Andrea Cozzi, Flavio Moroni, Guido Mannaioni, and Domenico E. Pellegrini-Giampietro*

NF-kappaB Dimers in the Regulation of Neuronal Survival
*Ilenia Sarnico, Annamaria Lanzillotta, Marina Benarese, Manuela Alghisi, Cristina Baiguera, Leontino Battistin, PierFranco Spano, and Marina Pizzi*

Oxidative Stress in Stroke Pathophysiology: Validation of Hydrogen Peroxide Metabolism as a Pharmacological Target to Afford Neuroprotection
*Diana Amantea, Maria Cristina Marrone, Robert Nisticò, Mauro Federici, Giacinto Bagetta, Giorgio Bernardi, and Nicola Biagio Mercuri*

Role of Akt and ERK Signaling in the Neurogenesis following Brain Ischemia
*Norifumi Shioda, Feng Han, and Kohji Fukunaga*

Prevention of Glutamate Accumulation and Upregulation of Phospho-Akt may Account for Neuroprotection Afforded by Bergamot Essential Oil against Brain Injury Induced by Focal Cerebral Ischemia in Rat
*Diana Amantea, Vincenza Fratto, Simona Maida, Domenicantonio Rotiroti, Salvatore Ragusa, Giuseppe Nappi, Giacinto Bagetta, and Maria Tiziana Corasaniti*

Identification of Novel Pharmacological Targets to Minimize Excitotoxic Retinal Damage
*Rossella Russo, Domenicantonio Rotiroti, Cristina Tassorelli, Carlo Nucci, Giacinto Bagetta, Massimo Gilberto Bucci, Maria Tiziana Corasaniti, and Luigi Antonio Morrone*

INDEX

## Volume 86

Section One: Hybrid Bionic Systems
EMG-Based and Gaze-Tracking-Based Man–Machine Interfaces
*Federico Carpi and Danilo De Rossi*

Bidirectional Interfaces with the Peripheral Nervous System
*Silvestro Micera and Xavier Navarro*

Interfacing Insect Brain for Space Applications
*Giovanni Di Pino, Tobias Seidl, Antonella Benvenuto, Fabrizio Sergi, Domenico Campolo, Dino Accoto, Paolo Maria Rossini, and Eugenio Guglielmelli*

Section Two: Meet the Brain
Meet the Brain: Neurophysiology
*John Rothwell*

Fundamentals of Electroencefalography, Magnetoencefalography, and Functional Magnetic Resonance Imaging
*Claudio Babiloni, Vittorio Pizzella, Cosimo Del Gratta, Antonio Ferretti, and Gian Luca Romani*

Implications of Brain Plasticity to Brain–Machine Interfaces Operation: A Potential Paradox?
*Paolo Maria Rossini*

Section Three: Brain Machine Interfaces, A New Brain-to-Environment Communication Channel
An Overview of BMIs
*Francisco Sepulveda*

Neurofeedback and Brain–Computer Interface: Clinical Applications
*Niels Birbaumer, Ander Ramos Murguialday, Cornelia Weber, and Pedro Montoya*

Flexibility and Practicality: Graz Brain–Computer Interface Approach
*Reinhold Scherer, Gernot R. Müller-Putz, and Gert Pfurtscheller*

On the Use of Brain–Computer Interfaces Outside Scientific Laboratories: Toward an Application in Domotic Environments
*F. Babiloni, F. Cincotti, M. Marciani, S. Salinari, L. Astolfi, F. Aloise, F. De Vico Fallani, and D. Mattia*

Brain–Computer Interface Research at the Wadsworth Center: Developments in Noninvasive Communication and Control
*Dean J. Krusienski and Jonathan R. Wolpaw*

Watching Brain TV and Playing Brain Ball: Exploring Novel BCL Strategies Using Real–Time Analysis of Human Intercranial Data
*Karim Jerbi, Samson Freyermuth, Lorella Minotti, Philippe Kahane, Alain Berthoz, and Jean-Philippe Lachaux*

Section Four: Brain-Machine Interfaces and Space
Adaptive Changes of Rhythmic EEG Oscillations in Space: Implications for Brain–Machine Interface Applications
*G. Cheron, A. M. Cebolla, M. Petieau, A. Bengoetxea, E. Palmero-Soler, A. Leroy, and B. Dan*

Validation of Brain–Machine Interfaces During Parabolic Flight
*José del R. Millán, Pierre W. Ferrez, and Tobias Seidl*

Matching Brain–Machine Interface Performance to Space Applications
*Luca Citi, Oliver Tonet, and Martina Marinelli*

Brain–Machine Interfaces for Space Applications—Research, Technological Development, and Opportunities
*Leopold Summerer, Dario Izzo, and Luca Rossini*

INDEX

## Volume 87

Peripheral Nerve Repair and Regeneration Research: A Historical Note
*Bruno Battiston, Igor Papalia, Pierluigi Tos, and Stefano Geuna*

Development of the Peripheral Nerve
*Suleyman Kaplan, Ersan Odaci, Bunyami Unal, Bunyamin Sahin, and Michele Fornaro*

Histology of the Peripheral Nerve and Changes Occurring During Nerve Regeneration
*Stefano Geuna, Stefania Raimondo, Giulia Ronchi, Federica Di Scipio, Pierluigi Tos, Krzysztof Czaja, and Michele Fornaro*

Methods and Protocols in Peripheral Nerve Regeneration Experimental Research: Part I—Experimental Models
*Pierluigi Tos, Giulia Ronchi, Igor Papalia, Vera Sallen, Josette Legagneux, Stefano Geuna, and Maria G. Giacobini-Robecchi*

Methods and Protocols in Peripheral Nerve Regeneration Experimental Research: Part II—Morphological Techniques
*Stefania Raimondo, Michele Fornaro, Federica Di Scipio, Giulia Ronchi, Maria G. Giacobini-Robecchi, and Stefano Geuna*

Methods and Protocols in Peripheral Nerve Regeneration Experimental Research: Part III—Electrophysiological Evaluation
*Xavier Navarro and Esther Udina*

Methods and Protocols in Peripheral Nerve Regeneration Experimental Research: Part IV—Kinematic Gait Analysis to Quantify Peripheral Nerve Regeneration in the Rat
*Luís M. Costa, Maria J. Simões, Ana C. Maurício and Artur S.P. Varejão*

Current Techniques and Concepts in Peripheral Nerve Repair
*Maria Siemionow and Grzegorz Brzezicki*

Artificial Scaffolds for Peripheral Nerve Reconstruction
*Valeria Chiono, Chiara Tonda-Turo, and Gianluca Ciardelli*

Conduit Luminal Additives for Peripheral Nerve Repair
*Hede Yan, Feng Zhang, Michael B. Chen, and William C. Lineaweaver*

Tissue Engineering of Peripheral Nerves
*Bruno Battiston, Stefania Raimondo, Pierluigi Tos, Valentina Gaidano, Chiara Audisio, Anna Scevola, Isabelle Perroteau, and Stefano Geuna*

Mechanisms Underlying The End-to-Side Nerve Regeneration
*Eleana Bontioti and Lars B. Dahlin*

Experimental Results in End-To-Side Neurorrhaphy
*Alexandros E. Beris and Marios G. Lykissas*

End-to-Side Nerve Regeneration: From the Laboratory Bench to Clinical Applications
*Pierluigi Tos, Stefano Artiaco, Igor Papalia, Ignazio Marcoccio, Stefano Geuna, and Bruno Battiston*

Novel Pharmacological Approaches to Schwann Cells as Neuroprotective Agents for Peripheral Nerve Regeneration
*Valerio Magnaghi, Patrizia Procacci, and Ada Maria Tata*

Melatonin and Nerve Regeneration
*Ersan Odaci and Suleyman Kaplan*

Transthyretin: An Enhancer of Nerve Regeneration
*Carolina E. Fleming, Fernando Milhazes Mar, Filipa Franquinho, and Mónica M. Sousa*

Enhancement of Nerve Regeneration and Recovery by Immunosuppressive Agents
*Damien P. Kuffler*

The Role of Collagen in Peripheral Nerve Repair
*Guido Koopmans, Birgit Hasse, and Nektarios Sinis*

Gene Therapy Perspectives for Nerve Repair
*Serena Zacchigna and Mauro Giacca*

Use of Stem Cells for Improving Nerve Regeneration
*Giorgio Terenghi, Mikael Wiberg, and Paul J. Kingham*

Transplantation of Olfactory Ensheathing Cells for Peripheral Nerve Regeneration
*Christine Radtke, Jeffery D. Kocsis, and Peter M. Vogt*

Manual Stimulation of Target Muscles has Different Impact on Functional Recovery after Injury of Pure Motor or Mixed Nerves
*Nektarios Sinis, Thodora Manoli, Frank Werdin, Armin Kraus, Hans E. Schaller, Orlando Guntinas-Lichius, Maria Grosheva, Andrey Irintchev, Emanouil Skouras, Sarah Dunlop, and Doychin N. Angelov*

Electrical Stimulation for Improving Nerve Regeneration: Where do we Stand?
*Tessa Gordon, Olewale A. R. Sulaiman, and Adil Ladak*

Phototherapy in Peripheral Nerve Injury: Effects on Muscle Preservation and Nerve Regeneration
*Shimon Rochkind, Stefano Geuna, and Asher Shainberg*

Age-Related Differences in the Reinnervation after Peripheral Nerve Injury
*Uroš Kovačič, Janez Sketelj, and Fajko F. Bajrović*

Neural Plasticity After Nerve Injury and Regeneration
*Xavier Navarro*

Future Perspective in Peripheral Nerve Reconstruction
*Lars Dahlin, Fredrik Johansson, Charlotta Lindwall, and Martin Kanje*

INDEX

## Volume 88

Effects Of Psychostimulants On Neurotrophins: Implications For Psychostimulant-Induced Neurotoxicity
*Francesco Angelucci, Valerio Ricci, Gianfranco Spalletta, Carlo Caltagirone, Aleksander A. Mathé, and Pietro Bria*

Dosing Time-Dependent Actions of Psychostimulants
*H. Manev and T. Uz*

Dopamine-Induced Behavioral Changes and Oxidative Stress in Methamphetamine-Induced Neurotoxicity
*Taizo Kita, Ikuko Miyazaki, Masato Asanuma, Mika Takeshima, and George C. Wagner*

Acute Methamphetamine Intoxication: Brain Hyperthermia, Blood–Brain Barrier, Brain Edema, and morphological cell abnormalities
*Eugene A. Kiyatkin and Hari S. Sharma*

Molecular Bases of Methamphetamine-Induced Neurodegeneration
*Jean Lud Cadet and Irina N. Krasnova*

Involvement of Nicotinic Receptors in Methamphetamine- and MDMA-Induced Neurotoxicity: Pharmacological Implications
*E. Escubedo, J. Camarasa, C. Chipana, S. García-Ratés, and D.Pubill*

Ethanol Alters the Physiology of Neuron–Glia Communication
*Antonio González and Ginés M. Salido*

Therapeutic Targeting of "DARPP-32": A Key Signaling Molecule in the Dopiminergic Pathway for the Treatment of Opiate Addiction
*Supriya D. Mahajan, Ravikumar Aalinkeel, Jessica L. Reynolds, Bindukumar B. Nair, Donald E. Sykes, Zihua Hu, Adela Bonoiu, Hong Ding, Paras N. Prasad, and Stanley A. Schwartz*

Pharmacological and Neurotoxicological Actions Mediated By Bupropion and Diethylpropion
*Hugo R. Arias, Abel Santamaría, and Syed F. Ali*

Neural and Cardiac Toxicities Associated With 3,4-Methylenedioxymethamphetamine (MDMA)
*Michael H. Baumann and Richard B. Rothman*

Cocaine-Induced Breakdown of the Blood–Brain Barrier and Neurotoxicity
*Hari S. Sharma, Dafin Muresanu, Aruna Sharma, and Ranjana Patnaik*

Cannabinoid Receptors in Brain: Pharmacogenetics, Neuropharmacology, Neurotoxicology, and Potential Therapeutic Applications
*Emmanuel S. Onaivi*

Intermittent Dopaminergic Stimulation causes Behavioral Sensitization in the Addicted Brain and Parkinsonism
*Francesco Fornai, Francesca Biagioni, Federica Fulceri, Luigi Murri, Stefano Ruggieri, Antonio Paparelli*

The Role of the Somatotrophic Axis in Neuroprotection and Neuroregeneration of the Addictive Brain
*Fred Nyberg*

INDEX

## Volume 89

Molecular Profiling of Striatonigral and Striatopallidal Medium Spiny Neurons: Past, Present, and Future
*Mary Kay Lobo*

BAC to Degeneration: Bacterial Artificial Chromosome (Bac)-Mediated Transgenesis for Modeling Basal Ganglia Neurodegenerative Disorders
*Xiao-Hong Lu*

Behavioral Outcome Measures for the Assessment of Sensorimotor Function in Animal Models of Movement Disorders
*Sheila M. Fleming*

The Role of DNA Methylation in the Central Nervous System and Neuropsychiatric Disorders
*Jian Feng and Guoping Fan*

Heritability of Structural Brain Traits: An Endo-phenotype Approach to Deconstruct Schizophrenia
*Nil Kaymaz and J. Van Os*

The Role of Striatal NMDA Receptors in Drug Addiction
*Yao-Ying Ma, Carlos Cepeda, and Cai-Lian Cui*

Deciphering Rett Syndrome With Mouse Genetics, Epigenomics, and Human Neurons
*Jifang Tao, Hao Wu, and Yi Eve Sun*

INDEX

## Volume 90

Part I: Introduction

Introductory Remarks on the History and Current Applications of TCS
*Matthew B. Stern*

Method and Validity of Transcranial Sonography in Movement Disorders
*David Školoudík and Uwe Walter*

Transcranial Sonography—Anatomy
*Heiko Huber*

Part II: Transcranial Sonography in Parkinsons Disease

Transcranial Sonography in Relation to SPECT and MIBG
*Yoshinori Kajimoto, Hideto Miwa and Tomoyoshi Kondo*

Diagnosis of Parkinson's Disease—Transcranial Sonography in Relation to MRI
*Ludwig Niehaus and Kai Boelmans*

Early Diagnosis of Parkinson's Disease
*Alexandra Gaenslen and Daniela Berg*

Transcranial Sonography in the Premotor Diagnosis of Parkinson's Disease
*Stefanie Behnke, Ute Schroder and Daniela Berg*

Pathophysiology of Transcranial Sonography Signal Changes in the Human Substantia Nigra
*K. L. Double, G. Todd and S. R. Duma*

Transcranial Sonography for the Discrimination of Idiopathic Parkinson's Disease from the Atypical Parkinsonian Syndromes
*A. E. P. Bouwmans, A. M. M. Vlaar, K. Srulijes, W. H. Mess AND W. E. J. Weber*

Transcranial Sonography in the Discrimination of Parkinson's Disease Versus Vascular Parkinsonism
*Pablo Venegas-Francke*

TCS in Monogenic Forms of Parkinson's Disease
*Kathrin Brockmann and Johann Hagenah*

Part III—Transcranial Sonography in other Movement Disorders and Depression

Transcranial Sonography in Brain Disorders with Trace Metal Accumulation
*Uwe Walter*

Transcranial Sonography in Dystonia
*Alexandra Gaenslen*

Transcranial Sonography in Essential Tremor
*Heike Stockner and Isabel Wurster*

VII—Transcranial Sonography in Restless Legs Syndrome
*Jana Godau and Martin Sojer*

Transcranial Sonography in Ataxia
*Christos Krogias, Thomas Postert and Jens Eyding*

Transcranial Sonography in Huntington's Disease
*Christos Krogias, Jens Eyding and Thomas Postert*

Transcranial Sonography in Depression
*Milija D. Mijajlovic*

Part IV: Future Applications and Conclusion

Transcranial Sonography-Assisted Stereotaxy and Follow-Up of Deep Brain Implants in Patients with Movement Disorders
*Uwe Walter*

Conclusions
*Daniela Berg*

INDEX

## Volume 91

The Role of microRNAs in Drug Addiction: A Big Lesson from Tiny Molecules
*Andrzej Zbigniew Pietrzykowski*

The Genetics of Behavioral Alcohol Responses in *Drosophila*
*Aylin R. Rodan and Adrian Rothenfluh*

Neural Plasticity, Human Genetics, and Risk for Alcohol Dependence
*Shirley Y. Hill*

Using Expression Genetics to Study the Neurobiology of Ethanol and Alcoholism
*Sean P. Farris, Aaron R. Wolen and Michael F. Miles*

Genetic Variation and Brain Gene Expression in Rodent Models of Alcoholism: Implications for Medication Development
*Karl Björk, Anita C. Hansson and W. olfgang H. Sommer*

Identifying Quantitative Trait Loci (QTLs) and Genes (QTGs) for Alcohol-Related Phenotypes in Mice
*Lauren C. Milner and Kari J. Buck*

Glutamate Plasticity in the Drunken Amygdala: The Making of an Anxious Synapse
*Brian A. Mccool, Daniel T. Christian, Marvin R. Diaz and Anna K. Läck*

Ethanol Action on Dopaminergic Neurons in the Ventral Tegmental Area: Interaction with Intrinsic Ion Channels and Neurotransmitter Inputs
*Hitoshi Morikawa and Richard A. Morrisett*

Alcohol and the Prefrontal Cortex
*Kenneth Abernathy, L. Judson Chandler and John J. Woodward*

BK Channel and Alcohol, A Complicated Affair
*Gilles Erwan Martin*

A Review of Synaptic Plasticity at Purkinje Neurons with a Focus on Ethanol-Induced Cerebellar Dysfunction
*C. Fernando Valenzuela, Britta Lindquist and Paula A. Zflmudio-Bulcock*

INDEX

## Volume 92

The Development of the Science of Dreaming
*Claude Gottesmann*

Dreaming as Inspiration: Evidence from Religion, Philosophy, Literature, and Film
*Kelly Bulkeley*

Developmental Perspective: Dreaming Across the Lifespan and What This Tells Us
*Melissa M. Burnham and Christian Conte*

REM and NREM Sleep Mentation
*Patrick Mcnamara, Patricia Johnson, Deirdre McLaren, Erica Harris,Catherine Beauharnais and Sanford Auerbach*

Neuroimaging of Dreaming: State of the Art and Limitations
*Caroline Kussé, Vincenzo Muto, Laura Mascetti, Luca Matarazzo, Ariane Foret, Anahita Shaffii-Le Bourdiec and Pierre Maquet*

Memory Consolidation, The Diurnal Rhythm of Cortisol, and The Nature of Dreams: A New Hypothesis
*Jessica D. Payne*

Characteristics and Contents of Dreams
*Michael Schredl*

Trait and Neurobiological Correlates of Individual Differences in Dream Recall and Dream Content
*Mark Blagrove and Edward F. Pace-Schott*

Consciousness in Dreams
*David Kahn and Tzivia Gover*

The Underlying Emotion and the Dream: Relating Dream Imagery to the Dreamer's Underlying Emotion can Help Elucidate the Nature of Dreaming
*Ernest Hartmann*

Dreaming, Handedness, and Sleep Architecture: Interhemispheric Mechanisms
*Stephen D. Christman and Ruth E. Propper*

To What Extent Do Neurobiological Sleep-Waking Processes Support Psychoanalysis?
*Claude Gottesmann*

The Use of Dreams in Modern Psychotherapy
*Clara E. Hill and Sarah Knox*

INDEX

## Volume 93

Underlying Brain Mechanisms that Regulate Sleep-Wakefulness Cycles
*Irma Gvilia*

What Keeps Us Awake?—the Role of Clocks and Hourglasses, Light, and Melatonin
*Christian Cajochen, Sarah Chellappa and Christina Schmidt*

Suprachiasmatic Nucleus and Autonomic Nervous System Influences on Awakening From Sleep
*Andries Kalsbeek, Chun-xia Yi, Susanne E. la Fleur, Ruud m. Buijs, and Eric Fliers*

Preparation for Awakening: Self-Awakening Vs. Forced Awakening: Preparatory Changes in the Pre-Awakening Period
*Mitsuo Hayashi, Noriko Matsuura and Hiroki Ikeda*

Circadian and Sleep Episode Duration Influences on Cognitive Performance Following the Process of Awakening
*Robert L. Matchock*

The Cortisol Awakening Response in Context
*Angela Clow, Frank Hucklebridge and Lisa Thorn*

Causes and Correlates of Frequent Night Awakenings in Early Childhood
*Amy Jo Schwichtenberg and Beth Goodlin-Jones*

Pathologies of Awakenings: The Clinical Problem of Insomnia Considered From Multiple Theory Levels
*Douglas E. Moul*

The Neurochemistry of Awakening: Findings from Sleep Disorder Narcolepsy
*Seiji Nishino and Yohei Sagawa*

INDEX

## Volume 94

$5\text{-HT}_6$ Medicinal Chemistry
*Kevin G. Liu and Albert J. Robichaud*

Patents
*Nicolas Vincent Ruiz and Gloria Oranias*

$5\text{-HT}_6$ Receptor Charactertization
*Teresa Riccioni*

$5\text{-HT}_6$ Receptor Signal Transduction: Second Messenger Systems
*Xavier Codony, Javier Burgueño, Maria Javier Ramírez and José Miguel Vela*

Electrophysiology of $5\text{-HT}_6$ Receptors
*Annalisa Tassone, Graziella Madeo, Giuseppe Sciamanna, Antonio Pisani and Paola Bonsi*

Genetic Variations and Association
*Massimo Gennarelli and Annamaria Cattaneo*

Pharmacokinetics of $5\text{-HT}_6$ Receptor Ligands
*Angelo Mancinelli*

INDEX

## Volume 95

Introductory Remarks: Catechol-O-Methyltransferase Inhibition–An Innovative Approach to Enhance L-dopa Therapy in Parkinson's Disease with Dual Enzyme Inhibition
*Erkki Nissinen*

The Catechol-O-Methyltransferase Gene: its Regulation and Polymorphisms
*Elizabeth M. Tunbridge*

Distribution and Functions of Catechol-O-Methyltransferase Proteins: Do Recent Findings Change the Picture?
*Timo T. Myöhänen and Pekka T. Männistö*

Catechol-O-Methyltransferase Enzyme: Cofactor S-Adenosyl-L-Methionine and Related Mechanisms
*Thomas Müller*

Biochemistry and Pharmacology of Catechol-O-Methyltransferase Inhibitors
*Erkki nissinen and Pekka T. Männisto*

The Chemistry of Catechol-O-Methyltransferase Inhibitors
*David A. Learmonth, László E. Kiss, and Patrício Soares-da-Silva*

Toxicology and Safety of COMT Inhibitors
*Kristiina Haasio*

Catechol-O-Methyltransferase Inhibitors in Preclinical Models as Adjuncts of L-dopa Treatment
*Concepció Marin and J. A. Obeso*

Problems with the Present Inhibitors and a Relevance of New and Improved COMT Inhibitors in Parkinson's Disease
*Seppo Kaakkola*

Catechol-O-Methyltransferase and Pain
*Oleg Kambur and Pekka T. Männistö*

INDEX

## Volume 96

The Central Role of $5\text{-HT}_6$ Receptors in Modulating Brain Neurochemistry
*Lee A. Dawson*

$5\text{-HT}_6$ Receptor Memory and Amnesia: Behavioral Pharmacology – Learning and Memory Processes
*Alfredo Meneses, G. Pérez-García, R. Tellez, T. Ponce-Lopez and C. Castillo*

Behavioral Pharmacology: Potential Antidepressant and Anxiolytic Properties
*Anna Wesołowska and Magdalena Jastrzbska-Wisek*

The 5-$HT_6$ Receptor as a Target for Developing Novel Antiobesity Drugs
*David Heal, Jane Gosden and Sharon Smith*

Behavioral and Neurochemical Pharmacology of 5-$HT_6$ Receptors Related to Reward and Reinforcement
*Gaetano Di Chiara, Valentina Valentini and Sandro Fenu*

5-$HT_6$ Receptor Ligands and their Antipsychotic Potential
*Jørn Arnt and Christina Kurre Olsen*

5-$HT_6$ Receptor Ligands as Antidementia Drugs
*Ellen Siobhan Mitchell*

Other 5-$HT_6$ Receptor-Mediated Effects
*Franco Borsini*

INDEX

## Volume 97

Behavioral Pharmacology of Orofacial Movement Disorders
*Noriaki Koshikawa, Satoshi Fujita and Kazunori Adachi*

Regulation of Orofacial Movement: Dopamine Receptor Mechanisms and Mutant Models
*John L. Waddington, Gerard J. O'Sullivan and Katsunori Tomiyama*

Regulation of Orofacial Movement: Amino Acid Mechanisms and Mutant Models
*Katsunori Tomiyama, Colm M.P. O'Tuathaigh, and John L. Waddington*

The Trigeminal Circuits Responsible for Chewing
*Karl-Gunnar Westberg and Arlette Kolta*

Ultrastructural Basis for Craniofacial Sensory Processing in the Brainstem
*Yong Chul Bae and Atsushi Yoshida*

Mechanisms of Nociceptive Transduction and Transmission: A Machinery for Pain Sensation and Tools for Selective Analgesia
*Alexander M. Binshtok*

Peripheral and Central Mechanisms of Orofacial Inflammatory Pain
*Barry J. Sessle*

The Role of Trigeminal Interpolaris-Caudalis Transition Zone in Persistent Orofacial Pain
*Ke Ren and Ronald Dubner*

Physiological Mechanisms of Neuropathic Pain: The Orofacial Region
*Koichi Iwata, Yoshiki Imamura, Kuniya Honda and Masamichi Shinoda*

Neurobiology of Estrogen Status in Deep Craniofacial Pain
*David A Bereiter and Keiichiro Okamoto*

Macroscopic Connection of Rat Insular Cortex: Anatomical Bases Underlying its Physiological Functions
*Masayuki Kobayashi*

The Balance Between Excitation And Inhibition And Functional Sensory Processing in the Somatosensory Cortex
*Zhi Zhang and Qian-Quan Sun*

INDEX

## Volume 98

An Introduction to Dyskinesia—the Clinical Spectrum
*Ainhi Ha and Joseph Jankovic*

L-dopa-induced Dyskinesia—Clinical Presentation, Genetics, And Treatment
*L.K. Prashanth, Susan Fox and Wassilios G. Meissner*

Experimental Models of L-DOPA-induced Dyskinesia
*Tom H. Johnston and Emma L. Lane*

Molecular Mechanisms of L-DOPA-induced Dyskinesia
*Gilberto Fisone and Erwan Bezard*

New Approaches to Therapy
*Jonathan Brotchie and Peter Jenner*

Surgical Approach to L-DOPA-induced Dyskinesias
*Tejas Sankar and Andres M. Lozano*

Clinical and Experimental Experiences of Graft-induced Dyskinesia
*Emma L. Lane*

Tardive Dyskinesia: Clinical Presentation and Treatment
*P.N. van Harten and D.E. Tenback*

Epidemiology and Risk Factors for (Tardive) Dyskinesia
*D.E. Tenback and P.N. van Harten*

Genetics of Tardive Dyskinesia
*Heon-Jeong Lee and Seung-Gul Kang*

Animal Models of Tardive Dyskinesia
*S.K. Kulkarni and Ashish Dhir*

Surgery for Tardive Dyskinesia
*Stephane Thobois, Alice Poisson and Philippe Damier*

Huntington's Disease: Clinical Presentation and Treatment
*M.J.U. Novak and S.J. Tabrizi*

Genetics and Neuropathology of Huntington's Disease: Huntington's Disease
*Anton Reiner, Ioannis Dragatsis and Paula Dietrich*

Pathogenic Mechanisms in Huntington's Disease
*Lesley Jones and Alis Hughes*

Experimental Models of HD And Reflection on Therapeutic Strategies
*Olivia L. Bordiuk, Jinho Kim and Robert J. Ferrante*

Cell-based Treatments for Huntington's Disease
*Stephen B. Dunnett and Anne E. Rosser*

Clinical Phenomenology of Dystonia
*Carlo Colosimo and Alfredo Berardelli*

Genetics and Pharmacological Treatment of Dystonia
*Susan Bressman and Matthew James*

Experimental Models of Dystonia
*A. Tassone, G. Sciamanna, P. Bonsi, G. Martella and A. Pisani*

Surgical Treatment of Dystonia
*John Yianni, Alexander L. Green and Tipu Z. Aziz*

INDEX

## Volume 99

Seizure and Epilepsy: Studies of Seizure-disorders in *Drosophila*
*Louise Parker, Iris C. Howlett, Zeid M. Rusan and Mark A. Tanouye*

Homeostatic Control of Neural Activity: A *Drosophila* Model for Drug Tolerance and Dependence
*Alfredo Ghezzi and Nigel S. Atkinson*

Attention in *Drosophila*
*Bruno van Swinderen*

The roles of *Fruitless* and *Doublesex* in the Control of Male Courtship
*Brigitte Dauwalder*

Circadian Plasticity: from Structure to Behavior
*Lia Frenkel and María Fernanda Ceriani*

Learning and Memory in *Drosophila*: Behavior, Genetics, and Neural Systems
*Lily Kahsai and Troy Zars*

Studying Sensorimotor Processing with Physiology in Behaving *Drosophila*
*Johannes D. Seelig and Vivek Jayaraman*

Modeling Human Trinucleotide Repeat Diseases in *Drosophila*
*Zhenming Yu and Nancy M. Bonini*

From Genetics to Structure to Function: Exploring Sleep in *Drosophila*
*Daniel Bushey and Chiara Cirelli*

INDEX

## Volume 100

Structural Properties of Human Monoamine Oxidases A and B
*Claudia Binda, Andrea Mattevi and Dale E. Edmondson*

Behavioral Outcomes of Monoamine Oxidase Deficiency: Preclinical and Clinical Evidence
*Marco Bortolato and Jean C. Shih*

Kinetic Behavior and Reversible Inhibition of Monoamine Oxidases—Enzymes that Many Want Dead
*Keith F. Tipton, Gavin P. Davey and Andrew G. McDonald*

The Pharmacology of Selegiline
*Kálmán Magyar*

Type A Monoamine Oxidase Regulates Life and Death of Neurons in Neurodegeneration and Neuroprotection
*Makoto Naoi, Wakako Maruyama, Keiko Inaba-Hasegawa and Yukihiro Akao*

Multimodal Drugs and their Future for Alzheimer's and Parkinson's Disease
*Cornelis J. Van der Schyf and Werner J. Geldenhuys*

Neuroprotective Profile of the Multitarget Drug Rasagiline in Parkinson's Disease
*Orly Weinreb, Tamar Amit, Peter Riederer, Moussa B.H. Youdim and Silvia A. Mandel*

Rasagiline in Parkinson's Disease
*L.M. Chahine and M.B. Stern*

Selective Inhibitors of Monoamine Oxidase Type B and the "Cheese Effect"
*John P.M. Finberg and Ken Gillman*

A Novel Anti-Alzheimer's Disease Drug, Ladostigil: Neuroprotective, Multimodal Brain-Selective Monoamine Oxidase and Cholinesterase Inhibitor
*Orly Weinreb, Tamar Amit, Orit Bar-Am and Moussa B.H. Youdim*

Novel MAO-B Inhibitors: Potential Therapeutic Use of the Selective MAO-B Inhibitor PF9601N in Parkinson's Disease
*Mercedes Unzeta and Elisenda Sanz*

INDEX

## Volume 101

General Overview: Biomarkers in Neuroscience Research
*Michaela D. Filiou and Christoph W. Turck*

Imaging Brain Microglial Activation Using Positron Emission Tomography and Translocator Protein-Specific Radioligands
*David R.J. Owen and Paul M. Matthews*

The Utility of Gene Expression in Blood Cells for Diagnosing Neuropsychiatric Disorders
*Christopher H. Woelk, Akul Singhania, Josué Pérez-Santiago, Stephen J. Glatt and Ming T. Tsuang*

Proteomic Technologies for Biomarker Studies in Psychiatry: Advances and Needs
*Daniel Martins-de-Souza, Paul C. Guest, Natacha Vanattou-Saifoudine, Laura W. Harris and Sabine Bahn*

Converging Evidence of Blood-Based Biomarkers for Schizophrenia: An update
*Man K. Chan, Paul C. Guest, Yishai Levin, Yagnesh Umrania, Emanuel Schwarz, Sabine Bahn and Hassan Rahmoune*

Abnormalities in Metabolism and Hypothalamic–Pituitary–Adrenal Axis Function in Schizophrenia
*Paul C. Guest, Daniel Martins-de-Souza, Natacha Vanattou-Saifoudine, Laura W. Harris and Sabine Bahn*

Immune and Neuroimmune Alterations in Mood Disorders and Schizophrenia
*Roosmarijn C. Drexhage, Karin Weigelt, Nico van Beveren, Dan Cohen, Marjan A. Versnel, Willem A. Nolen and Hemmo A. Drexhage*

Behavioral and Molecular Biomarkers in Translational Animal Models for Neuropsychiatric Disorders
*Zoltán Sarnyai, Murtada Alsaif, Sabine Bahn, Agnes Ernst, Paul C. Guest, Eva Hradetzky, Wolfgang Kluge, Viktoria Stelzhammer and Hendrik Wesseling*

Stem Cell Models for Biomarker Discovery in Brain Disease
*Alan Mackay-Sim, George Mellick and Stephen Wood*

The Application of Multiplexed Assay Systems for Molecular Diagnostics
*Emanuel Schwarz, Nico J.M. VanBeveren, Paul C. Guest, Rauf Izmailov and Sabine Bahn*

Algorithm Development for Diagnostic Biomarker Assays
*Rauf Izmailov, Paul C. Guest, Sabine Bahn and Emanuel Schwarz*

Challenges of Introducing New Biomarker Products for Neuropsychiatric Disorders into the Market
*Sabine Bahn, Richard Noll, Anthony Barnes, Emanuel Schwarz and Paul C. Guest*

Toward Personalized Medicine in the Neuropsychiatric Field
*Erik H.F. Wong, Jayne C. Fox, Mandy Y.M. Ng and Chi-Ming Lee*

Clinical Utility of Serum Biomarkers for Major Psychiatric Disorders
*Nico J.M. van Beveren and Witte J.G. Hoogendijk*

The Future: Biomarkers, Biosensors, Neuroinformatics, and E-Neuropsychiatry
*Christopher R. Lowe*

SUBJECT INDEX

## Volume 102

The Function and Mechanisms of Nurr1 Action in Midbrain Dopaminergic Neurons, from Development and Maintenance to Survival
*Yu Luo*

Monoclonal Antibodies as Novel Neurotherapeutic Agents in CNS Injury and Repair
*Aruna Sharma and Hari Shanker Sharma*

The Blood–Brain Barrier in Alzheimer's Disease: Novel Therapeutic Targets and Nanodrug delivery
*Hari Shanker Sharma, Rudy J. Castellani, Mark A. Smith and Aruna Sharma*

Neurovascular Aspects of Amyotrophic Lateral Sclerosis
*Maria Carolina O. Rodrigues, Diana G. Hernandez-Ontiveros, Michael K. Louis, Alison E. Willing, Cesario V. Borlongan, Paul R. Sanberg, Júlio C. Voltarelli and Svitlana Garbuzova-Davis*

Quercetin in Hypoxia-Induced Oxidative Stress: Novel Target for Neuroprotection
*Anand Kumar Pandey, Ranjana Patnaik, Dafin F. Muresanu, Aruna Sharma and Hari Shanker Sharma*

Environmental Conditions Modulate Neurotoxic Effects of Psychomotor Stimulant Drugs of Abuse
*Eugene A. Kiyatkin and Hari Shanker Sharma*

Central Nervous Tissue Damage after Hypoxia and Reperfusion in Conjunction with Cardiac Arrest and Cardiopulmonary Resuscitation: Mechanisms of Action and Possibilities for Mitigation
*Lars Wiklund, Cecile Martijn, Adriana Miclescu, Egidijus Semenas, Sten Rubertsson and Hari Shanker Sharma*

Interactions Between Opioids and Anabolic Androgenic Steroids: Implications for the Development of Addictive Behavior
*Fred Nyberg and Mathias Hallberg*

Neurotrophic Factors and Neurodegenerative Diseases: A Delivery Issue
*Barbara Ruozi, Daniela Belletti, Lucia Bondioli, Alessandro De Vita, Flavio Forni, Maria Angela Vandelli and Giovanni Tosi*

Neuroprotective Effects of Cerebrolysin, a Combination of Different Active Fragments of Neurotrophic Factors and Peptides on the Whole Body Hyperthermia-Induced Neurotoxicity: Modulatory Roles of Co-morbidity Factors and Nanoparticle Intoxication
*Hari Shanker Sharma, Aruna Sharma, Herbert Mössler and Dafin Fior Muresanu*

Alzheimer's Disease and Amyloid: Culprit or Coincidence?
*Stephen D. Skaper*

Vascular Endothelial Growth Factor and Other Angioglioneurins: Key Molecules in Brain Development and Restoration
*José Vicente Lafuente, Naiara Ortuzar, Harkaitz Bengoetxea, Susana Bulnes and Enrike G. Argandoña*

Index

## Volume 103

Lost and Found in Behavioral Informatics
*Melissa A. Haendel and Elissa J. Chesler*

Biological Databases for Behavioral Neurobiology
*Erich J. Baker*

A Survey of the Neuroscience Resource Landscape: Perspectives from the Neuroscience Information Framework
*Jonathan Cachat, Anita Bandrowski, Jeffery S. Grethe, Amarnath Gupta, Vadim Astakhov, Fahim Imam, Stephen D. Larson, and Maryann E. Martone*

The Neurobehavior Ontology: An Ontology for Annotation and Integration of Behavior and Behavioral Phenotypes
*Georgios V. Gkoutos, Paul N. Schofield, and Robert Hoehndorf*

Ontologies for Human Behavior Analysis and Their Application to Clinical Data
*Janna Hastings and Stefan Schulz*

Text-Mining and Neuroscience
*Kyle H. Ambert and Aaron M. Cohen*

Applying *In Silico* Integrative Genomics to Genetic Studies of Human Disease: A Review
*Scott F. Saccone*

Subject Index

## Volume 104

Cross Species Integration of Functional Genomics Experiments
*Jeremy J. Jay*

Model Organism Databases in Behavioral Neuroscience
*Mary Shimoyama, Jennifer R. Smith, G. Thomas Hayman, Victoria Petri, and Rajni Nigam*

Accessing and Mining Data from Large-Scale Mouse Phenotyping Projects
*Hugh Morgan, Michelle Simon, and Ann-Marie Mallon*

Bioinformatics Resources for Behavior Studies in the Laboratory Mouse
*Carol J. Bult*

Using Genome-Wide Expression Profiling to Define Gene Networks Relevant to the Study of Complex Traits: From RNA Integrity to Network Topology
*M.A. O'Brien, B.N. Costin, and M.F. Miles*

Genetic and Molecular Network Analysis of Behavior
*Robert W. Williams and Megan K. Mulligan*

Large-Scale Neuroinformatics for *In Situ* Hybridization Data in the Mouse Brain
*Lydia L. Ng, Susan M. Sunkin, David Feng, Chris Lau, Chinh Dang, and Michael J. Hawrylycz*

Opportunities for Bioinformatics in the Classification of Behavior and Psychiatric Disorders
*Elissa J. Chesler and Ryan W. Logan*

SUBJECT INDEX

## Volume 105

Optic Nerve Disease and Axon Pathophysiology
*Alireza Ghaffarieh and Leonard A. Levin*

Role of Electrical Activity of Neurons for Neuroprotection
*Takeshi Morimoto*

Molecular Control of Axon Growth: Insights from Comparative Gene Profiling and High-Throughput Screening
*Murray G. Blackmore*

Gatekeeper Between Quiescence and Differentiation: p53 in Axonal Outgrowth and Neurogenesis
*Giorgia Quadrato and Simone Di Giovanni*

Cyclin-Dependent Kinase 5 in Axon Growth and Regeneration
*Tao Ye, Amy K. Y. Fu, and Nancy Y. Ip*

Rho Signaling and Axon Regeneration
*L. McKerracher, Gino B. Ferraro, and Alyson E. Fournier*

Neuron-Intrinsic Inhibitors of Axon Regeneration: PTEN and SOCS3
*Xueting Luo and Kevin K. Park*

INDEX

## Volume 106

Neurotrophic Factors and the Regeneration of Adult Retinal Ganglion Cell Axons
*Alan R. Harvey, Jacob Wei Wei Ooi, and Jennifer Rodger*

MBS: Signaling Endosomes and Growth Cone Motility in Axon Regeneration
*Michael B. Steketee and Jeffrey L. Goldberg*

Intrinsic Mechanisms Regulating Axon Regeneration: An Integrin Perspective
*Richard Eva, Melissa R. Andrews, Elske H.P. Franssen, and James W. Fawcett*

The Role of Serotonin in Axon and Dendrite Growth
*Ephraim F. Trakhtenberg and Jeffrey L. Goldberg*

Inflammatory Pathways in Spinal Cord Injury
*Samuel David, Juan Guillermo Zarruk, and Nader Ghasemlou*

Combinatorial Therapy Stimulates Long-Distance Regeneration, Target Reinnervation, and Partial Recovery of Vision After Optic Nerve Injury in Mice
*Silmara de Lima, Ghaith Habboub, and Larry I. Benowitz*

From Bench to Beside to Cure Spinal Cord Injury: Lost in Translation?
*Andreas Hug and Norbert Weidner*

SUBJECT INDEX

## Volume 107

Neuromodulation: A More Comprehensive Concept Beyond Deep Brain Stimulation
*Clement Hamani and Elena Moro*

Computational Models of Neuromodulation
*Christopher R. Butson*

Neurophysiology of Deep Brain Stimulation
*Manuela Rosa, Gaia Giannicola, Sara Marceglia, Manuela Fumagalli, Sergio Barbieri, and Alberto Priori*

Neurophysiology of Cortical Stimulation
*Jean-Pascal Lefaucheur*

Neural Mechanisms of Spinal Cord Stimulation
*Robert D. Foreman and Bengt Linderoth*

Magnetoencephalography and Neuromodulation
*Alfons Schnitzler and Jan Hirschmann*

Current Challenges to the Clinical Translation of Brain Machine Interface Technology
*Charles W. Lu, Parag G. Patil, and Cynthia A. Chestek*

Nanotechnology in Neuromodulation
*Russell J. Andrews*

Optogenetic Neuromodulation
*Paul S. A. Kalanithi and Jaimie M. Henderson*

Diffusion Tensor Imaging and Neuromodulation: DTI as Key Technology for Deep Brain Stimulation
*Volker Arnd Coenen, Thomas E. Schlaepfer, Niels Allert, and Burkhard Mädler*

DBS and Electrical Neuro-Network Modulation to Treat Neurological Disorders
*Amanda Thompson, Takashi Morishita, and Michael S. Okun*

Neuromodulation in Psychiatric Disorders
*Yasin Temel, Sarah A. Hescham, Ali Jahanshahi, Marcus L. F. Janssen, Sonny K. H. Tan, Jacobus J. van Overbeeke, Linda Ackermans, Mayke Oosterloo, Annelien Duits, Albert F. G. Leentjens, and LeeWei Lim*

Ethical Aspects of Neuromodulation
*Christiane Woopen*

Subject Index

## Volume 108

Tissue Engineering and Regenerative Medicine: Past, Present, and Future
*António J. Salgado, Joaquim M. Oliveira, Albino Martins, Fábio G. Teixeira, Nuno A. Silva, Nuno M. Neves, Nuno Sousa, and Rui L. Reis*

Tissue Engineering and Peripheral Nerve Reconstruction: An Overview
*Stefano Geuna, S. Gnavi, I. Perroteau, Pierluigi Tos, and B. Battiston*

Bone Marrow Mesenchymal Stem Cell Transplantation for Improving Nerve Regeneration
*Júlia Teixeira Oliveira, Klauss Mostacada, Silmara de Lima, and Ana Maria Blanco Martinez*

Perspectives of Employing Mesenchymal Stem Cells from the Wharton's Jelly of the Umbilical Cord for Peripheral Nerve Repair
*Jorge Ribeiro, Andrea Gartner, Tiago Pereira, Raquel Gomes, Maria Ascensão Lopes, Carolina Gonçalves, Artur Varejão, Ana Lúcia Luís, and Ana Colette Maurício*

Adipose-Derived Stem Cells and Nerve Regeneration: Promises and Pitfalls
*Alessandro Faroni, Giorgio Terenghi, and Adam J. Reid*

The Pros and Cons of Growth Factors and Cytokines in Peripheral Axon Regeneration
*Lars Klimaschewski, Barbara Hausott, and Doychin N. Angelov*

Role of Inflammation and Cytokines in Peripheral Nerve Regeneration
*P. Dubový, R. Jančálek, and T. Kubek*

Ghrelin: A Novel Neuromuscular Recovery Promoting Factor?
*Raimondo Stefania, Ronchi Giulia, Geuna Stefano, Pascal Davide, Reano Simone, Filigheddu Nicoletta, and Graziani Andrea*

Neuregulin 1 Role in Schwann Cell Regulation and Potential Applications to Promote Peripheral Nerve Regeneration
*Giovanna Gambarotta, Federica Fregnan, Sara Gnavi, and Isabelle Perroteau*

Extracellular Matrix Components in Peripheral Nerve Regeneration
*Francisco Gonzalez-Perez, Esther Udina, and Xavier Navarro*

Subject Index

## Volume 109

The Use of Chitosan-Based Scaffold to Enhance Regeneration in the Nervous System
*Sara Gnavi, Christina Barwig, Thomas Freier, Kirsten Haarstert-Talini, Claudia Grothe, and Stefano Geuna*

Interfaces with the Peripheral Nerve for the Control of Neuroprostheses
*Jaume del Valle and Xavier Navarro*

The Use of Shock Waves in Peripheral Nerve Regeneration: New Perspectives?
*Thomas Hausner and Antal Nógrádi*

Phototherapy and Nerve Injury: Focus on Muscle Response
*Shimon Rochkind, Stefano Geuna, and Asher Shainberg*

Electrical Stimulation for Promoting Peripheral Nerve Regeneration
*Kirsten Haastert-Talini and Claudia Grothe*

Role of Physical Exercise for Improving Post-traumatic Nerve Regeneration
*Paulo A.S. Armada-da-Silva, Cátia Pereira, SandraAmado, and António P. Veloso*

The Role of Timing in Nerve Reconstruction
*Lars B. Dahlin*

Future Perspectives in Nerve Repair and Regeneration
*Pierluigi Tos, Giulia Ronchi, Stefano Geuna, and Bruno Battiston*

INDEX

## Volume 110

The Relevance of Metals in the Pathophysiology of Neurodegeneration, Pathological Considerations
*Kurt A. Jellinger*

Pantothenate Kinase-Associated Neurodegeneration (PKAN) and *PLA2G6*-Associated Neurodegeneration (PLAN): Review of Two Major Neurodegeneration with Brain Iron Accumulation (NBIA) Phenotypes
*Manju A. Kurian and Susan J. Hayflick*

Mitochondrial Membrane Protein-Associated Neurodegeneration (MPAN)
*Monika Hartig, Holger Prokisch, Thomas Meitinger, and Thomas Klopstock*

BPAN: The Only X-Linked Dominant NBIA Disorder
*T.B. Haack, P. Hogarth, A. Gregory, P. Prokisch, and S.J. Hayflick*

Neuroferritinopathy
*M.J. Keogh, C.M. Morris, and P.F. Chinnery*

Aceruloplasminemia: An Update
*Satoshi Kono*

Therapeutic Advances in Neurodegeneration with Brain Iron Accumulation
*Giovanna Zorzi and Nardo Nardocci*

The Neuropathology of Neurodegeneration with Brain Iron Accumulation
*Michael C. Kruer*

Imaging of Iron
*Petr Dusek, Monika Dezortova, and Jens Wuerfel*

The Role of Iron Imaging in Huntington's Disease
*S.J.A. van den Bogaard, E.M. Dumas, and R.A.C. Roos*

Lysosomal Storage Disorders and Iron
*Jose Miguel Bras*

Manganese and the Brain
*Karin Tuschl, Philippa B. Mills, and Peter T. Clayton*

Update on Wilson Disease
*Aggarwal Annu and Bhatt Mohit*

An Update on Primary Familial Brain Calcification
*R.R. Lemos, J.B.M.M. Ferreira, M.P. Keasey, and J.R.M. Oliveira*

INDEX

## Volume 111

History of Acupuncture Research
*Yi Zhuang, Jing-jing Xing, Juan Li, Bai-Yun Zeng, and Fan-rong Liang*

Effects of Acupuncture Needling with Specific Sensation on Cerebral Hemodynamics and Autonomic Nervous Activity in Humans
*Kouich Takamoto, Susumu Urakawa, Kazushige Sakai, Taketoshi Ono, and Hisao Nishijo*

Acupuncture Point Specificity
*Jing-jing Xing, Bai-Yun Zeng, Juan Li, Yi Zhuang, and Fan-rong Liang*

Acupuncture Stimulation Induces Neurogenesis in Adult Brain
*Min-Ho Nam, Kwang Seok Ahn, and Seung-Hoon Choi*

Acupuncture and Neurotrophin Modulation
*Marzia Soligo, Stefania Lucia Nori, Virginia Protto, Fulvio Florenzano, and Luigi Manni*

Acupuncture Stimulation and Neuroendocrine Regulation
*Jung-Sheng Yu, Bai-Yun Zeng, and Ching-Liang Hsieh*

Current Development of Acupuncture Research in Parkinson's Disease
*Bai-Yun Zeng, Sarah Salvage, and Peter Jenner*

Acupuncture Therapy for Stroke Patients
*Xin Li and Qiang Wang*

Effects of Acupuncture Therapy on Alzheimer's Disease
*Bai-Yun Zeng, Sarah Salvage, and Peter Jenner*

Acupuncture Therapy for Psychiatric Illness
*Karen Pilkington*

Acupuncture for the Treatment of Insomnia
*Kaicun Zhao*

Acupuncture for the Treatment of Drug Addiction
*Cai-Lian Cui, Liu-Zhen Wu, and Yi-jing Li*

Acupuncture Regulation of Blood Pressure: Two Decades of Research
*John C. Longhurst and Stephanie Tjen-A-Looi*

Effect and Mechanism of Acupuncture on Gastrointestinal Diseases
*Toku Takahashi*

INDEX

## Volume 112

An Introduction to the Clinical Phenomenology of Tourette Syndrome
*Davide Martino, Namrata Madhusudan, Panagiotis Zis, and Andrea E. Cavanna*

Functional Neuroanatomy of Tics
*Irene Neuner, Frank Schneider, and N. Jon Shah*

Functional Imaging of Dopaminergic Neurotransmission in Tourette Syndrome
*Bàrbara Segura and Antonio P. Strafella*

Nondopaminergic Neurotransmission in the Pathophysiology of Tourette Syndrome
*Patrick T. Udvardi, Ester Nespoli, Francesca Rizzo, Bastian Hengerer, and Andrea G. Ludolph*

Reinforcement Learning and Tourette Syndrome
*Stefano Palminteri and Mathias Pessiglione*

Genetic Susceptibility and Neurotransmitters in Tourette Syndrome
*Peristera Paschou, Thomas V. Fernandez, Frank Sharp, Gary A. Heiman, and Pieter J. Hoekstra*

Pharmacological Animal Models of Tic Disorders
*Kevin W. McCairn and Masaki Isoda*

Animal Models Recapitulating the Multifactorial Origin of Tourette Syndrome
*Simone Macrì, Martina Proietti Onori, Veit Roessner, and Giovanni Laviola*

Neuroendocrine Aspects of Tourette Syndrome
*Davide Martino, Antonella Macerollo, and James F. Leckman*

Clinical Pharmacology of Dopamine-Modulating Agents in Tourette's Syndrome
*Sabine Mogwitz, Judith Buse, Stefan Ehrlich, and Veit Roessner*

Clinical Pharmacology of Nondopaminergic Drugs in Tourette Syndrome
*Andreas Hartmann*

Antiepileptic Drugs and Tourette Syndrome
*Andrea E. Cavanna and Andrea Nani*

Clinical Pharmacology of Comorbid Obsessive–Compulsive Disorder in Tourette Syndrome
*Valeria Neri and Francesco Cardona*

Clinical Pharmacology of Comorbid Attention Deficit Hyperactivity Disorder in Tourette Syndrome
*Renata Rizzo and Mariangela Gulisano*

Emerging Treatment Strategies in Tourette Syndrome: What's in the Pipeline?
*C. Termine, C. Selvini, G. Rossi, and U. Balottin*

Tics and Other Stereotyped Movements as Side Effects of Pharmacological Treatment
*Marcos Madruga-Garrido and Pablo Mir*

INDEX

## Volume 113

Autism Spectrum Disorder and the Cerebellum
*Esther B.E. Becker and Catherine J. Stoodley*

Contribution of Long Noncoding RNAs to Autism Spectrum Disorder Risk
*Brent Wilkinson and Daniel B. Campbell*

Identifying Essential Cell Types and Circuits in Autism Spectrum Disorders
*Susan E. Maloney, Michael A. Rieger, and Joseph D. Dougherty*

Connecting Signaling Pathways Underlying Communication to ASD Vulnerability
*Stephanie Lepp, Ashley Anderson, and Genevieve Konopka*

MET Receptor Tyrosine Kinase as an Autism Genetic Risk Factor
*Yun Peng, Matthew Huentelman, Christopher Smith, and Shenfeng Qiu*

Transcriptional Dysregulation of Neocortical Circuit Assembly in ASD
*Kenneth Y. Kwan*

Motor Skill in Autism Spectrum Disorders: A Subcortical View
*Leanne Chukoskie, Jeanne Townsend, and Marissa Westerfield*

Orchestration of Neurodevelopmental Programs by RBFOX1: Implications for Autism Spectrum Disorder
*Brent R. Bill, Jennifer K. Lowe, Christina T. DyBuncio, and Brent L. Fogel*

Immune Dysregulation in Autism Spectrum Disorder
*Elaine Y. Hsiao*

Autism Susceptibility Genes and the Transcriptional Landscape of the Human Brain
*Shingo Miyauchi and Irina Voineagu*

INDEX

## Volume 114

Modern Concepts of Focal Epileptic Networks
*Premysl Jiruska, Marco de Curtis, and John G.R. Jefferys*

Neocortical Focus: Experimental View
*Igor Timofeev, Sylvain Chauvette, and Sara Soltani*

Malformations of Cortical Development and Neocortical Focus
*Heiko J. Luhmann, Werner Kilb, and Hans Clusmann*

Limbic Networks and Epileptiform Synchronization: The View from the Experimental Side
*Charles Behr, Margherita D'Antuono, Shabnam Hamidi, Rochelle Herrington, Maxime Lévesque, Pariya Salami, Zahra Shiri, Rüdiger Köhling, and Massimo Avoli*

Limbic Networks: Clinical Perspective
*Aylin Y. Reid and Richard J. Staba*

Modern Concepts of Seizure Modeling
*Christophe Bernard, Sebastien Naze, Timothée Proix, and Viktor K. Jirsa*

Mechanisms of Ictogenesis
*Thomas Blauwblomme, Premysl Jiruska, and Gilles Huberfeld*

Seizure Termination
*Frédéric Zubler, Andreas Steimer, Heidemarie Gast, and Kaspar A. Schindler*

Epileptic Focus and Alteration of Metabolism
*Jakub Otáhal, Jaroslava Folbergrová, Richard Kovacs, Wolfram S. Kunz, and Nicola Maggio*

Modern Techniques of Epileptic Focus Localization
*Lukas Martinkovic, Hrvoje Hecimovic, Vlastimil Sulc, Radek Marecek, and Petr Marusic*

From Treatment to Cure: Stopping Seizures, Preventing Seizures, and Reducing Brain Propensity to Seize
*Ivan Pavlov and Stephanie Schorge*

INDEX

## Volume 115

Environmental Alterations of Epigenetics Prior to the Birth
*Chiao-Ling Lo and Feng C. Zhou*

Transgenerational Epigenetics and Brain Disorders
*Nadia Rachdaoui and Dipak K. Sarkar*

The Epigenetic Landscape of Alcoholism
*Harish R. Krishnan, Amul J. Sakharkar, Tara L. Teppen, Tiffani D.M. Berkel, and Subhash C. Pandey*

Epigenetic Regulatory Mechanisms in Stress-Induced Behavior
*Sumana Chakravarty, Salil Saurav Pathak, Swati Maitra, Nitin Khandelwal, Karisetty Bhanu Chandra, and Arvind Kumar*

Epigenetics of Schizophrenia: An Open and Shut Case
*David P. Gavin and Christina Floreani*

Epigenetic Mechanisms in Autism Spectrum Disorder
*Adrian Zhubi, Edwin H. Cook, Alessandro Guidotti, and Dennis R. Grayson*

MicroRNAs and Ethanol Toxicity
*Rajesh C. Miranda*

INDEX

## Volume 116

Introduction to Sequencing the Brain Transcriptome
*Robert Hitzemann, Priscila Darakjian, Nikki Walter, Ovidu Iancu, Robert Searles, and Shannon McWeeney*

Analysis Considerations for Utilizing RNA-Seq to Characterize the Brain Transcriptome
*Christina Zheng, Sunita Kawane, Daniel Bottomly, and Beth Wilmot*

Data Integration and Reproducibility for High-Throughput Transcriptomics
*Michael Mooney and Shannon McWeeney*

Coexpression and Cosplicing Network Approaches for the Study of Mammalian Brain Transcriptomes
*Ovidiu Dan Iancu, Alexander Colville, Priscila Darakjian, and Robert Hitzemann*

Splicing in the Human Brain
*Ammar Zaghlool, Adam Ameur, Lucia Cavalier, and Lars Feuk*

Understanding Complex Transcriptome Dynamics in Schizophrenia and Other Neurological Diseases Using RNA Sequencing
*Xi Wang and Murray J. Cairns*

The Central Role of Noncoding RNA in the Brain
*Boris Guennewig and Antony A. Cooper*

Genetics of Gene Expression in CNS
*Robert W. Williams and Ashutosh K Pandey*

Transcriptomic Changes in Brain Development
*Allissa A. Dillman and Mark R. Cookson*

Gene Expression in the Addicted Brain
*Zhifeng Zhou, Mary-Anne Enoch, and David Goldman*

RNA-Seq Reveals Novel Transcriptional Reorganization in Human Alcoholic Brain
*Sean P. Farris and R. Dayne Mayfield*

INDEX

## Volume 117

Learning-Induced Structural Plasticity in the Cerebellum
*Hiroshi Nishiyama*

Cerebellar Mechanisms of Learning and Plasticity Revealed by Delay Eyelid Conditioning
*Michael D. Mauk, Wenke Li, Andrei Khilkevich, and Hunter Halverson*

Cerebellar Long-Term Potentiation: Cellular Mechanisms and Role in Learning
*Giorgio Grasselli and Christian Hansel*

The Ontogeny of Associative Cerebellar Learning
*John H. Freeman*

INDEX

## Volume 118

Neuroimmune Mechanisms of Alcohol and Drug Addiction
*Changhai Cui, David Shurtleff, and R. Adron Harris*

Neuroimmune Pathways in Alcohol Consumption: Evidence from Behavioral and Genetic Studies in Rodents and Humans
*Gizelle Robinson, Dana Most, Laura B. Ferguson, Jody Mayfield, R. Adron Harris, and Yuri A. Blednov*

Fetal Alcohol Spectrum Disorders and Neuroimmune Changes
*Paul D. Drew and Cynthia J.M. Kane*

Role of Microglia in Regulation of Ethanol Neurotoxic Action
*Lucy Chastain and Dipak K. Sarkar*

Functions of the Chemokine Receptor CXCR4 in the Central Nervous System and Its Regulation by μ-Opioid Receptors
*Bradley Nash and Olimpia Meucci*

Discovery of a Novel Site of Opioid Action at the Innate Immune Pattern-Recognition Receptor TLR4
*Jonathan Henry W. Jacobsen, Linda R. Watkins, and Mark R. Hutchinson*

Neuroimmune Basis of Methamphetamine Toxicity
*Jennifer M. Loftis and Aaron Janowsky*

Marijuana Use Brain Immune Mechanisms
*Guy A. Cabral and Melissa Jamerson*

Interactions of HIV and Drugs of Abuse: The Importance of Glia and Host Genetic Factors
*Kurt F. Hauser and Pamela E. Knapp*

Neuroimmune Basis of Alcoholic Brain Damage
*Fulton T. Crews and Ryan P. Vetreno*

Converging Actions of Alcohol on Liver and Brain Immune Signaling
*Gyongyi Szabo and Dora Lippai*

Opportunities for the Development of Neuroimmune Therapies in Addiction
*Lara A. Ray, Daniel Roche, Keith Heinzerling, and Steve Shoptaw*

Use of Addictive Substances and NeuroHIV
*Sulie L. Chang, Kaitlyn P. Connaghan, Yufeng Wei, and Ming D. Li*

INDEX

## Volume 119

Adenosine Receptor Neurobiology: Overview
*Jiang-Fan Chen, Chien-fei Lee, and Yijuang Chern*

Adenosine Receptor PET Imaging in Human Brain
*Masahiro Mishina and Kiich Ishiwata*

An Overview of Adenosine $A_{2A}$ Receptor Antagonists in Parkinson's Disease
*Peter Jenner*

Mode of Action of Adenosine $A_{2A}$ Receptor Antagonists as Symptomatic Treatment for Parkinson's Disease
*Akihisa Mori*

Adenosine Receptors and Dyskinesia in Pathophysiology
*Masahiko Tomiyama*

Clinical/Pharmacological Aspect of Adenosine $A_{2A}$ Receptor Antagonist for Dyskinesia
*Tomoyuki Kanda and Shin-ichi Uchida*

Interaction of Adenosine Receptors with Other Receptors from Therapeutic Perspective in Parkinson's Disease
*Nicolas Morin and Thérèse Di Paolo*

Effects of the Adenosine $A_{2A}$ Receptor Antagonist on Cognitive Dysfunction in Parkinson's Disease
*Shin-ichi Uchida, Takako Kadowaki-Horita, and Tomoyuki Kanda*

Clinical Nonmotor Aspect of $A_{2A}$ Antagonist in PD Treatment
*Masahiro Nomoto, Masahiro Nagai, and Noriko Nishikawa*

Adenosine Receptors and Huntington's Disease
*Chien-fei Lee and Yijuang Chern*

Adenosine Receptors and Epilepsy: Current Evidence and Future Potential
*Susan A. Masino, Masahito Kawamura, Jr., and David N. Ruskin*

Adenosine Receptor Control of Cognition in Normal and Disease
*Jiang-Fan Chen*

Adenosine Receptors in Cerebral Ischemia
*Alessia Melani, Anna Maria Pugliese, and Felicita Pedata*

Roles of Adenosine and its Receptors in Sleep–Wake Regulation
*Zhi-Li Huang, Ze Zhang, and Wei-Min Qu*

Involvement of Adenosine $A_{2A}$ Receptors in Depression and Anxiety
*Koji Yamada, Minoru Kobayashi, and Tomoyuki Kanda*

The Adenosine Neuromodulation System in Schizophrenia
*Daniel Rial, Diogo R. Lara, and Rodrigo A. Cunha*

INDEX

## Volume 120

The Story of "Speed" from "Cloud Nine" to Brain Gain
*Andrew Lees, Katrin Sikk, and Pille Taba*

Amphetamine-Type Stimulants: The Early History of Their Medical and Non-Medical Uses
*Nicolas Rasmussen*

Miracle or Menace?
*Mike Jay*

Psychostimulants: Basic and Clinical Pharmacology
*Andrew C. McCreary, Christian P. Müller, and Małgorzata Filip*

Epigenetic Mechanisms of Psychostimulant-Induced Addiction
*Anti Kalda and Alexander Zharkovsky*

Experimental Models on Effects of Psychostimulants
*Sulev Kõks*

Neurologic Complications of Psychomotor Stimulant Abuse
*Juan Sanchez-Ramos*

Neurobehavioral Sequelae of Psychostimulant Abuse
*Atbin Djamshidian*

Neuropsychiatric Adverse Effects of Amphetamine and Methamphetamine
*Jaanus Harro*

"Addicted to Euphoria": The History, Clinical Presentation, and Management of Party Drug Misuse
*Jenny Bearn and Matthew O'Brien*

"Natural Amphetamine" Khat: A Cultural Tradition or a Drug of Abuse?
*Nilesh B. Patel*

Methcathinone "Kitchen Chemistry" and Permanent Neurological Damage
*Katrin Sikk and Pille Taba*

"Legal Highs" – An Emerging Epidemic of Novel Psychoactive Substances
*Jolanta B. Zawilska*

Psychostimulants and Artistic, Musical, and Literary Creativity
*Iain Smith*

Opium as a Literary Stimulant: The Case of Samuel Taylor Coleridge
*Neil Vickers*

INDEX

## Volume 121

Alzheimer's Disease: Genomics and Beyond
*Fuhai Song, Guangchun Han, Zhouxian Bai, Xing Peng, Jiajia Wang, and Hongxing Lei*

The Potential of Proteomics in Understanding Neurodegeneration
*Ramavati Pal, Jan Petter Larsen, and Simon Geir Moller*

Proteomics Approach to Identify Biomarkers in Neurodegenerative Diseases
*Annapurna Nayak, Gregory Salt, Sunil K. Verma, and Uday Kishore*

Uncovering Neurodegenerative Protein Modifications via Proteomic Profiling
*Xavier Gallart-Palau, Aida Serra, and Siu Kwan Sze*

Comparative Proteomics for the Evaluation of Protein Expression and Modifications in Neurodegenerative Diseases
*Antonio Conti and Massimo Alessio*

INDEX

FSC
www.fsc.org
MIX
Papier | Fördert gute Waldnutzung
FSC® C083411

Kolibri 360 GmbH
Ferdinand-Jühlke-Straße 7
99095 Erfurt, Deutschland
produktsicherheit@kolibri360.de